Placement Learning in
Community
Nursing

A guide for students in practice

Jane Harris BNurs, MSc, Cert Ed, RN, DN, HV, RM, DNT, CPT,
Hon. Fellow of the Queen's Nursing Institute Scotland
Senior Lecturer, School of Nursing & Midwifery, University of Dundee,
Dundee, UK; Professional Advisor for Community Nursing and Education,
Scottish Government

Sheila Nimmo BSc, MEd, PG Dip Educational Research, RN, DN, CPT, RNT
Independent Consultant in Nurse Education, Dundee, UK

Series Editor:
Karen Holland BSc(Hons) MSc
CertEd SRN
Professorial Fellow, School of
Nursing, University of Salford,
Salford, UK

Student Advisor:
Philippa Sharp
Student Nurse, Division of
Nursing, University of
Nottingham, Nottingham, UK

With a contribution from:
Ian Murray BEd, Dip Nursing, Cert
Education, PG Dip, MPH, RMN, RGN
Educational Research, Deputy
Head of School of Nursing,
Midwifery and Health,
University of Stirling, UK

BAILLIÈRE
TINDALL

ELSEVIER

Edinburgh   London   New York   Oxford   Philadelphia   St Louis   Sydney   Toronto 2013

BAILLIÈRE TINDALL
ELSEVIER

ISBN 978-0-7020-4301-7

British Library Cataloguing in Publication Data
A catalogue record for this book is available from the British Library

Library of Congress Cataloging in Publication Data
A catalog record for this book is available from the Library of Congress

ELSEVIER your source for books, journals and multimedia in the health sciences

www.elsevierhealth.com

Working together to grow libraries in developing countries

www.elsevier.com • www.bookaid.org

The Publisher's policy is to use **paper manufactured from sustainable forests**

Printed in China

Contents

Contents

Series preface

Learning to become a nurse is a journey which sees the student engaging in both challenging and life-changing experiences as well as developing their skills and knowledge base in order to be able to practise as a competent and accountable practitioner. To be able to do this requires engagement with others in two different, yet complementary environments, namely the clinical setting and university, with the ultimate aim of learning the necessary knowledge and skills to be able to care for patients, clients and their families in whatever field of practice the student chooses to pursue. The clinical placement becomes the centre of this integrated learning experience.

Tracey Levett-Jones and Sharon Bourgeois (2007) point out, however, that 'there is plenty of evidence, anecdotal and empirical, to suggest that clinical placements can be both tremendous and terrible' but that it is at the same time 'one of the most exciting journeys of your life'. Whilst their book focuses on helping you through this journey in relation to the more 'general' aspects of learning and coping when undertaking your clinical experiences, this series of books sets out to help you gain maximum learning from specific placement-learning opportunities and placements.

The focus of each book is the actual nature of the placements, the client/patient groups you may encounter and the fundamentals of care they might require, together with the evidence-based knowledge and skills that underpin that care. Whilst the general structure of each book might be different, the underpinning principles are the same in each.

To ensure that the learning undertaken in university is linked to that in practice there will be reference to academic regulations, specific learning responsibilities (such as meeting with personal tutors, mentor-student relationships, placement expectations) and the importance of professional accountability.

Each book also outlines how your experiences in practice will help you achieve specific learning outcomes and competencies as specified by the United Kingdom (UK) Nursing and Midwifery Council (NMC). Although the books are primarily aimed at the UK student, the general principles underpinning the care practice described and the underpinning evidence base throughout are valid for all student nurses who are required by their respective international professional organisations to gain experience in a number of clinical environments in order to become competent to practice as a registered qualified nurse.

Nursing is a challenging and rewarding profession. The books in this series offer a foundation of knowledge and learning to support you on your professional journey and their content is based on the editors' and authors' experiences of engaging with students and colleagues in this learning experience. In addition, their content draws on personal experience of working with service users and carers as to what is best practice in caring for people at various stages of life and with various health problems. The ultimate aim is to enable you to use them as 'pocket guides' to learning in a range of clinical placements and specific planned placement learning opportunities, and to share their content with those who manage this learning experience in practice. We hope that you find them a valued resource and companion during your journey to becoming a qualified nurse.

Karen Holland
Series Editor

...MENT LEARNING IN
Community
Nursing

LIBRARY

Learning
Resource Centre

This book is dedicated to Malcolm James Nimmo, 1958–2006

Titles in this series:

Placement Learning in Cancer and Palliative Care Nursing
Penny Howard, Becky Chady
ISBN 978-0-7020-4300-0

Placement Learning in Community Nursing
Jane Harris, Sheila Nimmo
ISBN 978-0-7020-4301-7

Placement Learning in Medical Nursing
Maggie Maxfield, Michelle Parker
ISBN 978-0-7020-4302-4

Placement Learning in Mental Health Nursing
Gemma Stacey, Anne Felton, Paul Bonham
ISBN 978-0-7020-4303-1

Placement Learning in Older People Nursing
Julie McGarry, Philip Clissett, Davina Porock, Wendy Walker
ISBN 978-0-7020-4304-8

Placement Learning in Surgical Nursing
Karen Holland, Michelle Roxburgh
ISBN 978-0-7020-4305-5

Content Strategist: Mairi McCubbin
Content Development Specialist: Carole McMurray
Project Manager: Andrew Riley
Designer: Miles Hitchen
Illustration Manager: Jennifer Rose

Student foreword

Like most students, I have experienced a range of feelings on starting a new placement: the fears and excitement of what experiences you will have, who you are going to meet and work with, what you will learn and the responsibilities that come with being that bit further along in your training. These are all feelings that are part of our education and training and contribute to the student's growth as a nurse and as an individual. What is expected of you during a placement is another persistent anxiety, in particular how you can get the best from that specific placement and how you achieve the gold standard of truly incorporating theory into your practice in an effective and useful way.

Most placement experiences vary in length from introductory 2-week placements to full 18-week hub-and-spoke model placements. It can take a significant amount of the placement time to settle in, understand the way that particular clinical area works and develop an effective professional relationship with your mentor and other members of staff that enables you to learn and achieve.

This series of books makes the gap between what is taught in the university and what is practiced in clinical placements much smaller and less frightening. It provides guidance on achieving the Nursing and Midwifery Council (NMC) outcomes and proficiencies that are essential for becoming a registered nurse, using case studies and real examples to help you. Knowledge of what opportunities to seek in particular clinical areas and how best to achieve them helps considerably, especially when there is so much else to think about.

The series also provides a number of opportunities to recap essential knowledge needed for that area (very useful as lectures can seem a long time ago!). From student nurses setting out on that journey to those nearly ending, these books are a valuable resource and support and will help you overcome these sudden panic attacks when you suddenly think 'what do I do now?' Enjoy them, as I have enjoyed being able to have an opportunity to contribute to their development.

Philippa Sharp
Third-year student nurse
University of Nottingham

Introduction

Placement Learning in Community Nursing is one of a series of books which are designed as 'good companions', on hand to support your learning during each specific practice component of your nursing programme. This book will help to inspire and motivate you not only to make the most of your experience now, but also to use your learning from the community in different contexts in the future.

Often referred to as the 'community placement', the scope for learning in the community is wide and varied. Nursing students are allocated to community-based practice at various stages of the programme. This book aims to cater for your needs from first year, possibly with community as your first practice experience, to final year where community may be the setting for your management experience immediately prior to registration.

A number of factors make it challenging to describe the context and practice of community nursing. This is because different arrangements and service models for health and care delivery operate in each part of the UK; local variations within each country can make things look very different; there is constant change; and finally the sheer volume and complexity of information can at times seem overwhelming. Our intention here is to introduce you to some of the key themes and experiences you are likely to encounter and some of the general principles of nursing in the community that are relevant wherever you are based.

Mentors and other members of the care team who play an essential role in your

practice learning experience will also find this book useful.

You will feel better prepared to take an active role in your learning and together with your mentor identify opportunities and structure learning activities to ensure that your experience enables you to meet your learning outcomes. We have also made reference to the competencies associated with the Nursing and Midwifery Council standards and Essential Skills Clusters to assist you.

We encourage you to work through the activities that you will find in each chapter and take opportunities to discuss your answers with your mentor, peers and others who are supporting you during your placement. The principles of evidence based practice are highlighted throughout the book and you are guided to further reading and relevant websites at the end of each chapter to enhance your learning.

Placement learning in Community Nursing is organized in 4 sections.

Section 1: Preparation for the community practice learning environment

The chapters in Section 1 include information about the community which will develop your understanding of this diverse environment and help you to feel prepared for your experience as a nursing student. Chapter 1 explores the health and social care context of community nursing, the agencies that provide services in the UK and the importance of public health. Chapter 2 introduces a wide range of settings where people live or receive care and support and the roles of the practitioners who are involved. Chapter 3 explores what is different about learning in the community; what to expect and what's expected of you as a student. Chapter 4 discusses the learning strategies that support effective learning, such as being prepared for the placement and adopting a proactive and reflective approach.

Section 2: Placement Learning Opportunities

In Section 2, we explore service users' possible experience of community care and how the community nursing service works to meet the needs of individuals, families and communities. There is a focus on person-centred approaches that demonstrate partnership, and co-production with service users, their carers and health and care providers, and organisations. Similar to Section 1, several learning activities are included to enable you to develop your knowledge and understanding and consider the application of theory to practice. You may also find some of the references and websites useful for further reading. Chapter 5 explores the role of the community nurse in assessing and addressing need, not only for individuals and families, but for communities. Chapter 6 focuses on the safe and effective management of long-term conditions, how people are enabled and supported to live as independently as possible at home and the role that informal carers play in the home environment. Infection prevention and control are discussed in Chapter 7, demonstrating how core principles are applied in the community setting with particular reference to wound management in the community. Chapter 8 discusses in

detail the range of mental health problems experienced by people living in the community, the role of the community nurse and other practitioners in providing treatment and support and the learning from this context that students can apply across a range of settings.

Section 3: Professional Issues

A range of professional issues that are particularly important in community nursing have been selected for Section 3. These issues are not unique to community nursing but there is valuable and life-long learning available here for students when they experience the impact that issues such as effective communication can have on keeping vulnerable children safe, or enabling someone to stay at home and avoid hospitalisation. Communication skills in community practice are discussed in Chapter 9, highlighting different ways in which communication styles, methods and technologies are used to support individuals and families in the community. Chapter 10 discusses leadership skills, teamwork and management and explores how the nursing student can develop experience and competencies during a community placement. Quality and clinical effectiveness are explored in Chapters 11 and 12 and the different aspects of medicine management in the community is discussed.

Section 4: Consolidating learning

Possibly, more than any other component of practice learning that you will experience during your programme, practice learning in the community will offer the most variety, opportunity and challenge. This book will by no means have covered everything that you need to know but it has introduced you to some of the key aspects of nursing in the community. The two chapters in this final section aim to help you consolidate the knowledge and understanding you have gained from previous chapters, the further reading and from your practice experience to date.

We have included scenarios and situations that you are likely to come across in the community to enable you to draw on your knowledge and experience and test your learning. You will find it helpful to reflect back on some of the theory within the previous chapters and to use opportunities to discuss your answers with your mentor.

Acknowledgements

We would like to thank series editor Karen Holland and the editorial team at Elsevier for their valuable advise and support.

We would particularly like to thank and acknowledge the following colleagues who have contributed to chapters within this text.

Joan Cameron, PhD, MSc, RGN, RM Senior Lecturer, Lead Midwife for Education, University of Dundee; Karen Shewan, AHP Lead for Bolton PCT and AHP Professional Advisor Primary Care, Scottish Government; Jo Smith BSc, RGN,RM, SCPHN Lecturer Practitioner, University of Stirling; Jan Thompson, Senior Nurse, Learning Disabilities, NHS Ayrshire and Arran.

Finally our thanks are also due to the students who shared some of their experiences of practice learning in the community.

Section 1. Preparation for practice placement experience in the community

1 The context of community nursing

CHAPTER AIMS

- To explore the health and social care context of community nursing
- To clarify the meaning of primary, secondary and community care
- To discuss the importance of public health

Introduction

The context of nursing in the community is the backdrop for how and where people live their lives, their health and wellbeing, their relationships with others and the communities in which they live. Factors which influence this are many and varied but a common theme is constant change. Therefore changes in the political agenda, patterns of health and disease, the age structure of the population, services and technology and people's expectations of health and social care are all part of the rich context of nursing in the community. The hospital context is certainly touched by these factors, but in the community, they shape the way that nurses practice and respond to healthcare needs on a daily basis. This chapter gives a brief overview of factors which determine the context. It starts by looking at the political agenda which, not surprisingly, is dominated by the health of the population and the challenges of providing a healthcare system which is effective and affordable.

Social policy

In order to understand the part that community nursing plays within the wider health and social care context, it is helpful to clarify the way in which services are structured and delivered in the UK. This is largely determined by government policy and comes under the 'umbrella' term, 'social policy'.

⟩ Activity

If you have already studied social policy in your curriculum it would be a good idea now to look over your university notes. If social policy is new to you or you would like to refresh your interest, Hudson et al (2008) provide a short overview which you will find readable and engaging. It includes current debates and uses examples from other countries.

Hudson J, Lowe S, Kühner S (2008) The short guide to social policy. Policy Press, Bristol.

Nursing students sometimes find the study of social policy challenging and have difficulty appreciating its relevance to nursing practice, particularly from the perspective of a hospital ward. In a community setting social policy comes alive. It is the blueprint for how we live, work and play and for how the most vulnerable members of our society are protected and cared for. While you are in the community, you will see how social policy applies to society on a daily basis but before we look at this in more detail, try the following exercise; you may be surprised how much we take for granted in our own lives.

 Activity

Hudson et al (2008) refer to the 'five pillars' of social policy (Figure 1.1).

- Reflect for a moment on your own family life in relation to the five pillars.
- Make a list of the ways in which social policy influences or has influenced your life.

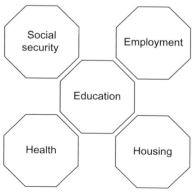

Figure 1.1 The five pillars of social policy.

Even a basic grasp of social policy makes it easier to understand health and health inequalities in society and within communities. Social policy is a complex area and political parties, academics, professionals and individuals have different views on the provision of welfare and the role of the state. Social policy is very relevant to nursing and health care and the National Health Service, used by most people at some point in their lives, is one of the most important areas. (See the National Archives website for actual documents from the setting up of the Welfare State and other social policy issues over time in the UK: http://www.nationalarchives.gov.uk/pathways/citizenship/brave_new_world/welfare.htm).

The UK is renowned for its welfare state which came into being after the Second World War. Essentially, the Welfare State was a package of social policies introduced to eradicate the five 'Giant Evils': squalor, ignorance, want, idleness and disease, which were identified by William Beveridge in his report to the British Parliament in 1942. The plans proposed in the Beveridge report are the foundation for the welfare state as it is in the UK today. Table 1.1 shows examples of current social policy related to Beveridge's five Giant Evils. Personal and social services are also fundamental to welfare provision and often go hand in hand with other social policy such as health, social security and housing.

Social policy is underpinned by different ideologies and these are apparent in the ways in which political parties express their views and the types of social policy that governments develop and implement. Traditionally, political parties that are positioned to the left of the centre of the political spectrum, e.g. the Labour Party, advocate more state intervention in the provision of welfare than those to the right of centre, e.g. the Conservative party. A good example of this difference was the

Table 1.1 Social policy today	
Beveridge's Five Giant Evils	**UK Social policy today**
1. Want	Social Security system, e.g. retirement pension and benefits such as unemployment benefit, housing, maternity
2. Disease	National Health Service
3. Squalor	State-funded housing
4. Ignorance	Pre-school to further and higher education
5. Idleness	Commitment to full employment

conservative policy in the 1980s known as the 'right to buy', which gave council house tenants the opportunity to buy the house they rented. As there was no corresponding policy to build more state funded housing, the effect was to drastically reduce the stock of good quality and reasonably priced rented housing to those who needed it.

Welfare provision in the UK

In the UK, we have a mixed economy of welfare, which means that welfare is provided by organisations including the state. These are categorised into three sectors:
1. The Public sector, e.g. National Health Service, local authority social services
2. The Private sector, e.g. private hospitals, nursing homes and care homes
3. The Third sector, e.g. voluntary and non-profit organisations

The mixed economy of welfare is very evident in health and care services with public, private and voluntary or third sector providers involved in providing a wide range of services. In the community particularly organisations within each of the three sectors often work closely together to offer the best possible care package, particularly to people who have complex needs.

The public sector

Public sector services are those provided by the government or the state. The range and quantity of services varies between countries but most provide what are considered to be fundamental services to support the economic and social wellbeing of individuals and society as a whole. Examples of public sector services include police, defence, roads and transport infrastructure, education, health and social security. You will be aware from regular reporting in the media that the nature and extent of support that the state should or does provide is a source of constant political and academic debate. However, despite the actions of successive governments, the overarching principles in aiming to guarantee a minimum standard of income, health and education for all are consistent, as are the challenges in achieving these. It is important that nurses together with other members of the care team are familiar with the range of services and benefits that people are entitled to receive. Community practitioners must be well informed so that they are in a position to advise people and signpost them to the most appropriate support.

The four United Kingdom (UK) countries

In 1997, the Labour Government began a process of devolution, which led to the establishment of a Scottish Parliament, a Northern Ireland Assembly and a Welsh Assembly, now the Welsh Parliament. These bodies have a range of primary legislative powers, which means they can pass their own laws on topics devolved from

Westminster such as health and education. They also have secondary powers to vary some other laws that are not devolved. Decisions which remain with the Westminster Parliament are known as reserved powers and these include defence and social security.

Devolution has therefore resulted in each country running its own services, shaped by its own legislation and the needs of the population, and influenced by the political ideology of the government. Table 1.2 summarises devolved health-related topics by UK country.

Table 1.2 Devolved health-related topics by UK Country			
Topic	**Scottish Parliament**	**Northern Ireland Executive**	**Welsh Government**
Health	Responsible for running the NHS in Scotland with primary and secondary powers; reserved powers include genetics, abortion, safety of medicines, embryology	Responsible for running the NHS in Northern Ireland with primary and secondary powers (reserved powers as for Scotland)	Responsible for running the NHS in Wales with primary and secondary powers, but with exceptions in the same areas as Northern Ireland and Scotland
Social services	Responsible for social services in Scotland with primary and secondary legislative powers	Responsible for social services in Northern Ireland with primary and secondary powers	Responsible for social services in Wales with primary and secondary powers
Social security	No responsibility	Primary and secondary legislative powers (social security benefits rates and qualifying conditions are similar to those in other parts of the UK)	No responsibility
Economic policy	Scottish Parliament has some limited powers to vary tax rates	No responsibility	No responsibility
Local government and housing	Primary and secondary powers. Its responsibilities include control of local government finance	Local government and housing	Primary and secondary legislative powers. It decides on the overall funding for local authorities

The National Health Service

The National Health Service (NHS) came into being in 1948 and has evolved to meet the changing health and care needs of the population. It is described as 'free at the point of the delivery', which means that apart from a few services such as dental services, service users do not pay up front. However, the NHS is not a free service, as people pay for it indirectly as taxpayers, irrespective of how much they use it. Currently, NHS funding is generated from UK-wide taxation. The Westminster government decides the proportion of tax revenue that it allocates to the NHS and then, through a formula, how much is allocated to each of the four UK countries. The NHS is the world's largest publicly funded health service.

As health is a devolved responsibility, the administration in each UK country has the authority to legislate and manage their NHS in a different way. This means that although the underlying principles of the NHS remain the same, the services that people receive vary depending on where they live in the UK. One example of this variation is the charge for prescriptions in different UK countries. NHS Wales was the first to abolish prescription charges in 2007. NHS Northern Ireland followed in 2010 and NHS Scotland in 2011. In England, there are no plans to abolish prescription charges which are currently set at £7.40 per item.

 Activity

> Spend a few minutes browsing each of the websites noted in Table 1.3. What are the messages? Can you identify similarities? Which sites do you think people find most useful? Look in more detail at the website for the country where you work.

Despite its name, the NHS is no longer the unified and national UK health service that it was at the outset. Strictly speaking, the term NHS now only refers to the NHS in England. The health service has developed a different identity, structure and name in each country, although a similar level and type of service is provided based on the original principles of the NHS.

Devolution has enabled social policy to shape services that match the needs of people and communities in different parts of the country. The overarching aims are to improve the health of everyone wherever they live, prevent ill health and provide the best quality services to those who need

Table 1.3 National Health Service websites

Country	Population in millions[a]	Name of service	Web address
England	51.8	NHS	http://www.nhs.uk/Pages/HomePage.aspx
Northern Ireland	1.7	HSC (Health & Social Care in Northern Ireland)	http://www.hscni.net/
Scotland	5.1	NHS Scotland	http://www.show.scot.nhs.uk
Wales	2.9	NHS Wales	http://www.wales.nhs.uk

[a]Population estimates mid-2009/2010 Office for National Statistics. Online. Available at: http://www.statistics.gov.uk/STATBASE/Product.asp?vlnk=15106

them. The expectations of service users and service providers are changing, most notably in a move away from a paternalistic system where the health service provides and the user passively receives services.

Sharing information and getting people involved is a key theme in all countries and this is clearly reflected in government websites. The internet provides an ideal forum for giving people information, advice and encouragement to take more responsibility for their health by keeping healthy, addressing minor health needs themselves and accessing appropriate services when necessary. In addition, patient and public involvement forums and membership on NHS Trust Boards and in community health partnerships and councils involve people in decision-making and shaping their local health services in the future.

 Activity

Watch the national TV news or listen to the national radio news and pick out items that refer to social policy, e.g. health, social care. Try answering these questions:

■ Are you sure to which UK country the policy or debate relates or to which members of society?

■ How clear is the message?

■ Would you be able to clarify the message for someone in the community who might be concerned or confused?

■ Who could you ask for further information of advice?

Health and social care policies designed to shift the balance from secondary to primary care are a common theme in healthcare reform in all four UK countries. The potential of services provided close to home has been recognised as being comprehensive, co-ordinated, what people want and less costly, whereas secondary care services are increasingly being viewed as costly, fragmented and to be used only when a local solution is not available. The importance of the contribution of community nursing to this agenda is articulated in health policy across the UK and, although nurses are not expected to be experts in all areas of social policy, they should be familiar with the aspects that affect those for whom they provide services.

 Activity

The following are examples of policy documents relating to community nursing in each of the four UK countries. Find and read through the policy documents in the country that relates to your practice. These are available on the government websites listed at the end of the chapter.

England (Department of Health)

Transforming Community Services

■ 6 Transformational guides

■ 43 Indicators for Quality Improvement in the Community

Wales (Welsh government)

Community Nursing Strategy for Wales

Scotland (Scottish government)

Modernising Nursing in the Community

Northern Ireland

■ Redesign of Community Nursing Project

■ Review of District Nursing (DHSSPSNI 2011)

Social services

Social services are provided by local authorities or local councils. They include a wide range of services for children or families in need, people with disabilities, emotional or psychological difficulties or financial or housing problems and older people who need help with daily living activities. Services include residential care, day care and home care. Central to social services are those provided by social workers such as assessment, planning and coordinating services and resources often from other agencies and, crucially, their role in the safety and protection of vulnerable children and adults and direct involvement in supporting people with complex personal issues.

As in healthcare, there is a focus on providing services that enable people, as far as possible, to do things for themselves rather than the service doing things for them. The term social care rather than social service is becoming more commonly used to reflect this. The Department of Health describes social care as:

> *the wide range of services designed to support people to maintain their independence, enable them to play a fuller part in society, protect them in vulnerable situations and manage complex relationships.*
> Department of Health (2006)

The demand for services is increasing rapidly as life expectancy increases and people require more help and support to maintain their independence and quality of life. The largest amount of local authority expenditure apart from education is on social care. Political debate in each country focuses on how best social care can be funded to meet increasing demand. This raises questions about the balance between the role of the state, the individual and the family in funding social care, whether there should be national consistency or local flexibility, whether adults of all ages should be subject to the same funding model and whether public funds should be targeted primarily on the basis of need or at those least able to pay. Devolution has led to different systems for

the provision and funding of social care in different parts of the UK.

Essentially, social care is funded by each UK government, as part of its total allocation to local councils or local authority organisations, council tax revenues and user charges. Third sector organisations also subsidise and provide a range of services. Users can be charged for some aspects of social care based on their assets and income. This system operates differently in each country.

In Scotland, people over the age of 65 who are in need of assistance are assessed by the social services department of the local authority. If they require care at home, there is no charge for personal care such as washing and dressing but there are charges for non-personal care such as cleaning, shopping, preparing meals or receiving meals on wheels. This does not affect entitlement to Attendance Allowance or the care component of the Disability Living Allowance, which people may then use to pay for these non-personal services. Where care is required from a registered nurse, this is funded by the NHS. Means testing is applied in Scotland where people are under 65, or over 65 and assessed as needing residential care. For those over 65, this only relates to the costs of accommodation (also known as 'hotel costs') in the care or nursing home. Nursing care provided as part of a care package in residential care is funded for by the NHS. However, although the costs for personal care appear free, entitlement to benefits (Attendance Allowance or the care component of the Disability Living Allowance) is foregone to pay for this. Similar systems operate in other parts of the UK.

Scotland has the only system which provides free personal care for older people. A new 10-year social services strategy for Wales was published in February 2011, laying the foundations for a national care service. Northern Ireland has a fully integrated health and social care system and other parts of the UK are looking at integration models to improve the quality, efficiency and effectiveness of health and social care services.

Reform of health and social services

Proposed reform in all four countries recognises the value of joining up health and social care provision to improve communication and offer a more streamlined service. Priorities that are common are based on improving quality by ensuring services are safe, effective and centred on the individual's needs. These include:

- Improving prevention and health promotion services
- Addressing inequalities
- Improving access to services
- Empowering and enabling people to take more responsibility for health and self-care.

In England, the government's Health and Social Care Act (DH 2012) proposes to introduce more choice for service users and more competition between providers. It proposes to give patients more information about the performance of services and choice as to where they are treated. And rather than Primary Care Trusts (PCTs) commissioning services on behalf of GPs, local GP consortia would commission services directly.

The impact of policy on shaping services

 Activity

The proposals outlined in the Health and Social Care Act (DH 2012) signalled radical changes to the NHS in England and consequently proved controversial. Extensive debate delayed the passage of the Bill through parliament and, at time of writing, there

are likely to be a number of amendments before it achieves Royal Assent and becomes law. Follow the link below to the parliament website and find out more about the future of the NHS in England: http://services. parliament.uk/bills/2010–11/ healthandsocialcare.html

Private sector health and social care

Not everyone uses the services to which they are entitled free of charge from the NHS. People choose private health care for a number of reasons, namely, choice of hospital and when they can receive treatment, no waiting lists, choice of consultants and specialists and the perception that private hospitals are cleaner, more comfortable and better equipped. Not all conditions and treatments are covered in the private sector and as much of the practice is carried out by NHS doctors, there is often no difference in the standard of care. Nurses employed in the private sector also work or have worked in the NHS. They may be employed on a permanent or agency basis to provide care in private hospitals or nursing homes or to care for patients at home. Most private patients pay through medical insurance and for many, this is provided as part of an employment package.

Other private provision in the community includes social care, also delivered in both a person's home and in residential care homes and nursery provision for pre-school children.

Third sector

Health and social care is also provided by third sector organisations. The name 'third sector' has become recognised

Continued

internationally as a positive and inclusive term to describe organisations that are: non-profit; non-government; non-statutory; voluntary; club; religious orders; community; society; association; co-operative; foundation; friendly society; church; union and charity. These non-government and not-for-profit organisations rely on donations to support paid staff and the work of volunteers. They make a major contribution in many areas including community health services, rural areas, education, housing, sport and recreation.

 Activity

Find out about a local third sector organisation in the area where you live that has an impact on health, e.g. a voluntary group or society.

- How accessible was the information?
- How accessible is the group itself and the service it offers?
- Is the remit of the group clear to the user?
- How does the group support individuals or the local community?

Third sector organisations vary widely in size and scope. Some are large national bodies that receive grants from the government and others are small local groups that are formed by the local community and work for the local community. Some third sector organisations contribute directly to the clinical and social care of people at home and may deliver the service which actually provides the most benefit to the patient and family. The Marie Curie nursing service provides nursing care overnight, not only offering respite for the family, but often making the difference in enabling the patient to stay at home at the end of their life.

Recently, there has been considerable interest in the potential for the third sector to play a much more important role in society and the economy. The UK government is promoting the value of the civil society which has the third sector at its core, in improving health and wellbeing.

Informal, unpaid care

Publically funded or organised health and social care is a small proportion of the care and support that is provided in the community. People receive care at home from unpaid voluntary carers, such as friends, family members and neighbours, without sometimes even coming to the attention of the statutory services. It is often this care that makes the difference between someone being able to remain at home rather than being admitted to hospital or long-term residential care. Carers UK estimate that there are currently 6 million carers in the UK, a number which is set to rise to approximately 9 million in 2037. This gives an indication of the enormous contribution that informal carers make to society and the impact they have on reducing pressure on often overstretched statutory services.

Carers are represented across all ages, socioeconomic, minority and ethnic communities in society. Young carers caring for parents; parents caring for young children; older parents caring for children who are now adults or becoming older adults themselves; plus all the partners, friends, neighbours and family members who dedicate time to caring, need to be supported themselves. Many carers juggle family life, career and caring for their relative with very little support and this is known to lead to poor health and a break down in their ability to continue caring. In a report to the Department of Health, Pickard (2008) has estimated that by 2017, we will reach the tipping point when the numbers of older people needing care will overtake the numbers of family members of working age currently available to meet that demand.

Recent government policies acknowledge that involving carers at all stages of planning and delivery of statutory services ensures services are flexible, appropriate and support a whole family approach. In turn, the quality of life for carers will be improved and as a consequence, the quality of life of their relatives. For example, The Unpaid Carers Policy Branch, in the Scottish Government, is working with carers, national carers organisations and with other partners to improve the recognition of carers' needs and to promote the rights and interests of unpaid carers in Scotland. The role of carers in England has been recognised in the new public health strategy.

 Activity

It is often the third sector organisations that carers find most supportive and for some carers, local and national carers groups are a lifeline. A further discussion regarding the role of carers is included in Chapter 5.

Visit the Carers UK website (http://www.carersuk.org/) and read about how this national organisation works for and with carers across the country.

What does community mean?

The term 'community' means something different to different people, depending on their perspective. Before exploring this in more detail, try the following short exercise which will start you thinking about what community means to you.

 Activity

Write down the first five things that *you* would include in a description of the term 'community'.

The Latin word for community, *commūnitās*, from *commūnis*, meaning common, gives us the word community. We use the word community to describe 'common' in the sense of the context to mean something shared. Here are some of the ways in which 'community' is used:

- The people living in one locality
- A group of people having cultural, religious, ethnic or other characteristics in common, e.g. *the Muslim community*
- A group of nations having certain interests in common, e.g. the European Community
- The public in general – society
- Common ownership or participation (*community spirit*)
- Social equality, togetherness, solidarity
- Similarity or agreement; community of interests.

In Chapter 3, we look at the people who make up a community. In the context of nursing, 'community' describes a setting, the place where nursing care is delivered outside the hospital environment and also a way of nursing. However, rather than referring to hospital and community, the NHS defines services in three tiers: primary, secondary and tertiary care, with community nursing as part of primary care.

Secondary care is provided by a wide range of health professionals in specialist teams in district general hospitals and large teaching hospitals to people who require inpatient care or investigations and treatments as outpatients. Tertiary care refers to the most specialised services and is delivered in a limited number of very specialist hospital units, which are often regional or national centres, for example cardiac transplant units. Primary care is provided in the community and is usually the primary or first contact that people have with the health service. This first contact could be an appointment with the GP or general practice nurse to discuss a health issue; an appointment with a dentist for a check-up; a visit to the optician for an eye test or advice from the local pharmacist.

These practitioners normally work for the NHS as independent contractors, which means they are not directly employed by the NHS.

Community nurses such as district nurses, health visitors and community mental health nurses are directly employed by the NHS and consequently, a distinction is made between primary care and community care because of the way services are funded and managed. In practice, primary care and community care services work as a primary care team, which also includes community physiotherapists and occupational therapists, together with social workers.

This way of thinking tends to place secondary and tertiary services at the centre and primary care and community care on the periphery as three distinct entities. However, it is more accurate and realistic to think in terms of primary, secondary/tertiary and community care as overlapping and integrating services that are all part of the community, as Figure 1.2 illustrates.

Also within the community are a host of other services and organisations that work across and with primary, secondary and community care, for example other primary contacts such as the phone line services, NHS Direct (England), NHS Direct – Wales, NHS 24 (Scotland) or walk-in centres or minor injuries unit, all the social services and other statutory services such as education, housing and the police and the voluntary services and independent sector.

Primary and community care services constitute a much larger part of the health service than secondary care but it does not always appear this way. This is mainly because of the way we think about the NHS in the UK, where much of the attention focuses on emergency and acute hospital care not only in the news but also in television dramas and documentaries. Not only are more services provided in the community but also more people use primary care than secondary care services. In the example from Scotland, shown in Figure 1.3, general practice, pharmacy, health visiting and district nursing and hospital outpatients' services accounted for the largest number of patient contacts. Hospital inpatient services had a relatively low number of patient contacts.

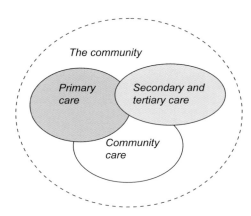

Figure 1.2 Integrating care in the community.

Activity

Figure 1.3 shows an example of care activity in Scotland in 2006/2007. Primary and community care activity is shown on the left and activity for secondary care on the right. The shaded areas indicate services with the most patient contacts. Is there anything you find surprising about the highest and lowest levels of activity?

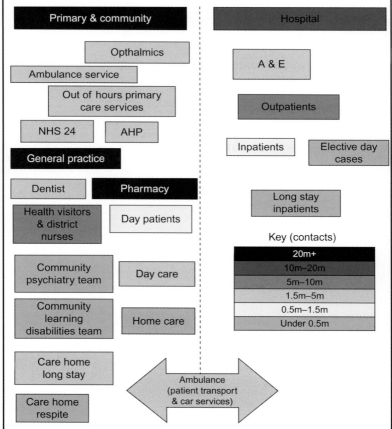

Figure 1.3 Care activity in Scotland in 2006/2007. (Reproduced with permission from Scottish Health and Care Activity 2006/07. Source: ISD Scotland: http://www.scotland.gov.uk/resource/doc/933/0060072.doc)

The Department of Health estimates that 90% of people's contact with the NHS in England is with primary care services with GPs and practice nurses seeing over 800 000 people a day.

Planning services to meet the needs of the population

Changes in the birth and death rates and the number of people entering and leaving the UK not only change the size of the population but also the structure in terms of age, sex, ethnicity, employment and distribution of people in different parts of the country. Table 1.4 shows statistics from the Office for National Statistics.

They are examples of the type of information that is collated and made easily accessible to planners, practitioners, entrepreneurs and others. Population statistics give an indication of trends; the way in which the structure of the UK population is changing and importantly underpin policy and planning both in the public and private sector.

Public health

This chapter so far has focused on the organisation of structures and services that support people in need, fill gaps and aim to solve health problems. This is just one part of the picture and without the

---

Table 1.4 Population statistics

In 2009, an estimated 61.8 million people were resident in the UK – an increase of 2.7 million since 2001. The main driver of population increase in the UK is the difference between births and deaths

In 1983, there were 0.6 million people aged 85 and over (1% of the total population), which by 2008 had more than doubled to 1.3 million

Between 2008/2009 and 2009/2010, provisional net migration increased from 166 000 to 226 000 due to a decrease in emigration

The total fertility rate in the UK has risen from a record low of 1.63 children per woman in 2001, to 1.96 children per woman in 2008

It is projected that by 2033, the number of people aged 85 and over will rise to 3.3 million, or around 5% of the population

The most common country of last residence for long-term immigrants to the UK in 2009, was India

Between 1971 and 2009, the proportion of the UK population aged under 16 decreased from 25.5% to 18.7%, while the proportion aged 75 and over increased from 4.7% to 7.8%

It is estimated that the number of residents aged 90 and over increased by 12% between 2002 and 2009; from 388 200 to 436 500

Between 2001 and 2008, the estimated number of people resident in the UK born in central and eastern European Accession countries rose from 114 000 to 689 000; in 2008, accounting for 10% of the total foreign-born population of the UK and 1% of the total UK population

It is projected that the number of UK residents aged 65 and over will be larger than the number aged under 16 years by 2018

Life expectancy at birth in the UK has risen steadily to 77.4 years for men and 81.6 years for women in 2006–2008

It is projected that by 2021, over one-third of all households will be single person households	The average age of the population in the UK has increased from 36 years in 1992, to 40 years in 2009	In 2009, an estimated 93% of UK residents were British citizens, and 89% had been born in the UK

Office for National Statistics (2011) Social Trends 41.

other, improving health and life chances in the first place, these systems would be unable to cope.

There have been numerous definitions of public health but essentially, they are based on the same principles, preventing illness and improving the health and wellbeing of whole communities and populations, rather than focusing on individuals. Wanless (2004) defines public health as 'the science and art of preventing disease, prolonging life and promoting health through the organised efforts and informed choices of society, organisations, public and private, communities and individuals'. This definition is reflected in government policies and campaigns such as immunisation programmes, tobacco and alcohol legislation, healthy eating campaigns, cancer screening programmes, maternity and child health provision and environmental legislation.

 Activity

The United Nations World Health Organization's (WHO) definition of health has given direction to public health for many years.

Explore the World Health Organization's website and find out about its core public health functions: http://www.who.int/about/role/en/index.html

One of the core principles of the World Health Organization is improving the health of populations. Over the past few

years, there is increasing evidence that the most effective way to improve health and wellbeing and reduce health inequalities is to focus support on the early years of life starting before a child is born. 'Fair Society, Healthy Lives: The Marmot Review' (Department of Health 2010) provides an overview of the current health status and health inequalities in England. The report was developed through a systematic review of the literature and also engaging with people living in communities and learning from their experiences and insights.

 Activity

Access 'Fair Society, Healthy Lives: The Marmot Review' at: http://www.marmotreview.org/. Consider the list of 12 headline indicators on page 85 of the Marmot report and reflect on the impact the indicators (e.g. parental substance misuse) may have on infants, children or young people's lives. Make a note of your findings.

The Marmot report is large and would take you a long time to read, however it will be helpful to read pages 85–91, on lessons to be learned from current strategy targets and indicators. By reading this section you will be able to gain an understanding of where much of public health nursing practice derives from. Public health nursing practice is based on current evidence on what we know about our population's health and wellbeing needs.

The Marmot Review reflects the circumstances in England. However, there are parallels in all UK countries and the aims and principles of addressing health inequalities can be applied elsewhere. Thinking again about communities as groups that share something in common, understanding how these communities develop and relate to each other within society is important for those who plan and deliver health and care services.

If you are studying in Scotland, Northern Ireland or Wales, you will find it useful to explore the government's approach to public health and addressing inequality. Links to the government's websites can be found in the resource section at the end of the chapter.

There is no doubt that the health of the nation is improving overall but the differences in factors which we know determine health continue to widen and so do inequalities in health (Marmot Review 2010). This means that the life expectancy, health and wellbeing of people who experience poor social, economic and environmental circumstances, particularly from birth are considerably worse than those who do not.

Traditional public health approaches that have focused on cause and effect relationships have been effective in many areas, for example the compulsory wearing of seatbelts has reduced the number of fatalities and severity of injury from road traffic accidents, and immunisation programmes have reduced and, in some cases, eradicated communicable diseases. However, for some people and communities, so strong is the influence of adverse life circumstances that traditional approaches have had limited impact on health improvement. This has led to interest in different approaches which look at factors that support and promote health in the broadest sense, rather than the deficits and problems that cause ill health.

One model is an asset-based approach, which aims to mobilise the assets, capacities or resources available to individuals and communities which could enable them to gain more control over their lives and circumstances (Morgan et al 2010). Central to the approach is helping to create the right conditions for people in disadvantaged communities to be in control of their lives, rather than telling them what to do. This person-centred way of working with people as active participants rather than passive recipients of health or social care allows them to feel empowered, build on their strengths and assets and helps them to do things for themselves. Foot and Hopkins (2010) describe assets as any of the following:

- Practical skills, capacity and knowledge of local residents
- Passions and interests of local residents that give them energy for change
- Networks and connections – known as 'social capital' – in a community, including friendships and neighbourliness
- Effectiveness of local community and voluntary associations
- Resources of public, private and third sector organisations that are available to support a community
- Physical and economic resources of a place that enhance wellbeing.

Activity

Are you aware of any activities or services that have developed in the community in which you live or in your community practice learning environment, as a result of the strengths and assets of local individuals or groups?

Examples may be a breakfast club for school children provided by a local church, a football team for young people with mental health problems organised with the help of a community development worker or a fresh fruit and vegetable co-operative making fresh produce available to the local community at cost price.

An overview of the evidence on asset-based approaches for health improvement has been published in a short briefing paper by the Glasgow Centre for Population Health (2011).

Summary of learning points from this chapter

- The health and social care context shapes the way services develop in different parts of the UK
- Primary, secondary and community care overlap and integrate and are all part of the community
- Public health approaches are fundamental to improving the health of individuals, communities and populations.

References

Department of Health, 2006. Our health, our care, our say: a new direction for community services. DH, London.

Department of Health, 2010. Fair Society, Healthy Lives: A strategic review of health inequalities in England post-2010. The Marmot Review. DH, London.

Department of Health, 2012. Health and Social Care Act. The Stationary Office, London.

Department of Health, Social Services and Public Safety Northern Ireland, 2011. A District Nursing Service for Today and Tomorrow. A review of district nursing in Northern Ireland. DHSSPSNI, Belfast.

Foot, J., Hopkins, T., 2010. A glass half-full: how an asset approach can improve community health and well-being. Improvement and Development Agency, London.

Glasgow Centre for Population Health, 2011. Asset based approaches for health improvement: Redressing the balance. Briefing Paper 9. Concepts Series, Glasgow.

Hudson, J., Lowe, S., Kühner, S., 2008. The short guide to social policy. Policy Press, Bristol.

Morgan, A., Davies, M., Ziglio, E., 2010. Health assets in a global context: theory, methods, action: investing in assets of individuals, communities and organisations. Springer, London.

Office for National Statistics, 2011. Social Trends 41. Online. Available at: http://www.statistics.gov.uk/Articles/Social_trends/social-trends-41-population.pdf (accessed November 2011).

Pickard, L., 2008. Informal care for older people provided by their adult children: projections of supply and demand to 2041 in England. Report to the Strategy Unit and Department of Health. PSSRU Discussion Paper 2515.

Wanless, D., 2004. Securing good health for the whole population: Final Report. Department of Health, London.

Further reading

Fatchett, A., 2012. Social policy for nurses. Polity Press, Cambridge.

Fyffe, T., 2009. Nursing shaping and influencing health and social care policy. Journal of Nursing Management 17 (6), 698–706.

Maslin-Prothero, S.E., Masterson, A., Jones, K., 2008. Four parts or one whole: The National Health Service (NHS) post-devolution. Journal of Nursing Management 16 (6), 662–672.

National Institute for Clinical Excellence, 2008. Public Health Guidance: Community engagement to improve health. NICE, London.

Watkins, D., Cousins, J., 2009. Public health and community nursing; frameworks for practice, 3rd ed. Elsevier, Edinburgh.

Williamson, G., Jenkinson, T., Proctor-Childs, T., 2010. Contexts of contemporary nursing practice, 2nd ed Learning Matters Ltd, Exeter.

Websites

Transforming Community Services, http://www.dh.gov.uk/en/Healthcare/TCS/index.htm.

The NHS Information Centre, England's national source of health and social care information. http://www.ic.nhs.uk/.

National Patient Safety Agency (NPSA) informs, supports and influences organisations and people working in the health sector to improve safety in patient care. The agency is an arm's length body of the Department of Health and through three divisions covers the health service across the UK: http://www.npsa.nhs.uk/corporate/about-us/.

NHS Choices: Background to the NHS, http://www.nhs.uk/NHSEngland/thenhs/about/Pages/overview.aspx.

Local Government Improvement and Development (Formerly IDeA), http://www.idea.gov.uk/idk/core/page.do?pageId=1.

Government websites

Scotland, http://www.scotland.gov.uk.
England, http://www.direct.gov.uk.
Northern Ireland, http://www.northernireland.gov.uk.
Wales, http://wales.gov.uk/splash?orig=/.

2

Introduction to community settings, services and roles

CHAPTER AIMS

- To describe the settings where services are provided in the community
- To discuss community nursing roles
- To introduce the student to the roles of the wider primary health and social care team

Introduction

This chapter helps to familiarise you with some of the settings, services and personnel that you will come across in the community during your clinical placement experience. It also touches upon the history of community nursing and the ways in which community nursing roles have developed. Roles continue to change and develop, not only in nursing but across all professional groups and agencies in response to the needs of people and communities, policy changes, initiatives in service delivery and direction from professional bodies, for example the Nursing and Midwifery Council (NMC).

Unlike the hospital environment where service provision is fairly straightforward, and housed in one place, the vast array of different healthcare settings, services and providers in the community may seem overwhelming at first. However, not only does the setting help to shape the nature and range of services that you will come across in the community but it also has a profound effect on the approach to care, the relationship between the service user and the practitioner and how practitioners use their skills and knowledge. The different providers and practitioners' roles are discussed in more detail later in the chapter but first we look at settings and some of the services they offer.

Care settings in the community

In Chapter 1, we described the setting for primary, secondary and community care as being part of the community. One way of helping to understand how services are organised and delivered in primary and community care and to overcome some of the complexity, is to group together those that have something in common. Figure 2.1 shows how settings can be grouped into three categories: clinical, community and home settings.

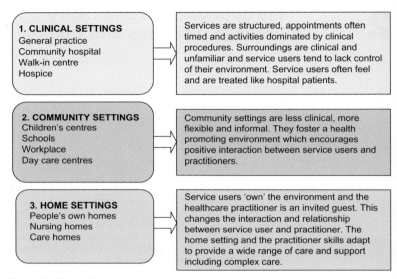

1. CLINICAL SETTINGS
General practice
Community hospital
Walk-in centre
Hospice

Services are structured, appointments often timed and activities dominated by clinical procedures. Surroundings are clinical and unfamiliar and service users tend to lack control of their environment. Service users often feel and are treated like hospital patients.

2. COMMUNITY SETTINGS
Children's centres
Schools
Workplace
Day care centres

Community settings are less clinical, more flexible and informal. They foster a health promoting environment which encourages positive interaction between service users and practitioners.

3. HOME SETTINGS
People's own homes
Nursing homes
Care homes

Service users 'own' the environment and the healthcare practitioner is an invited guest. This changes the interaction and relationship between service user and practitioner. The home setting and the practitioner skills adapt to provide a wide range of care and support including complex care.

Figure 2.1 Care settings in the community.

Clinical settings in the community

General practice

The doctor's surgery, health centre, medical centre and medical practice are all used to describe the General Practitioner's (GP) base. GPs are medical practitioners who choose to work in the community setting with patients and their families, rather than in a hospital. GPs provide a wide spectrum of services from those offered by single handed or small group GP practices, some in remote and rural areas, to large Health Centres, where a number of practices and their practice teams share premises and provide a comprehensive range of services. Core general medical services include consultation, examination, diagnosis and treatment, family health advice, vaccinations, prescriptions and referrals.

GP health centres

The first GP health centres opened in England in 2008, as part of a wider programme to improve access to GP services, particularly in parts of the country that had fewer GPs and greater health challenges. Apart from the general medical services offered at most GP practices and health centres, GP health centres offer additional services that would normally be provided elsewhere such as maternity, dentistry, physiotherapy and minor surgery. Described in the press as 'super surgeries', GP health centres have a strong focus on promoting health, particularly for hard-to-reach groups, and on reducing health inequalities. Most centres open from 8 am to 8 pm, 7 days a week, and anyone can use the additional services and stay registered with their local family doctor. Appointments can be pre-booked or patients can walk in without an appointment. Health Trusts in England determine the types of services offered based on local needs and local health improvement plans.

Minor injuries units

Minor injuries units (MIU) are community-based facilities that provide an alternative to attending an accident and emergency (A&E) department, if the person's injury is not serious. This frees up time for A&E staff to deal with more serious and life-threatening conditions. MIUs are usually nurse-led and attendees do not have to be registered with a particular GP. As appointments are not necessary and they are close to where people live, MIUs are convenient and save everyone time and unnecessary travel.

Treatment room services

Treatment room services are usually provided for people living and registered with a GP in a particular locality. The nurse completes a full and comprehensive assessment at the person's first visit to the treatment room to ensure the most appropriate care and treatment is delivered. Treatment room nurses are usually qualified to prescribe a variety of products used in the delivery of care.

NHS walk-in centres

NHS walk-in centres have become well established in England, treating approximately 3 million patients a year, and offering a complementary service to traditional GP and A&E services. They are based in local communities and provide on-site treatment for people with minor illnesses or injuries. They may be run by independent companies but are managed by Primary Care Trusts and they provide an NHS service. Most centres are open long hours and for 365 days a year. Walk-in centres are available for everyone to use, regardless of where they live or the GP they are registered with. Appointments are not necessary. They are usually managed by nurses but in some centres there is also access to doctors. They are not designed for treating long-term conditions or immediately life-threatening problems but they offer convenient access to a range of treatments for the following types of minor conditions:

- Infections and rashes
- Fractures and lacerations
- Emergency contraception and advice
- Gastric upsets
- Cuts and bruises
- Burns and strains.

Community hospital

A community hospital is a local hospital, unit or centre providing healthcare facilities and resources that are accessible by the local community. GPs usually provide the medical care in liaison with hospital consultant, nursing and allied health professional colleagues as necessary.

Most of the original community hospitals pre-dated the NHS and provided inpatient beds for the people living in the locality. Often in small towns, they were funded by local benefactors and some were built as war memorials to commemorate local service men and funded by families and the local community. Consequently, there is often still a strong sense of local ownership, community pride and identity, which contributes to what can be described as 'social capital'; the idea that communities working together create benefits for the whole community and for individuals. Community hospitals enable positive links and networks with and between carers and carer organisations, voluntary organisations, care providers in the social, private and care home sectors and local businesses, and are well placed to respond to new opportunities to work with and for the community. They are very well placed to promote a multidisciplinary, multisectoral approach to health care and have the potential to provide 24-hour, 7-days-a-week local access to a wide range of services. In most areas, nurses are employed to work specifically in the community hospital, although there are examples in some rural areas where district nurses are involved on a rotational basis.

The range of services that rural or urban community hospitals offer differs according to local arrangements for healthcare provision and depending on the needs of the locality. The following are some examples of the services that might be available at a community hospital, although most would focus on providing a selection of these:

- Intermediate managed care provided by GPs
- Consultant long-stay beds
- Nurse-led services
- Out-of-hours and emergency triaging services
- Outpatient and specialist clinics with visiting consultants
- Pre-admission and routine testing
- Day surgery
- Palliative care
- Rehabilitation
- Treatment for patients who cannot be cared for at home but who do not require the specialist care provided by a district hospital
- Convalescence or step down care
- Primary care midwifery services.

The term community hospital is often associated with the traditional model of a small local hospital in a small town providing an inpatient service which is scaled down from the large acute and specialist hospital miles away in the city. It is probably more relevant these days to refer to community-based centres which may or may not include inpatient beds, depending on the identified needs of the area. Not only do community hospitals or community-based centres have an important role to play in rural areas, urban areas can also benefit from locally based services, and there is

potential to make a real difference to inner city areas with significant health needs.

The following are three examples of community-based centres in urban settings:

1. A '24-bed urban community-based facility' offers GPs an alternative to admission to the acute sector for medically stable older people. It provides nurse-led, GP-supported care with a focus on the promotion of independence through rehabilitation and co-ordinated health and social care.
2. A 'community treatment centre' provides healthcare for local people in the centre of their community. As well as providing a range of diagnostic services and outpatient clinics, including paediatrics, it also offers rehabilitation assessment for older people and services, such as dietetics, physiotherapy, midwifery and community dentistry. Co-located services include social work, psychiatric nursing, voluntary services and school nursing. There are no inpatient beds.
3. A 'general practice urgent care centre' is a healthcare services facility commissioned by a teaching Primary Care Trust. The centre, operated by an independent provider of health and social care services, is located within a multicultural inner city community. The centre is open every day from 8 am and 8 pm and offers a range of comprehensive healthcare services to registered patients and a walk-in service for the treatment of minor injuries and illnesses, without having to make an appointment. Services include doctor's certificates, repeat prescriptions, treatment of minor injuries and illnesses, follow-up care, emergency contraception, vaccinations and immunisations, contraceptive services, cervical screening services, child health surveillance services, maternity services, chronic disease management (e.g. asthma, diabetes), lifestyle advice and smoking cessation.

Hospice

A hospice can be defined as a place or setting but it is actually much more than that. Since Dame Cecily Saunders' work in the 1950s and 1960s and the development of the modern hospice, it is more accurately defined as an approach to care. The aim of hospice care is to enhance the quality of life for the person who is dying and for their family. Care focuses on helping to control pain and relieve symptoms and to enable people to remain as positive, alert and active for as long as possible. Attention is given to meeting the person's social, spiritual and emotional needs and care is delivered with compassion to maintain the person's dignity, control and choice.

Hospice care teams include palliative medicine consultants and palliative care nurse specialists, together with a range of expertise provided by physiotherapists, occupational therapists, dieticians, pharmacists, complementary therapists, social workers and those able to give spiritual and psychological support.

Care in the hospice

The hospice offers a homely environment with the flexibility to meet the individual needs of people and their families. Most people prefer to stay at home for as long as they can and may be admitted to the hospice for a short time to get difficult symptoms under control or in the advanced stages of their illness.

Home care

Hospice home care nurses are specialist palliative care nurses who work alongside the community palliative care team, the GP and the district nursing team, and liaise with palliative care staff in secondary care. Hospice home care nurses often do not provide clinical hands on care but provide advice and support to the person, their carers and the primary care team.

Day care

Day care facilities usually offer a range of opportunities for assessment and review of people's needs and enable the provision of physical, psychological and social interventions within a context of social interaction, support and friendship. Creative activities, complementary therapies and hair dressing are often available and help to boost the person's self-confidence in safe and familiar surroundings.

Hospice outpatient service

In some hospices, outpatient clinics are available for people who are being cared for at home. This may include the option for a consultant appointment at the hospice rather than at the hospital or a clinic appointment with the physiotherapist, social worker, welfare advisor, complementary therapist and other hospice services.

Activity

Before continuing further, write down the nurse-led services that you are aware of in your local community and perhaps you or members of your family have used. What was your experience of these services?

Nurse-led services

Nurse-led services are a feature of the clinical settings described so far. In fact without the knowledge and skills of nurses in these settings and their competence to assess, diagnose, treat and prescribe, it is unlikely that services would have developed at all.

Laurent et al (2005) undertook a review of the substitution of doctors by nurses in primary care. Although there was limited research evidence, the review indicated that appropriately trained nurses can produce care of the same high quality and achieve equally good health outcomes for patients

Table 2.1 Examples of nurse-led clinics in the community

Asthma and COPD	Minor injuries
Family planning	Minor illness
Diabetes	Childhood immunisation
Cervical smears	Heart disease and stroke
Well person clinic	Travel health
Smoking cessation	Leg ulcer clinic

as doctors and at a lower cost. In many cases, it is not necessary to see a GP, so in areas where it is hard to recruit doctors or in some rural, remote and inner city areas where GP services are more difficult for people to access, nurse-led clinics and services offer a more accessible alternative. Not surprisingly, nurse-led services in primary care have flourished since the 1990s and tend to be either specialised and defined by the activities that are performed (there are some examples in Table 2.1) or more generalist in nature, such as nurse-led walk-in centres or minor injuries units.

Community settings

Childcare and pre-school education

There is a wide range of provision in the community for both childcare and pre-school education. Private nurseries, registered child minders and workplace crèches offer day care for young children of working parents together with informal and family carers who look after children in their own homes. Local community playgroups, family centres and Sure Start children's centres enable children and their parents and carers to meet together in a positive and informal environment. All 3–5-year-old children in the UK are entitled to free nursery education and this is provided in day nurseries, private nursery schools, nursery classes attached to primary schools and by accredited child minders. Members of the health visiting team have contact with the individual child and family wherever the child is cared for. They contribute to health promoting activities working alongside staff and offer services within settings such as children's centres.

Sure Start children's centres

Sure Start is a government initiative introduced in England in 1998. Sure Start children's centres aim to provide a 'one stop shop' for children and their parents bringing together the different support agencies which offer a range of services and advice from pregnancy to school age. Each children's centre is developed to meet the needs of the local community and, although core services must be offered at all centres, additional services vary according to local needs. Examples of core and additional services are shown in Table 2.2.

The different organisations offering these services work in partnership to offer the best support to all children and families in the community that the centre serves. The overall aim is to help children, especially those who may be disadvantaged in some way, get the best start in life. In Scotland, the aims of the Sure Start programme are now being used to take forward the Early Years Framework, which increases the focus on prevention, early identification and early intervention by agencies working together for the individual child and family.

Table 2.2 Sure Start children's centre services

Core services	Additional services
Child and family health services including health visitors and breast-feeding support	Dental health, dietician, physiotherapy
Childcare and early learning facilities or advice on local childcare options	Parenting classes Smoking cessation
Parenting advice and access to specialist services for families such as speech therapy or healthy eating advice	Advice, support and short-term breaks for children with learning difficulties or disabilities
Links to local Jobcentre Plus offices and training providers	English language tuition when English is not the family's first language

School

School health services are provided in a range of education settings for school age children including mainstream primary and secondary schools, schools for children with special needs, independent and private schools and in the home for children who are home educated. Looked after children, children excluded from school and young people within the youth offending system, also receive school health services. Teams include school nurses, support workers and community medical officers and they are backed up by specialist services such as mental health, family planning, drug and alcohol services and specialist community children's nurses supported by a range of services. All schools have a named school nurse who provides a first point of contact between the school and other services, and who is responsible for offering every child a programme of health assessment, screening, immunisations and health promotion. Most school nurses are based within health centres or clinics, with a small number based within schools, usually for children with special needs.

Day care centres for adults

Day care centres are run by local authorities, the NHS, voluntary organisations and private companies such as care homes. They can be in purpose built centres, community centres and halls, often in smaller towns and villages, and in residential care homes or in nursing homes. Based on the assessment of a person's needs, day care aims to give people the skills they need to live as independently as possible, helps them to remain living safely at home rather than in a residential or nursing home and helps to minimise avoidable admission to hospital. It also enables carers to have a break from caring. Transport is usually available as part of the service and is often provided by volunteers from the local community. A range of services is offered at day care centres, including some or all of the following:

- Access to a variety of health and care services such as the district nurse, podiatrist, social worker, optician and care assistants to help with bathing
- Employment schemes for people with learning disabilities or people with mental health problems can offer employment opportunities to people who may otherwise have difficulty finding work
- Rehabilitation and enablement – the opportunity to re-learn skills that have been lost through illness or disability or to learn new skills to cope with changing circumstances

- Social interaction – meeting and mixing with others, sharing stories and experiences, making friends
- Stimulation – leisure activities such as painting sessions, singing, chess, bingo, mobile library, cookery, internet
- Information and advice
- A cooked meal.

In many areas, lunch clubs based in local facilities provide a hot meal and offer social interaction and support for older people. They are often run by volunteers and funded by members and local voluntary groups.

Community pharmacies

Community pharmacies are situated in cities, towns and villages across the UK. They include large chains with shops on every high street, premises in supermarkets and large retail outlets and small independently owned pharmacies in small communities. Many are open long hours when other healthcare professionals are unavailable. Consultation rooms are now available in many community pharmacies allowing pharmacy staff to undertake procedures such as blood pressure checks in private and discuss personal issues with people without being overheard by other customers.

They can be found in some of the most deprived communities, which offer very little else in terms of health care. Based in the heart of the community, community pharmacists are probably the most easily accessible of all healthcare providers and are consequently well placed to focus on the most hard-to-reach and vulnerable families in their community. (See more about the services that are offered in community pharmacies later in the chapter.)

The workplace

The workplace can be simply defined as a place where people work. Shops, factories and offices immediately spring to mind but the variety is endless. Later in the chapter,

the role of the occupational health nurse is discussed but here, the workplace is discussed within the context of occupational health.

Occupational health is about the relationship between the workplace environment, the activities associated with the job and the health of the person who does the job. Occupational health is therefore important in all settings where people work, including industry, health and social care, education, retail and business, whether this is the public, private or voluntary sector. Employers have a legal duty to care for their employees.

Developments in occupational health and safety legislation have made a very positive impact on working conditions and many of the industrial diseases such as asbestosis in asbestos miners and industrial deafness in factory workers have practically disappeared. However, there are new challenges for workplace health resulting from new technology, societal change and changes in our expectations of work and the working environment. These make occupational health services as important as ever, as organisations strive to optimise staff performance and productivity, reduce sickness absence levels and help employers care for and understand the needs of their employees. There is a focus on enhancing staff morale and promoting a healthy working culture. The occupational health services provided cater to the needs of all employees in the organisation. The effect that a job has on an employee depends on the nature of the job and the individual's personality and coping strategies. People who work in manual jobs are more at risk of injury resulting from accidents or musculoskeletal complaints such as back pain. Emotional and stress-related problems are more likely to be associated with more autonomous and managerial roles which carry a heavy burden of responsibility and where people are under pressure to meet tight deadlines.

Activity

Choose one of the large employers in your community practice area, e.g. large supermarket, a factory, a call centre, a university, a private business, a hospital. Think about the wide variety of jobs that will be undertaken by people who work for this organisation and the health issues that could be associated with them. Make a list of the types of issues an occupational health service may need to address.

Ask your mentor if you can arrange to spend a day (often referred to as an insight day or a spoke placement) with an occupational health nurse and find out about the services that are available to support the health and wellbeing of their staff.

In large organisations, most occupational health services are led by either an occupational health nurse, or an occupational health doctor, with other members of the team providing consultancy advice as needed. The day-to-day running of the occupational health service is often undertaken by a manager who is an occupational health nurse. Other members of the multidisciplinary occupational health team include physiotherapists; ergonomists, who specialise in the design of equipment and the workplace environment, toxicologists and clerical staff. Table 2.3 shows the types of services offered within occupational health.

Legal duties in relation to health and safety at work apply to all employers, including very small organisations. There is an occupational health advice service for small businesses and GPs provided by the Department of Work and Pensions, which focuses on physical and mental health issues that affect individual employees at work. The advice services provide small business owners and managers with early and easy access to high quality and professional occupational health advice, tailored to their needs.

Home and residential settings

Person's own home

The setting which is most associated with the work of community nurses is the person's home. 'Home' may be a flat, a house, a hostel, a room, permanent, temporary or mobile. For most of us, home is more than just a place. 'A man's home is his castle'; 'Home is where the heart is'; 'Home sweet home', are all expressions that reflect the strength of feeling that people have about their home. Comfort, security, stability and familiarity are things that most of us want in a home and if we share it with others, we expect love, friendship and companionship.

But of course, home may not be associated with positive feelings and for some, it is the root of their health and social problems. Living conditions may be inappropriate for people's needs or aspirations, uncomfortable, poorly maintained, cold, damp and remote from amenities, family and friends. People may feel isolated, vulnerable, subjected to abuse or neglect, overwhelmed by financial problems and feel unable to cope. The environment in which we live has a profound effect on our relationships, self-esteem and mental and physical health at all stages of our lives.

A research study looking at the environmental housing conditions on the health and wellbeing of children conducted by the Social Care Institute for Excellence (SCIE), in 2005, reported the following key messages:

- More than 1 million children live in housing in England that it considered sub-standard or unfit to live in

Table 2.3 Occupational health services

Pre-employment screening	Occupational health assessment is often used to ensure that the person can safely work in an environment that is suitable for them or so that the employer can consider appropriate adjustments to help reduce the risk of health and safety issues developing over time. In some jobs the law or regulation requires individuals to be assessed before they start work
Fitness assessment	People with health problems affecting their fitness for work may be assessed and regularly monitored and the appropriate support made available
Support	Occupational health services aim to support employees when they become ill by following best practice on rehabilitation and making reasonable adjustments for people with a disability
Address specific health issues	Specific health issues include, stress, back pain and repetitive strain injury or work-related upper limb disorders, bullying, discrimination and harassment by other staff, managers or members of the public, such as patients or customers, manage harmful substances safely, environmental issues such as vibration, temperature, light and noise
Health improvement	Health promoting activities may focus on the specific needs of the workplace, e.g. smoking, drug and alcohol use, disease prevention and control, e.g. coronary heart disease and obesity, mental health and wellbeing and work–life balance. In addition, travel advice, vaccinations and immunisations and fitness programmes may be provided
Health surveillance	This includes regular screening as required by health and safety regulations in addition to those statutory screening when working with lead, ionising radiation and asbestos
Absence reviews	Independent assessment of people who have been absent from work usually for prolonged periods of time help to identify possible solutions. Rehabilitation programmes, counselling and advice to both management and the individual can support a staged return to work
Provide information and advice	Managers, employees and trade unions often require information about the workplace practices and policies of the organisation. Occupational health teams also advise organisations on the development and implementation of policy in-line with regulatory and legal requirements and provide training for staff, e.g. moving and handling
Treatment centres	Large organisations can find it more cost-effective to provide on site services such as physiotherapy, dental care and counselling services

- On the whole, the research indicates that there is an association between homes with visible damp or mould and the prevalence of asthma or respiratory problems among children
- Dampness and mould has also been found to be associated with exacerbated symptoms among children with asthma or wheezing illness
- Poor-quality housing can have an adverse effect on children's psychological wellbeing
- Parents and children both complain of the social stigma of living in bad housing
- Overcrowding and cooking with gas may cause respiratory infections in pre-term infants
- Interventions such as installing or improving heating systems, has been found to be effective in alleviating the potentially adverse effects of damp on the health of children SCIE (2005).

Nursing home and residential care home

Nursing and residential care homes provide help and support for people unable to remain in their own home, even when a comprehensive support package is in place. The terms 'residential care home' and 'nursing home' are often used interchangeably and although there are similarities, they are not the same. Both settings provide accommodation, meals, care and support from staff 24 hours a day. The nursing home or residential care home may be owned and managed by the NHS, local authority, private company or voluntary organisation.

Residents are registered with a local GP who will visit them when they require medical care and advice. The main difference between the two is the complexity of the care needs of the individual. The care and services in residential care homes are provided by trained care staff. Qualified nurses are employed within some care homes often as managers but also may be part of the care team, providing nursing care and supervising care staff. However, district nurses have access to care homes and visit in response to referrals from the care home manager or GP. Nursing homes have qualified nursing staff on duty 24 hours a day to support needs that are too complex to be met within residential care homes.

All nursing homes and residential care homes must be inspected, registered and regulated by the national independent regulator of health and social care. Each country has its own regulator. In England, the regulator is the Care Quality Commission.

Activity

The independent health and social care regulatory bodies for the four UK countries are shown below. Choose the one that applies to you and spend 10 minutes reading about their role. Then select one from another UK country and see how they compare.

England

Care Quality Commission: http://www.cqc.org.uk/

Wales

Commission for Social Care Inspection Wales: http://wales.gov.uk/cssiwsubsite/newcssiw/publications/?lang=en

Northern Ireland

The Regulation and Quality Improvement Authority (RQIA): http://www.rqia.org.uk/home/index.cfm

Scotland

Social Care and Social Work Improvement Scotland (SCSWIS) known as The Care Inspectorate: http://careimprovementscotland.org/

There are differences in the ways in which the four regulators are structured and discharge their duties. However, their overall aim is the same: to ensure the safety and wellbeing of vulnerable people who use services in local authorities, businesses, charities and voluntary organisations in the community. Regulation, inspection, review and support are methods used to encourage compliance with care standards and promote continuous quality improvement.

Sheltered housing

Sheltered housing provides older people and people with disabilities with safe, independent living. Usually sheltered housing consists of flats or small houses, supervised by a manager or warden and part of a complex with a communal area, where people can meet and socialise. The warden keeps regular contact with the residents and can be called through an alarm system in an emergency. People may own or rent their home in a sheltered housing complex, depending on whether it is provided by the local authority, housing association, voluntary organisation or private company. Generally, any personal care or services such as meals on wheels that residents require is provided by social services or community nurses but there are sheltered housing complexes that provide additional care services, for example, extra care housing, assisted living, very sheltered housing, close care and continuing care environments and care villages.

The clinical, community and home settings described here are just some examples of the places where people receive care and support in the community. You will come across many more during your period of practice learning in the community. However, the focus of your practice learning experience is the health needs of the individuals and the families that you meet, regardless of the setting.

If you keep them at the centre, the providers and services fit into place around them and it becomes clear how their health needs are addressed.

 Activity

Figure 2.2 shows the five main health and care providers and includes some examples of the services they offer. Make a list of the services that you have used or are likely to use while you are a university student. Where would these services fit into this model?

Primary care services across the UK are estimated to deal with over 90% of patient contacts with the NHS. Most of these contacts are visits to the GP or practice nurse, so it is highly likely that you will use the NHS in this way. You may have contact with the wider primary care team by using NHS community services and visiting a walk-in centre or if you have young children you will be in contact with a health visitor. Some complementary therapies are provided by the NHS but most are provided by private companies. You may have chosen to pay for homeopathy or aromatherapy or had private dental treatment. A large national charity may have provided you with support and advice for a long-term condition such as Diabetes UK or you may have benefited from social support from a local voluntary group. Finally, you may use local authority health and exercise facilities at the local leisure centre.

Service provision

The way in which the settings and services have been described in this chapter could give the impression that they are separate entities. The fact is that the organisations that provide health and care services do not work in isolation but in partnership.

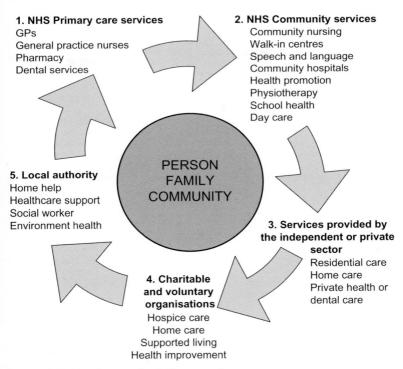

1. NHS Primary care services
GPs
General practice nurses
Pharmacy
Dental services

2. NHS Community services
Community nursing
Walk-in centres
Speech and language
Community hospitals
Health promotion
Physiotherapy
School health
Day care

PERSON
FAMILY
COMMUNITY

5. Local authority
Home help
Healthcare support
Social worker
Environment health

3. Services provided by the independent or private sector
Residential care
Home care
Private health or dental care

4. Charitable and voluntary organisations
Hospice care
Home care
Supported living
Health improvement

Figure 2.2 Health and care services in the community.

NHS primary care services and community services work together as a primary care team and rely on partnerships, working with the local authority, independent and voluntary sector organisations, depending on the outcomes they want to achieve.

The complex care needs of older people in the community often require a package of care which involves all providers. Sure Start children's centres are based on bringing a wide range of services and facilities together to offer a comprehensive service which has been shown to be much more effective than services delivered separately. For many, health and social care organisations such as Health Trusts and local authorities integration, rather than partnership, is the next step.

Many people live safely and independently at home managing the challenges associated with ageing or a long-term condition or disability with the support of a family member, neighbour or friend. Their medical care needs may be met by their GP and their contact with other health services such as community nursing may be minimal or not required. In many cases, it is the local authority social services departments that arrange the services which enable people to stay in their own home and avoid admission to hospital or a move to a care home.

Practical solutions such as providing equipment and home adaptations and help with daily tasks including, bathing and washing, getting in and out of bed, shopping, preparing meals, cleaning and transport, often make the most difference. Provision of services is based on assessment of need and where this is complex, a care plan will include a number of services provided by the NHS community services, such as home nursing, health promotion, continence advice, chiropody, occupational therapy, physiotherapy and the provision of equipment, such as wheelchairs and special beds. Other agencies can also provide cash for people to arrange their own services and manage care, e.g. employ a private carer to help with getting up and dressing, meals on wheels, a place at a day care centre run by a voluntary group.

Services differ in their characteristics because of the people they serve and also the type of provider organisation. Different solutions suit different service users, even within the same locality, and so reflect a personalised approach to care. The analysis of relevant and accurate information from local and national sources enables services to be planned at a strategic level. However, a local health needs assessment or a community profile builds up a picture of the health needs of the community in a particular area, often down to the level of the practice population and from there, services are adapted to meet the local needs. (Chapters 3 and 5 discuss health needs and assessment and community profiling in more detail.)

The roles of practitioners in NHS primary care services

General practitioner

The general practitioner (GP) is a medical doctor who provides primary care, offering health education and preventative care but also managing a wide range of acute and chronic medical conditions. The GP is usually the first point of contact that patients have with NHS services. General practitioners are not employed by the NHS. When the NHS first started in 1948, along with the dentists, pharmacists and opticians, they negotiated with the government to keep their independent contractor status. This meant that they worked under a contract for services with their health board or authority and this situation remains more or less the same today. The majority of GPs have a contract with their Primary Care Trust/Foundation Trust or Health Board, but in some areas, GPs are directly employed by the practice or the health authority to provide a range of services (shown below). A new national contract was introduced in 2004 and most practices operate under this, which is governed by the General Medical Services (GMS) Regulations, while a smaller proportion operate under local variations of the national contract. Changes to the national contract are negotiated every year with the British Medical Association (BMA) and this applies across all four UK countries. Primary medical services specified within a contract may include:

- 'Essential services', which form the core level of service that patients would expect their GP to provide, e.g. management of long-term conditions, health promotion advice, referral to specialist services
- 'Additional services', which consist of a number of further services that general practice usually provides to patients, e.g. cervical screening, contraceptive services, vaccinations/immunisations, child health surveillance, maternity services, minor surgery
- 'Enhanced services', which are either essential or additional services, delivered to a higher standard or further services beyond these, e.g. more specialised services.
- 'Out-of-hours services' are commissioned separately.

By far the largest proportion of a general practice's income is known as *the global sum* based on a formula including patient numbers and the provision of core services. This funds fees and services within the practice. The Quality & Outcomes Framework (QOF) payments are also an important source of income for practices. Previously, GPs' resources and rewards were based on the number of patients they treated rather than the quality of the care. QOF indicators are based on best available evidence in relation to aspects of care, including record-keeping, assessment, diagnosis and management.

Here are some examples of QOF indicators for coronary heart disease:

- CHD5: The percentage of patients with coronary heart disease whose notes have a record of blood pressure in the previous 15 months
- CHD6: The percentage of patients with coronary heart disease in whom the last blood pressure reading is 150/90 or less
- CHD10: The percentage of patients with coronary heart disease who are currently treated with a beta blocker.

The QOF contains 134 indicators in four domains: clinical, organisational, patient experience and additional services (additional services are clinical services that not all practices provide, such as maternity services). Community nurses and practice nurses in particular make a significant contribution to practices achieving their QOF targets.

Dental service

Dental care is focused on prevention and educating people of all ages to care for their mouths and their teeth. Two types of dentist practice in the community: general dental practitioners and community dentists.

General dental practice

General dental practitioners are based in the dental surgeries that we are familiar with, in high streets all over the country. They may practise under the NHS or privately but most dentists offer a combination of both NHS and private services. People are free to register with the dental practice of their choice, depending on vacancies on the dentist's list, locality and personal preference. For many people however, practices that provide NHS treatment are most attractive as private dental care can be expensive.

In the past, the mainstay of the dentist's role was treating tooth decay, minor dental and facial injuries and correcting dental irregularities, particularly in children. The role is now much wider and dentists are well placed to prevent disease and promote health. They can advise on behaviours that cause dental and oral disease such as poor mouth hygiene, poor diet, smoking and alcohol consumption, and identify early signs of oral disease and cancer, and refer people to specialist services quickly. NHS treatment for adults is paid for under a fee per item basis, which means the dentist receives a set amount for each procedure they carry out. Dental treatment for children incurs a monthly payment for each child on the dentist's list and a fee for each item of treatment.

Community dental service

Community dentists work for the NHS in a variety of settings, including, schools, people's homes, nursing homes and in community clinics. Oral health promotion is an important part of their role but they also provide the range of dental services that would be provided by the NHS and offered in general practice. The community dental service provides dental care to people who have difficulty accepting mainstream dental treatment. This may result from a physical, sensory, cognitive or developmental disability, where dental management is complicated because of a person's medical condition or children who are excessively anxious about attending a dentist. Community dentists also have a public health role and carry out dental surveys to monitor dental disease in the local community.

Pharmacist

Two types of pharmacist practice in the community: the community pharmacist and the primary care pharmacist.

Community pharmacist

Community pharmacists were known in the past as chemists, dispensing prescriptions written by doctors and selling a range of over-the-counter medicines. However, their role has changed radically over recent years and they have developed expertise in clinical roles traditionally undertaken by doctors, including prescribing, and have adopted a more integrated approach to working as members of the primary care team.

There is an NHS pharmacy contract for each UK country but the core or essential services and additional services are similar. Examples of these services are listed in Table 2.4 but try the activity in the next box before reading about them.

 Activity

You may be familiar with the role of the pharmacist in a hospital setting but what kind of services do you think a community pharmacist offers? Time spent with a community pharmacist is a very valuable learning experience. Discuss with your mentor how this could be arranged. However, community pharmacies are businesses and they may not be able to accommodate all students with an interest in learning about their role.

Primary care pharmacists

Most primary care pharmacists are employed by the NHS Primary Care Trust or Health Board and have either an operational or strategic role. Operational roles are usually based in the GP practice and involve a large amount of patient contact, for example: running anticoagulant, pain management and medication review clinics; providing pharmaceutical care to people living in care homes; liaison with hospitals on discharge planning issues – and many are qualified to prescribe. The pharmacist works closely with GPs, practice nurses and other healthcare professionals as part of the primary care team and may provide prescribing advice, education to other prescribers and pharmacy clinical governance co-ordination. Some primary care pharmacists work exclusively for one GP practice, others cover a number of practices and a few are employed directly by the GP. The term 'practice pharmacist' is often used to describe this role.

Primary care pharmacists with a strategic role focus on areas such as the planning of pharmaceutical services, budget setting, developing local drug formularies and clinical guidelines, as well as making the best use of resources allocated for medicines.

The roles of community nurses

Community nurse

The Nursing and Midwifery Council (NMC) define and set standards of education and practice for eight disciplines of community nursing:

1. District nursing
2. Public health nursing: health visiting
3. Public health nursing: school nursing
4. Public health nursing: occupational health nursing
5. Community mental health nursing
6. Community children's nursing
7. General practice nursing
8. Community learning disabilities nursing.

Table 2.4 Services provided by community pharmacists

Examples of essential services	Examples of additional services
Dispensing medicines and devices according to a prescription written by a doctor or non-medical prescriber and dispensing repeat prescriptions directly instead of person requesting it from their GP first.	Emergency out of hours services to provide medicines for the terminally ill.
Health promotion advice and practical help on keeping healthy, e.g. smoking cessation advice, diet and exercise.	Emergency hormonal contraception services.
Advise on minor ailments and supply medicines from a limited formulary, including medicines which you can buy over-the-counter from the pharmacy.	Anticoagulation monitoring and phlebotomy.
Work with community nurses and others.	Screening services (e.g. chlamydia, high blood pressure).
Signpost people to other services, self-care organisations or information resources.	Minor ailments services to reduce waiting times in GP practices.
Dispose of unwanted medicines.	Medicines use review to help people get the most out of their medicines.
	Supervising consumption of methadone.
	Needle exchange schemes for drug users.

Until 2004, the NMC approved preparation for all eight disciplines was the community specialist practitioner qualification (SPQ). The SPQ continues to be the route of preparation for general practice nursing, community mental health nursing, community learning disabilities nursing, community children's nursing and district nursing. Successful completion of the SPQ is recorded on the nursing part (Part 1) of the NMC register. However, preparation for specialist community public health nursing has replaced the specialist practice qualification leading to health visiting; school nursing and occupational health nursing. Specialist community public health nurses: health visitors, school nurses, occupational health nurses, as well as sexual health advisors and health protection nurses, are eligible to enter Part 3 of the NMC register (Part 2 of the NMC register applies to midwifery).

District nurse

District nurses lead in the delivery of high quality community nursing in the home. Home may be the person's house, flat or caravan or it may be in sheltered accommodation, a care home or relative's home. Some district nurses also work in treatment rooms, day centres and, in some areas, contribute to the care provided in community hospitals. The role of the district nurse has developed considerably over the years and continues to change in response to the changing needs of the community. Most notable changes include the increasing number of older people who require support to remain independent and safe at home; home-based complex care, which requires the very skilled nursing and highly technical interventions that would once have only been available to hospital inpatients; and the emphasis on promoting self-care and providing preventative and anticipatory care, which empowers people to take more responsibility for their own health and wellbeing.

Activity

District nurses have been described as the 'specialist generalists' of the community nursing team. Can you think why this is?

Essentially district nurses are the experts or specialists in the provision of direct clinical care to people in their own homes. The skills they use are more than an adaptation of hospital clinical skills to a different setting. Their role is very broad and rather like a GP, they can be involved in caring for people with any type of health issue, from minor illness and injury to any acute or long-term condition. Although district nurses generally provide care for adults, some are also involved in caring for children and their families. It is not easy to summarise their role but the following is an overview of the range of the district nurses' responsibilities.

- Assessing the healthcare needs of patients and families, planning care in partnership with them, respecting their dignity, choices and rights as a visitor in their home
- Promoting care approaches, which enable people to maintain their independence, remain at home safely and avoid unnecessary hospital admissions and readmissions. Examples include predicting care needs by using

anticipatory care plans and promoting self-care and carer involvement, helping them to learn how to care for themselves
- Professional accountability for the care provided by the skill mix team
- Providing education, information and advice and teaching patients and carers practical techniques and the use of equipment for self-caring
- Communicating, collaborating and working in effective partnerships with other professions and agencies across the health, social care and voluntary sectors, to secure and maintain the most suitable and effective care packages for individuals and their families
- Managing the skill mix team and other resources such as budgets, to achieve efficiency in the service and maximise patient contact time
- Leading the skill mix team: improving capacity and capability and educational support
- Selecting and delivering evidence-informed care and interventions that are patient-centred, effective and manageable in the person's home environment
- Monitoring and evaluating care and making adaptations to the care plan to ensure that the person and the family have the care and support they need to achieve the best health outcomes and quality of life
- Care or case management for people with complex health needs, resulting from long-term conditions such as respiratory disease, diabetes, chronic wounds, heart failure
- Follow-up care for recently discharged hospital inpatients and longer-term care for chronically ill patients who may be referred by many other services, as well as working collaboratively with GPs in preventing unnecessary or avoidable hospital admissions.

Activity

Understanding how the role and contribution of individual members of the skill mix team support a service or a person's care plan is very important. Consequently, spending time with and learning from a healthcare support worker is just as important as spending time with the specialist nurse or consultant nurse in the team.

When you plan your programme with your mentor, find opportunities to gain insight from all members of the team, not only about their current role but about the preparation and experience that they required.

Public health nursing: health visitor

A health visitor can be a registered nurse or midwife who has successfully completed an NMC approved post-registration programme of preparation for the role. Health visitors and most school nurses are recognised by the Nursing and Midwifery Council (NMC) as having a specialist qualification and are registered on Part 3 of the register 'Specialist Public Health Nurses'. The NMC set standards for practice, which enable practitioners to contribute safely and effectively in maintaining and improving the health of the public and communities therefore assuming accountability for public protection.

Health visitors work with individuals, families and communities in a range of settings, including people's homes, GP surgeries, children's centres, clinics and anywhere that improves access for service users. The health visitor's role is to improve and promote health, prevent ill health and to protect vulnerable groups. Health visitors may be involved in giving advice to older people, co-ordinating health promotion clinics such as smoking cessation or childhood immunisation and organising drop-in sessions and support groups. The health visitor role is to provide a universal preventative service and also focus on vulnerable babies, children and families. Every family with children under the age of 5 years has a named health visitor. Although most of their involvement is with children in this age group, they continue to provide support through the school years. Contact with the family often begins in the antenatal period, when support and preparation for parenthood is offered in partnership with the community midwife. Health visitors develop a rapport with the family, which continues through the child's development to school age. The health visitor monitors the child's development, encourages positive parenting, regularly assesses the child's health and advises on topics such as infant feeding, sleeping, weaning and immunisation. Health visitors work within skill mix teams, which include registered nurses, healthcare support workers, nursery nurses, nurse consultants and as part of the wider community nursing and primary care team. They work closely with families who are at risk, such as homeless families, and have a significant role in child protection. Health visitors often provide the lead from a health perspective in cases of actual or suspected child abuse or neglect as part of an interagency approach including health, social work, education and the police.

Public health nursing: school nurse

The school nurse is involved with the overall health improvement of school-age children. This work includes health surveillance programmes and promoting healthy lifestyles in schools and protection for vulnerable children and young people of school age. School nurses' responsibilities also include immunisation and vaccination programmes, promoting positive parenting, offering support and counselling to promote positive mental health in young people and playing a key role in the organisation of multidisciplinary care for children with complex medical needs.

Evidence demonstrates that to achieve positive outcomes for all children, the balance of care needs to shift from crisis intervention to an early intervention focus. This shift in focus is most successful in the early years. Health visitors, school nurses and those who work as part of the team are pivotal to this process. Their role is key in the co-ordination and delivery of the core universal service, as set out in national policy (e.g. Health for all Children 4, Scottish Government 2005); the promotion of health and wellbeing, surveillance and screening and facilitation of early intervention where appropriate. The Healthy Child programme is the public health early intervention and prevention programme in England.

Health promotion, prevention and early intervention

Public health nurses provide a core service to all children and families. The programme usually begins when children are 11 days old, when the responsibility for health promotion, health screening and health support is transferred from the midwife. The service is sometimes referred to as a universal service, which means something that is offered to all. Health visitors work closely with midwives so that care and support is consistent and any identified needs of the child or family are shared. The core service in each area includes evidence-based health promotion information that is shared and discussed with children and their families, developmental screening and assessment of children's health and wellbeing needs.

You will have the opportunity to follow your mentor as they provide this service. You will also have the opportunity to observe other practitioners involved in providing universal services to children, for example GPs and perhaps general practice nurses who are often involved in providing the immunisation programme

Frameworks for practice in public health nursing

There are times when children and young people need additional help and support to reach their full potential. It is well recognised that to be able to effectively assess, plan and implement care and support for children, practitioners need to work with both other agencies, parents and children themselves. Frameworks for practice aim to ensure that services provided to children are consistent, timely and appropriate for children and young people's needs, for example by improving the information that is shared by practitioners. Frameworks for practice have been developed in each country to improve services provided to children and families by identifying the principal positive outcomes that should be achieved by all children. You will find that each country has worded the main outcomes slightly differently, however in general, they suggest similar outcomes across the UK. The Scottish example is provided in Table 2.5 and shows some of the activities that health visitors and school nurses may be involved in to help children and young people achieve their full potential (Scottish Government 2011).

Child development

Health visitors and school nurses work with infants, children, young people and their families to assess, promote and support child development in many different ways. There are a number of definitions of child development, however most authors

Table 2.5 Health visiting and school nursing activities

Wellbeing indicators(Scottish Government 2011)	Health visiting and school nursing activities
Safe	
Protected from abuse, neglect or harm at school and in the community	Child protection
Healthy	
Having the highest attainable standards of physical and mental health, access to suitable healthcare and support in learning to make healthy and safe choices	Immunisations, health screening, health promotion
Nurtured	
Having a nurtured place to live, in a family setting with additional help if needed or, where this is not possible, in a suitable setting	Support with parenting, e.g. parenting groups; support to young people to make choices in their lives, e.g. school sessions on risk-taking
Active	
Having opportunities to take part in activities such as play, recreation or sport, which contribute to healthy growth and development both at home and in the community	Support and advice on child growth and development, e.g. healthy weight programmes
Respected	
Having the opportunity along with carers to be heard and involved in decisions which affect them	Group activities in school or attending meetings when planning care for children and young people
Responsible	
Having opportunities and encouragement to play active and responsible roles in their schools and communities and, where necessary, having the appropriate guidance and supervision and being involved in decisions that affect them	Co-ordinating and implementing care plans for individual children and young people
Included	
Having the help to overcome social, educational, physical and economic inequalities and being accepted as part of the community in which they live and learn	As above and public health work

describe child development as a whole concept where different areas of development contribute to the full potential children can achieve. The areas include physical, cognitive, emotional and psychosocial development. Children grow, develop and learn throughout their lives from birth and infancy to adulthood. A child's development can be measured through social, physical and cognitive developmental milestones. If children fail to develop properly, they may be unable to reach their full potential. Health visitors, school nurses and other staff who work with children and young people have an overall aim of helping all children to meet their full potential in all of the areas of child development. A child or young person's development can be influenced in many ways; in the past, there have been debates on whether children were affected by nature (i.e. the genetic influences) or nurture (i.e. parental influences). It is now recognised that both nature and nurture are equally important. Children's development can be influenced by genetic and biological factors and equally, their family situation or the external environment that surrounds them (Aldgate et al 2006).

Child protection

Child protection is everyone's responsibility, however as health visitors and school nurses work closely with all children and young people, they play a fundamental role.

Community mental health nurse

Community mental health (CMH) nurses work with children, adults and older adults in a wide variety of community settings, including the person's own home, outpatient department, GP surgery, health centre and community hospital. Some CMH nurses specialise in working with older people, children or people with drug or alcohol problems. They work closely with other members of the community mental health team and in partnership with psychiatrists, social workers, occupational therapists, clinical psychologists and pharmacists, and deliver multiprofessional person-centred services. A specific community role was established in the 1950s for mental health nurses, when they were called community psychiatric nurses (CPNs), a term which is still used today in some areas. The approach to care has developed in-line with the closure of the large psychiatric hospitals and institutions that were common until the1970s and CMH teams work in close partnership with service users who would once have had limited prospects of living independently in the community. The CMH nurse's role has changed considerably since then, moving from a more custodial role, with the emphasis on treatment, to a community-based approach focusing on prevention, maintaining wellbeing, recovery and rehabilitation. The following are some of the ways in which the CMH

 Activity

You may have the opportunity to observe the role of the health visitor or school nurse in child protection. Discuss the role with the practitioner and your mentor. You may also have the opportunity to spend some time with other practitioners involved in child protection, e.g. child protection advisors or the social worker. Access NSPCC Inform, which contains child protection resources for anyone working to safeguard children, and access the child protection guideline in your practice area. NSPCC Inform: http://www.nspcc.org.uk/Inform/informhub_wda49931.html

nurse supports people with mental health problems in the community:

- Assessment involving listening and interpreting a person's concerns and needs and care planning with the person to ensure the most appropriate and effective solutions are found
- Acting as a key worker, liaising with relatives and CMH team members, co-ordinating care and attending regular meetings to review and monitor patients' care plans
- Providing care for people experiencing acute mental distress or who have an enduring mental illness
- Providing evidence-based psychological therapies including cognitive behaviour therapy (CBT) for depression and anxiety preparing and participating in group and/or one-to-one therapy sessions, both individually and with other health professionals
- Assisting people to manage their medicines and monitoring their effectiveness and side-effects. Some CMH nurses are qualified to prescribe and initiate some treatments or alter the timing and dosage of medication
- Visiting people in their home to monitor progress, assessing their behaviour and psychological needs and identifying whether and when patients are at risk of harming themselves or others
- Encouraging people to retain or regain their social networks, take part and get involved in community activities, clubs groups and occupational therapy
- Helping people to talk through their problems and giving them and their families practical advice and support.

In addition to the professions already mentioned in the community mental health team, outreach workers, mental health support workers, art therapists and psychotherapists also play an important role. Peer support workers who have lived experience of mental illness support and whose role has been positively evaluated by Scottish Government Social Research

(2009), complement the CMH with new skills and knowledge. Specialist old-age psychiatry teams may include other professionals such as speech therapists or physiotherapists who may visit people in their own homes.

General practice nurse

General practice nurses are based alongside GPs in general practices, surgeries and health centres. They work in close collaboration with members of the practice team including GPs, the practice manager, practice pharmacist and the wider primary care team, which includes the community nurses and allied health professionals. In larger practices, there may be several general practice nurses sharing duties and responsibilities but often specialising in certain areas, for example, travel health, contraception and sexual health but in smaller practices, the general practice nurse may work alone and take on many roles. The role of the nurse in general practice is wide ranging and varied and depends very much on the skills and competencies of the nurse and the role determined by the needs of the practice population. The following are some of the activities that characterise general practice nursing:

- First point of contact for people contacting the practice with health problems. This may be by telephone triage where the practice nurse prioritises problems and allocates appropriate appointments, depending on the urgency of the person's problem
- A lead role in screening and secondary prevention programmes, running smoking cessation programmes and cervical screening clinics
- Treating minor injuries and minor illnesses, including dressing wounds and ear syringing
- Prescribing medicines for patients they treat. Many practice nurses are qualified independent and supplementary

prescribers (this is described in more detail in Chapter 11)

- Running clinics such as family planning, travel health, immunisation
- Providing nurse-led services for the management of people with long-term conditions such as asthma, COPD and diabetes.

Some general practice nurses have further developed their skills and knowledge through postgraduate study and practice as nurse practitioners at an advanced level. This enables them to assess patients and make initial diagnoses and initiate and monitor treatment in a similar way to a GP. It is not always straightforward to arrange learning in practice time with a member of the general practice nurse team. One reason for this is that they are employed directly by general practitioners. This means that there may be limited time for teaching and supervising students built into their clinical practice hours, which are essential for them to manage their workload. In some areas you may spend a day or part of a day with a practice nurse but in others, a much longer time may be allocated. Some practice nurses are qualified to mentor nurse students but this is not commonplace. There is so much to learn from time spent with the general practice nurse, so if the time allocated appears to be limited, discuss this with your mentor and be proactive in negotiating time for learning in this important area of community nursing.

Community children's nurse

Community children's nurses care for children with a wide range of acute nursing needs, long-term conditions and complex healthcare requirements. They provide a skilled nursing resource to children and their families, other health professionals and the community as a whole. The emphasis on care at home has increased and for most children, this is provided by the family in a supportive partnership with local community children's

nursing services as part of a wider multiprofessional and multiagency children's team. Not only do community children's nurses assess the needs of the child but they assess the particular needs of the family and ensure effective links with health, education and social services, enabling the child to be well supported at home and in other community settings such as playgroups, nurseries, schools and residential and respite care settings. As children with increasingly significant health problems are surviving through childhood and into adulthood, children's services aim to enable them to lead as full, enjoyable and active a life as possible, to achieve the best possible health outcomes and the best possible quality of life for themselves and their family. Children's community nurses play an important role in supporting this aim by both delivering care and also facilitating and organising care by supervising and developing others such as the family and other members of the healthcare team.

Depending on local arrangements, community children's nursing services may be based in the acute hospital, with specialist nurses providing an outreach service from the hospital unit to children at home. In other areas, there is a dedicated community-based service, staffed by community children's nurses with close links with the specialist hospital service. There are also examples where district nurses work with other members of the primary care team to provide care for children at home. The arrangements often reflect the needs of the child, for example a child who is in the acute stage of an illness will be managed very closely by the hospital consultant and any respite spent at home with their family would be supported by hospital outreach nurses or hospital-based community children's nurses. A child living at home with a long-term condition is likely to have infrequent contact with the acute hospital services and be involved with the community children's nurses as part of a

comprehensive child-centred multiagency team that, in many areas, includes the following:
- Community paediatricians
- Child development service
- School health
- Children and young adults mental health services
- Social services
- Education and training (schools and colleges)
- Child protection service
- Child health records
- Physiotherapy
- Occupational therapy
- Speech therapy
- Paediatric audiology
- Parent partnership

A child and family-centred approach is evident in all aspects of the community children's nurse's role:
- Assessment, referral, early intervention and care delivery, preventing hospital admission, facilitating early discharge where possible and arranging periods of respite where appropriate
- Planning care with the child and family to support recovery from acute episodes of illness or injury or to provide flexible and responsive plans to care for children with long-term and very complex healthcare needs
- Providing families with information, education and the skills to manage care at home and in social and recreational settings, giving children and families the reassurance and confidence to care effectively and independently and enable them to network with other families to promote peer support and reduce feelings of isolation
- A health improvement and health protection role with the child, family and community
- Promoting the health of all family members and supporting the child and family in reducing the impact of illness or disability

- Caring for families, supporting and providing interventions that relieve the physical and psychological stress associated with full-time caring
- Enabling children with complex needs to be part of mainstream activities, for example providing support and training to carers, teachers and school nurses in main stream schools to enable them to care for children who are dependent on technology such as oxygen therapy and enteral feeding
- Providing palliative and end of life care to the child dying at home and offering appropriate support to families following bereavement
- Promoting effective links and integrated working with the primary and care team and community-based services and children's hospital services.

Community learning disabilities nurse

The role of the community learning disabilities nurse involves working in partnership with the person with learning disabilities and often their family to promote health and wellbeing, independence and social inclusion. Health needs may be complex with physical and mental health problems making it even more challenging for the person with learning disabilities to cope. Learning disabilities' nurses are the specialists in providing care for people of all ages and in a variety of community settings.

Approximately 1.5 million people in the UK are affected by learning disabilities. Although many people lived within the community, often with the support of parents, long-term institutional care was traditionally provided for people with learning disabilities in large institutions often in remote areas and removed from mainstream society. The gradual closure of these institutions in response to government policy introduced in 1971, has been successful in shifting the balance of care to the community, where most people now live either in their own homes or in smaller more homely residential settings.

Learning disabilities nurses are now almost exclusively based in community settings where people with learning disabilities live and work. These include schools, day centres, adult education centres, the workplace, people's own homes, family homes, sheltered housing, independent living and supported living homes, treatment and assessment services and challenging behaviour units. They work as part of the primary care and community nursing team or in specialist teams such as, child health, mental health or forensic services. The role is consequently wide and varied, but in general includes the following:

- Using a range of specialist skills to provide clinical care for people who have co-existing complex health problems such as sight and hearing loss, complex behavioural needs, epilepsy, physical disability and depression
- Supporting families and working in partnership to assess health and care needs, plan and deliver care, providing information, education and practical advice
- Supporting people to be as confident and independent as possible in life, education and at work
- Advocating on behalf of people with learning disabilities and promoting access to health and other services
- Providing health education and health promotion to people and their carers
- Liaising with other agencies and co-ordinating services
- Developing services to meet the needs of people with learning disabilities, their families and employers
- Working with adults with learning disabilities that have families themselves

- Educating and supporting other members of the health and social care team to care for people with a learning disability both in the statutory and voluntary sectors.

◢ Activity

Successive government policy has aimed to reduce the stigma and discrimination associated with learning disabilities and to remove barriers to people leading economically and socially fulfilled lives.

Access the Foundation for People with Learning Disabilities website. This is a good example of an independent or third sector organisation that works to increase inclusion for people with learning disabilities by working with them, their families and the people who support them. Foundation for People with Learning Disabilities: http://www.learningdisabilities.org.uk/our-work

Community nurses normally work in skill mix teams which are discipline specific, for example district nursing teams. Staff working at all levels of the Career Framework may comprise a skill mix team, including unregistered staff or healthcare assistants, registered nurses or staff nurses who have not completed the post-registration specialist community nurse qualification and specialist nurses. This type of discipline-specific team will be a team within the wider community nursing team. Teamwork and leadership in the community are discussed in more detail later. However, apart from the eight branches of community nursing, there are many other nurses working in the community some of whom have developed specialist roles on the basis of their community-nurse background, for example a nurse in the role of a child protection advisor is likely to be a qualified health visitor and a specialist nurse in palliative care nurse may have a background in district nursing.

Other nursing roles in the community

Community matron

Community matrons not only provide nursing care to people in the community who have very complex care needs but they also act as case managers co-ordinating care and support across a wide range of different agencies and providers. They specialise in supporting people who might otherwise be admitted to hospital or to residential care because of long-term conditions or a combination of health problems such as, chronic obstructive pulmonary disease (COPD), hypertension, diabetes, heart failure, dementia, Parkinson's disease, motor neurone disease and multiple sclerosis. As case managers, community matrons act as a single point of contact which helps to avoid overlaps and omissions in care. They work in partnership with service users and their carers so that they are better informed and better prepared to participate more actively in their care.

Using a case management approach aims to prevent avoidable hospital admission and keep people safe and cared for at home for as long as possible. Where hospital admission is necessary, community matrons can reduce length of stay by liaising closely with hospital staff, advising on appropriate care for the patient and planning and co-ordinating services in the community in preparation for discharge. (The NHS and Social Care Long Term Conditions Model (DH 2007) described in Chapter 5, shows the level of intervention of the community matron at Level 3 high complexity case management.)

Community specialist nurses

Specialist nurses aim to ensure that people with specific conditions receive the most appropriate care and services wherever care is delivered. They may be community-based, sometimes with hospital in-reach responsibilities or hospital-based with an outreach function. Roles vary according to the nature of the service with some specialist nurses being more involved in direct patient care than others with a more advisory and educational role. Examples of specialist nurse roles include:

Respiratory or COPD nurses

Often part of a multidisciplinary team, including physiotherapist and occupational therapist, respiratory nurses visit people who have respiratory disease at home or in GP surgeries to offer clinical support and management of symptoms, education and advice to support self-care.

The team offers clinical support, management, education programmes and advice to patients and their families. It aims to improve the quality of life for patients with respiratory disease.

Tissue viability nurses

Tissue viability nurses are usually involved in developing and delivering educational programmes, developing guidelines, policies and care pathways for the management and prevention of chronic wounds. They visit people at home to assess and manage complex wounds such as postoperative wounds, pressure ulcers, leg ulcers and fungating wounds.

Heart failure nurses

Heart failure nurses aim to manage and improve symptoms of the person with heart failure, keeping them out of hospital and comfortable at home. They offer advice and education for self-care, referral to other members of the multidisciplinary team and support for carers.

Other specialist nursing roles include: continence nurse, lymphoedema specialist nurse, diabetes specialist nurse, HIV specialist.

Community control of infection team

Control of infection is an important and integral part of health and social care, regardless of the setting. Infection control includes the prevention and management of infections, using research-based knowledge. In the community, infection control applies to a wide range of environments, including a person's home, children's centres, residential care home, schools, pharmacies and general practice. Community infection control teams include specialist infection control nurses whose work includes: standard precautions, outbreak management, review and development of infection control policies, surveillance, infection control audits, specialist advice, education and training, involvement in new build and refurbishment projects, contact tracing and acting as a resource for staff and members of the public.

Community midwife

The midwife is the expert in normal pregnancy, birth and postnatal care and skilled in recognising complications and referring care to specialists and obstetricians as soon as necessary. Community midwives provide maternity care in settings that are appropriate and accessible to women and their families, GP surgeries, the home environment, community centre or children's centre, shopping centres, birth centre and on occasions within the hospital. Sometimes they are attached to the hospital and are based there but they can be GP attached and based in the surgery or health centre. They usually work in teams and aim to provide continuity of care from pre-birth to when the mother and baby no longer require their support. Midwives can provide

the first point of contact for women and they are encouraged to contact the midwife or GP as soon as they know they are pregnant.

Services provided by the community midwife
Antenatal care

Community midwives provide antenatal care which monitors the health and wellbeing of the woman and the progress of her pregnancy and helps women and their partners prepare for parenthood. Women are offered an initial booking appointment when they are between 8 and 12 weeks' pregnant. This includes a comprehensive assessment of the woman's social, psychological, physical condition and obstetric history, helps to identify any potential risk and enables choices to be offered and discussed. This is an important time for the midwife to give information and give the woman time to discuss issues including keeping well in pregnancy, diet and nutrition, maternity benefits, antenatal screening tests and options for antenatal care and birth.

Antenatal appointments provide continuous care throughout the pregnancy and are offered at intervals and at important stages, focusing on the needs of the woman and her pregnancy. NICE Guidance CG62 (2008) recommends 10 appointments for women expecting their first baby and seven appointments for subsequent pregnancies. Where additional care is required, women are more closely monitored in the community or referred to hospital-based obstetric services.

Unless there are risks to the health of the woman or the pregnancy, most antenatal care takes place in the community. If a home birth is planned, then all care usually takes place there. Another alternative is shared care between the hospital and the community midwife and GP. Some women require specialised consultant care during pregnancy and this may consist of a combination of visits to the hospital antenatal clinic, the GP and the community midwife. Community midwives have open access to obstetricians, or the antenatal day unit when women in their care require investigation and/or inpatient care.

 Activity

> The format and timing of antenatal care provision has changed in the last few years in response to NICE Clinical Guideline 62 published in 2008. This has resulted in fewer routine antenatal appointments but the introduction of a more efficient, effective and evidence informed approach. This guidance has been adopted UK-wide.
>
> Whether or not you have an opportunity to observe the community midwife giving antenatal care, you will learn about what a woman can expect from antenatal appointments with her midwife, and the priorities of antenatal care by reading the following short reference guide: The Quick Reference Guide: Antenatal care, routine care for the healthy pregnant woman http://www.nice.org.uk/nicemedia/live/11947/40110/40110.pdf

Care for labour and childbirth

Community midwives provide care for women in labour at home and can also provide care to women delivering their baby in hospital or a midwifery-led unit or birth centre. Community midwives are experts in preparing women and their families for home birth, adapting the home environment and helping women to give birth naturally and without the interventions associated with hospital birth. Home birth is one option for women who are healthy and having an uncomplicated pregnancy. Alternatives include birth at a

midwifery-led unit, birth centre or GP unit. These community settings differ in name but essentially, they provide a homely alternative to hospital delivery units. They offer more choice, privacy, flexible approaches to family members being present at the birth, birthing pools, massage, flexible furniture and a relaxed atmosphere. The community midwife must manage any complication or emergency situation that may arise in a community setting and care for the woman and/or her baby during the transfer to hospital. The community midwife may also accompany the mother and baby home afterwards if all is well.

 Activity

> You may be spending time with a community midwife who is preparing for a home birth. With the consent of the woman and her family and of course the community midwife, there may be an opportunity for you to attend. Discuss this with your mentor/the community midwife. Remember you would have to be on-call and available 24/7 and committed to being available when the woman goes into labour.

Postnatal care

Postnatal care ensures that a woman has made a recovery from pregnancy and birth, the baby is well, and the family is adjusting. The community midwife monitors physical recovery, psychological wellbeing, advises on infant feeding, provides breast-feeding support and advises the woman about rest and exercise. A midwife is required by law not only to be present at delivery but also to supervise the care of the woman and her baby for a period of not less than 10 days after the end of labour and for a period of time determined by her professional judgement thereafter. Therefore, the community midwife will continue to visit the family after a home birth or following the birth of the baby in hospital when the care of the woman and baby is transferred back to the community midwife. The frequency of visits depends on the midwife's assessment but normally after 10 days, this supervisory care usually transfers to the health visitor who will support the family throughout the rest of the baby's childhood. The community midwife can still be contacted if problems arise in the first weeks, which cannot be addressed by the health visitor. In some areas, community midwives offer postnatal care in a clinic settings and prioritise home visits for women who are unable to attend.

The community midwife's role also involves working closely with other members of the primary care team, including GPs, health visitors, social workers, community mental health nurses and school nurses. They deliver classes during the antenatal period such as parent craft and exercise classes and are involved in initiatives working with groups such as women from specific ethnic minority groups, pregnant teenagers, teenage parents and women with problems such as substance misuse.

⚡ Activity

Member states of the European Union have agreed professional standards of training for nurses. The inclusion of maternity care in programmes of preparation for adult nursing is an EU Directive requirement. Make sure you are aware and understand what the university expects of you in relation to this. You may have specific guidance and learning outcomes in this area. If you are in doubt, discuss this with your mentor.

Allied health professionals (AHPs)

AHPs are a mixed group of autonomous healthcare practitioners who are able to accept self-referrals from the public and from other health professionals, including community nurses. They can diagnose, treat and discharge clients and they are increasing being encouraged to use their skills to promote health and prevent illness. Some AHPs are based in community clinics or community hospitals, or they may be based in an acute hospital and deliver services in an outreach model. In general, the approach that all AHPs have in common is to support and promote rehabilitation or re-ablement and a return to or the maintenance of independence. Since AHPs are usually in limited supply in the community, most are keen to provide training for other health workers and encourage appropriate referrals. The type of AHP services available vary from area to area and may be delivered in different ways, for example in a remote and rural setting.

There may not be opportunities for you to spend time with all the AHPs described in Table 2.6 but use the questions in the boxes below to make the most of any learning opportunities that are available to you.

Table 2.6 Examples of Allied health professionals working in the community

Dietitians	Physiotherapists
Occupational therapists	Podiatrists
Orthoptists	Speech and language therapists

Dieticians

Dieticians work with people to promote nutritional wellbeing, prevent food-related problems and treat disease with diet therapy. They work with all age groups and client groups and deliver services in a variety of settings including health centres, GP surgeries, care/nursing homes, the client's home, community centres, schools, community hospitals and day centres. Some specialise in particular areas of work such as home enteral feeding/nutritional support, but in remote and rural areas, they are often more generalist and cover many clinical areas. They are increasingly involved with more preventative work in the local community and you may find them or their support workers doing community development type work such as running 'cook and taste' sessions. Dieticians are usually involved in or lead on prevention and treatment of obesity in children and adults, and these services are usually delivered in a community setting.

 Activity

- Find out what nutrition and dietetic services are available in your placement area.
- How do they support and complement the work of community nurses?
- Thinking about nutritional support, especially of the frail elderly – how do they contribute to keeping people out of hospital by encouraging good nutrition?

Occupational therapists

Occupational therapists help people to overcome physical, psychological or social problems arising from illness or disability. They concentrate on what people are able to achieve rather than on their disabilities.

They work with children and adults and deliver services mainly in clinics, care/nursing homes, the client's home, community hospitals, day centres, intermediate care centres and special schools. They have a key role in intermediate care services such as rapid response teams and rehabilitation/intermediate care at home. They are the only AHPs who are also employed by social services, where they are involved with assessment for and provision of special equipment and home adaptations and home care re-ablement.

 Activity

- Find out what occupational therapy services are available in your placement area.
- How do they support and complement the work of community nurses?
- How do they facilitate early supported discharge of people from hospital back to their homes and help to prevent hospital admissions?
- What is their role for children with special needs?

Orthoptists

Orthoptists assess and manage a range of eye problems, mainly those affecting the way the eyes move, such as squint (strabismus) and lazy eye (amblyopia). Most of their work is in acute hospitals in ophthalmology departments, but you may come across them in the community providing screening in schools or clinics.

Physiotherapists

Physiotherapists treat the physical problems caused by accidents, illness and ageing, particularly those that affect the muscles, bones, heart, circulation and lungs. They work with children and adults and deliver services mainly in clinics, care/nursing homes, the person's home, community hospitals, day centres, intermediate care centres and special schools. Along with occupational therapists they have a key role in intermediate care services such as rapid response teams and rehabilitation/intermediate care at home. They also have a key role in treatment of COPD and can help to prevent hospital admissions for people with chronic respiratory disease. They also work closely with GPs and are able to diagnose and treat most of the musculoskeletal problems that people traditionally consult their GP about, for example back pain. In some areas, people are encouraged to go direct to the physiotherapy service rather than the GP. They are then triaged to the appropriate service. Some physiotherapists work in partnership with local authority leisure services to promote exercise and fitness. Physiotherapists use a variety of treatments including manipulation and acupuncture. An important part of treatment is giving advice and exercises for the person to do, to prevent or reduce future problems.

Activity

■ Find out what physiotherapy services are available in your placement area.
■ How do they support and complement the work of community nurses?
■ How do they facilitate early supported discharge of people from hospital back to their own homes and help to prevent hospital admissions?
■ What is their role for children with special needs?
■ Is there a direct referral system in operation for musculoskeletal conditions?

Podiatrists

Also known as chiropodists, podiatrists specialise in keeping feet in a healthy condition. They play a particularly important role in helping older people to stay mobile and therefore independent. Most of their work in the community is with adults and older people. They deliver services mainly in clinics, care homes and nursing homes, the client's home and community hospitals, but also practise in day centres and intermediate care centres. Podiatrists often work closely with community nurses in detection, prevention and treatment of wounds of the foot and lower leg and can provide a specialist service to people with diabetes. Some podiatrists specialise in orthotics where they work closely with physiotherapists in gait analysis and provision of insoles or special footwear.

Activity

■ Find out what podiatry services are available in your placement area.
■ How do podiatrists support and complement the work of community nurses?
■ How are general foot care services (including toenail cutting) provided?

Speech and language therapists

People who have problems with communication, including speech defects, or with chewing or swallowing, benefit from the service offered by the speech and language therapist. They work with children and adults and deliver services mainly in clinics, residential care homes and nursing homes, the client's home, community hospitals and schools. They work closely with education departments and deliver speech and language therapy for children and their families and teachers, in mainstream and special schools. They also work closely with dieticians to support people with swallowing problems and can help to prevent hospital admissions or support early discharge.

Activity

- Find out what speech and language therapy services are available in your placement area.
- How do they support and complement the work of community nurses?
- How do they work in partnership with the local education sector?

Local authority services

Environmental health

Environmental health officers are employed by the local authority and have a wide and varied role in protecting the health and safety of the community. Their role is to advise on food safety and commercial kitchen design, pest control and waste disposal. They inspect premises where food is prepared and sold such as shops, pubs and restaurants, and advise on hygiene and safety and enforce the requirements of the Food Safety Act 1990. They have an important public health role and work in partnership with nurses and doctors in health protection agencies and public health departments to protect and promote public health and investigate outbreaks. They are also involved in educating the public about infectious diseases. Environmental health officers also work with occupational health teams, assess risk, monitor safety standards in the workplace and investigate accidents. They have responsibility for aspects of housing standards, for example monitoring sanitation arrangements, checking that legal fire escapes are in place and ensuring repairs are carried out by landlords. They are also

responsible for the control of pollution such as air quality and other nuisances such as noise.

Social worker

The primary responsibility of the social worker is the protection and promotion of the welfare and wellbeing of children, vulnerable adults and communities. A social worker works with and alongside an individual or family, often in a crisis situation to help them find solutions to help themselves. Developing an effective helping relationship with people who use services is central to the role of the social worker in order to ensure better outcomes. For some people, creating a long-term supportive relationship with social work services may be an appropriate response to managing risk and promoting the wellbeing of vulnerable children or adults. Social workers work in a variety of statutory, voluntary and private settings supporting individuals, families and groups within the community. Settings may include the service users' home, schools, hospitals, health centres and residential care. Young people and their families are often the focus of the social workers role but they also work with the following individuals and groups:

- Young offenders
- Older people
- People with mental health conditions
- People who abuse alcohol and drugs
- School non-attenders
- People with learning and physical disabilities.

In England, social workers tend to specialise in either children's or adults' services. In other parts of the UK social workers also work in specialties such as children's services, mental health or older adult services but some have more generic roles and work with people and families of all ages. Here are some examples of the role:

- Offer information and counselling support to service users and their families

- Take referrals from both individuals and other professionals such as hospital doctors, GPs, district nurses and psychologists
- Carry out holistic assessment of social care needs working in partnership with the client and family
- Organise and manage packages of support, liaising with and making referrals to other agencies to enable service users to lead the fullest lives possible
- Work in ways which integrate different health and social care teams
- Engage in multidisciplinary teams meetings and case conferences
- Maintain accurate records and prepare reports for legal action
- Give evidence in court
- Conduct interviews with service users and their families to assess and review their situation.

Social workers are distinct from most other members of the health and social care team in having responsibility for statutory tasks discharged to them by the local authority. The aim of this aspect of their role is to ensure the protection of vulnerable individuals and the public. The statutory tasks of the social worker relate to the following areas:

- Care and protection, e.g. undertaking child protection investigations
- Criminal justice, e.g. providing parole reports for a parole board
- Childcare provision, e.g. the monitoring, supervision and review of foster parents
- Children who are looked after and accommodated, e.g. assessment and recommendation about whether a child should be accommodated away from home
- Mental health, e.g. application of mental health legislation to assess people for involuntary admission to hospital.

Home help or home carer

Local authority social service departments are responsible for assessing people's need

for community care services and arranging or providing these services. An assessment of care needs is carried out and this may be in conjunction with a district nurse if the person also has healthcare needs. The home carer provides personal services such as:

- personal hygiene
- assistance with eating
- continence management
- assistance with medication
- assistance getting in/out of bed
- assistance with dressing.

Non-personal care services are provided by a home help and include housework, collecting pensions and prescriptions, shopping, preparing meals and making beds.

Many areas provide Emergency Care at Home services. A home care co-ordinator arranges for a support worker to assist with washing and dressing, preparing hot meals, monitoring and supporting people in taking their medicines. The service aims to prevent unnecessary admission to hospital or where appropriate, enable earlier discharge by providing practical support on a short-term basis. These services operate 24 hours a day, 7 days a week but if the person requires longer-term care, a referral will be made to another service.

Nursing in prisons

In England and Wales, prison nurses are generally employed by the NHS and work as part of the team in primary care, although some nurses are employed directly by the prison service. Those working in the NHS may rotate around settings, working some shifts in the community and some in prison health care. In Scotland, the prison health service became part of the NHS in 2011 and prison nurses are becoming established within primary care.

Nursing roles in prison reflect nurses' roles in other primary care settings and include elements of adult, mental health and learning disabilities nursing and in some prisons, there are roles for advanced nurse practitioners and specialist nurses. In general, the health needs of offenders also reflect those of the wider population. However, many offenders have had limited contact with health services prior to prison and effective management of long-term physical and mental health conditions may be more complex. More specific health issues commonly include addictions, sexual health, blood-borne viruses and communicable diseases.

Nursing in prisons has been compared with nursing in general practice but with greater emphasis on addressing mental health and problems associated with addictions and in addition, dealing with challenging behaviour. Promoting and improving health and preventing illness is an important role for all nurses but requires particular focus in prison health care, where offenders have previously had very limited access to this.

 Activity

'Offender' is the term used for someone who has come into contact with the criminal justice service because they have committed or are suspected of committing a crime. The majority of offenders have had limited access to the healthcare services and facilities that most of us take for granted because of their lifestyle and low expectations of themselves and society as a whole. Expressions such as 'excluded people' and 'hard-to-reach communities' are used to describe offenders, asylum seekers and refugees, homeless people, gypsy and traveller communities and sex workers. The people in these groups and communities have health needs that involve primary and community care services with community nurses playing a leading part in some

Continued

initiatives. The RCN have a put together an online resource to support practice with excluded people and hard to reach communities. Spend 30 minutes accessing the RCN website and reading about the ways in which community nurses and other members of the community team are supporting people in these groups. RCN website: http://www.rcn.org.uk/development/practice/social_inclusion

Summary of learning points from this chapter

- The range of settings where services are offered in the community is extensive and varied
- Organisations that provide health and care services do not work in isolation but in partnership with each other
- The roles of community practitioners are unique but complementary, and students will be able to gain an understanding of their roles through placement learning experiences in the various types of settings.

References

Aldgate, J., Jones, D., Rose, W., Jeffrey, C., 2006. The developing world of the child. Jessica Kinglsey publishers, London.

Department of Health, 2007. Policy and guidance: health and social care topics: long term conditions. DH, London.

Laurent, M., Reeves, D., Hermens, R., et al., 2005. Substitution of doctors by nurses in primary care. Cochrane Database of systematic reviews (2), CD001271.

National Institute for Health and Clinical Excellence, 2008. Antenatal care (CG62). NHS, London.

Scottish Government, 2005. Health for all children 4: Guidance on implementation in Scotland. Scottish Executive, Edinburgh.

Scottish Government Social Research, 2009. Evaluation of the delivering for mental health peer support worker pilot scheme. Scottish Government, Edinburgh.

Scottish Government, 2011. A Consultation on the common core skills, knowledge, understanding and values of the children's workforce in Scotland. Scottish Government, Edinburgh.

Social Care Institute for Excellence, 2005. Briefing 19. What is the impact of environmental housing conditions on the health and well-being of children? SCIE, London.

Further reading

Barr, O., 2006. The evolving role of community nurses for people with learning disabilities: changes over an 11-year period. Journal of Clinical Nursing 15 (1), 72–82.

Barrett, A., Latham, D., Levermore, J., 2007. Defining the unique role of the specialist district nurse practitioner. Part 2. British Journal of Community Nursing 12 (11), 522–526.

Blackman, A., 2009. The male community nurse. British Journal of Community Nursing 14 (11), 481–486.

Carnegie, E., Kiger, A., 2010. Developing the community environmental health role of the nurse. British Journal of Community Nursing 15 (6), 298–305.

Chilton, S., Bain, H., Clarridge, A., et al., 2012. Textbook of community nursing. Hodder Arnold, London.

Ebbett, S., 2005. General practice, the NHS & the practice nurse. Practice Nurse 29 (6), 15–22.

Hallet, C.E., Pateman, B.D., 2000. The 'invisible assessment': the role of the staff nurse in the community setting. Journal of Clinical Nursing 9, 751–762.

Holland, K., Hogg, C., 2010. Cultural awareness in nursing and health care: an introductory text, 2nd ed. Arnold, London.

Luker, K., Orr, J., McHugh, G.A., 2012. Health visiting: a rediscovery, 3rd ed. Wiley-Blackwell, London.

Naidoo, J., Wills, J., 2009. Foundations for health promotion, 3rd ed. Bailliere Tindall, London.

O'Shea, L., 2009. Community placements in nurse training. Practice Nurse 37 (8), 39–40.

Queens Nursing Institute, 2009. 2020 Vision: Focusing on the future of district nursing. QNIS, Edinburgh.

Trigg, E., Mohammed, T. (Eds.), 2010. Practices in children's nursing: guidelines for hospital and community, 3rd ed. Elsevier, Edinburgh.

Upton, D., 2010. The student nurse survival guide to health promotion. Pearson Education, Harlow.

Websites

The Modernising Nursing in the Community website was launched by the Scottish Government in January 2012 and contains a wide range of useful information and resources: www.mnic. nes.scot.nhs.uk.

Refer to the following website, which offers an explanation of different roles within the NHS: www.nhscareers.nhs.uk/ career.shtml.

The standards of proficiency underpin the 10 key principles of public health nursing. You can look the standards up at: www.nmc-uk.org/Educators/ Standards-for-education/Standards-of-proficiency-for-specialist-community-public-health-nurses.

Department of Health, Social Services and Public Safety, 2010. Healthy child healthy future. A framework for the universal child health promotion programme in Northern Ireland: Pregnancy to 19 years. www.dhsspsni.gov.uk/healthychildhealthyfuture.pdf.

Scottish Government, 2011. Getting it right for every child. www.scotland.gov.uk/Topics/People/Young-People/gettingitright.

Health, Work and Well-being is a cross-government initiative to protect and improve the health and wellbeing of working age people: www.dwp.gov.uk/health-work-and-well-being/about-us.

The Health Protection Agency (HPA) supports and advises the NHS, local authorities, emergency services, the Department of Health and others in its aim of improving public health, www.hpa.org.uk.

Transforming Community Services, Community indicators for quality improvement. www.dh.gov.uk/en/Publicationsandstatistics/Publications/PublicationsPolicyAndGuidance/DH_126110.

3

Practice learning in the community: what to expect

CHAPTER AIMS

- To highlight some of the differences between practice learning in the community and practice learning in hospital settings
- To discuss what is expected of the student to ensure a successful and positive learning experience
- To discuss the learning opportunities available in the community

Introduction

Chapters 1 and 2 should have started to build up your knowledge and understanding of the community, the diverse roles of nurses and other practitioners and agencies, and the range of services that they provide for people of all ages and social groups. Chapters 3 and 4 focus on what you can expect from practice learning in the community and how to get the most out of your experience.

The approaches to care and ways of working differ, depending on the community care setting and the care provider. However, these differences should not be viewed as barriers or lines of demarcation between settings.

A person-centred approach to care is about the person and their care pathway, which should be seamless between primary and secondary care and between different providers of health and social care in the community. The learning environment in the community will certainly feel very different to the hospital learning environment, not only because of what you can learn here but also how you learn. This chapter looks at some of these differences and gives you some insight into what you can expect.

 Activity

> The Nursing and Midwifery Council define community practice learning very broadly:
>
> *Any practice learning undertaken or related to care or health promotion activities outside of the hospital environment.*
>
> NMC (2010)
>
> Make a list of what you expect to learn in the community that you don't think you would learn in a hospital environment.

The scope of learning opportunities in the community is wide and varied. A few examples include: health assessment of the newborn; health education for young people in schools; complex care for people living at home with long-term conditions; clinics for smoking cessation; specialist services; management of chronic wounds; child protection; supportive care for people with mental health problems – the list is endless.

The student's experience will depend on the learning experiences on offer in the locality and the learning outcomes that need to be achieved during the placement. However, with your mentor, an appropriate range of experience tailored to meet essential skills and outcomes can be identified. (Chapter 4 looks in more detail at learning outcomes and we focus on nursing practice in the community later in this chapter.)

The first two chapters have given an overview of roles and services in the community. Some differences in provision between hospital and community are obvious and others not so clear. To consider this in a more *focused* way, the following case study illustrates how overall aims for a patient (Mr Jackson) are the same but the approach and the emphasis in the hospital and community is different.

■ Case study

Mr Jackson is 88, was widowed last year and lives alone. He fell at home recently and spent 3 weeks in hospital. While he was in hospital, his nursing care plan focused on improving his mobility and nutritional status, so that he could return home with a reduced risk of falling. (The focus is on 'doing things with or for him'.)

The most important part of Mr Jackson's nursing care plan now that he is back home is supporting him to achieve a level of self-care that enables him to live safely at home, where he wants to be and out of residential care. (The focus is on supporting him to 'do things for himself', to enable him to stay in his own home.)

What makes the community setting different?

In Chapters 1 and 2, community was discussed as a context for health and social care and the practitioners that provide services there. But nursing in the community is about the people who live in the community and who are the users or potential service users. Wherever nurses practice, they have contact with people from a diverse range of backgrounds. However, in a hospital, the context itself can restrict expressions of individuality and diversity. In the community, people are at home in their own world and this is where the wide spectrum of diversity is experienced and expressed.

As society becomes increasingly multicultural, nurses must be sensitive and responsive to a wide range of differing beliefs, traditions and practices in relation to health, illness and life events such as birth and death.

It is a privilege to visit anyone's home but as a student on a community placement, home visits and opportunities to get to know families from different ethnic and cultural backgrounds are invaluable experiences for learning and understanding the beliefs and traditions of other cultures. Holland and Hogg (2010) discuss cultural understanding and lack of prejudice as fundamental in ensuring quality and equality of healthcare provision. However, these core elements do not only apply to cultural diversity but also relate to age, gender, disability, religion, belief, political, social and health status, sexual orientation, lifestyle and health behavioural factors. Depending on the community profile of your placement area, community practice learning can offer learning experiences to develop your knowledge and understanding of people's health needs and beliefs that would not be available in other practice settings.

For example community nurses are often successful in engaging people that are described as 'hard to reach' by traditional health services, by providing services for homeless people, travelling families, refugees and asylum seekers.

Activity

Chambers and Ryder (2009) discuss compassion and dignity in nursing practice and ask readers to reflect on a number of questions throughout their book.

Think carefully about the following questions and answer them as honestly as you can:

- Have you ever judged somebody, based purely on their appearance, life choices or circumstances?
- Are you aware of your own biases and prejudices?
- In your practice, how can you challenge these attitudes in yourself and others?
- How do you stop these impacting on your role as a nurse?

Table 3.1 Extract from the Code: Standards of conduct, performance and ethics for nurses

Standard
1   You must treat people as individuals and respect their dignity
2   You must not discriminate in any way against those in your care
3   You must treat people kindly and considerately
4   You must act as an advocate for those in your care, helping them to access relevant health and social care, information and support
11 You must make arrangements to meet people's language and communication needs
12 You must share with people, in a way they can understand, the information they want or need to know about their health

NMC (2008)

The NMC (2008) makes clear that the care of people is a nurse's first concern, treating them as individuals and respecting their dignity. A number of standards in the NMC Code apply, including those shown in Table 3.1.

As more services are delivered in the community, acute hospitals concentrate on the provision of specialist care and services such as surgery and acute events. Many of the examples in Table 3.2 reflect this shift in the balance of care. They also reflect the importance of promoting health, addressing inequality, preventing illness and empowering people to take more responsibility for their health. This is not to say that these issues are not important in secondary care or that some

of the services listed in Table 3.2 are not provided there. Rather, that the community setting facilitates this way of working and consequently, a greater emphasis is given. A good example of this is 'person-centred care'. This has been described by Innes et al (2006) as care that focuses on the people using the service; promotes independence and autonomy; provides reliable and flexible services; enables users and carers to choose the services they need; and tends to be provided by teams of health and social care providers working in partnership. Of course, person centredness is an ambition of quality care wherever it is given but care in the community lends itself particularly to this approach.

Table 3.2 Characteristics of care in the community

More services that do things *with* people rather than *to* people. Service users have more autonomy, are offered choice and treated as partners in their care. People choose their general practice, dentist and pharmacist. NHS online and phone line services inform and give people a voice to request what they need, negotiate and share decision-making about the care and support that suits them best

A range of practitioners, not just doctors, provide first point of contact services. Nurses, pharmacists, physiotherapists and others assess, diagnose and treat people with health problems who present at clinics and walk-in centres

Partnership, integration and teamwork across health and social care providers to deliver complex care packages to people in their own homes

A public health approach to improving the health of whole communities

Services that focus entirely on health improvement, such as smoking cessation

Services that are focused on prevention such as immunisation, cervical screening

Long-term, continuing care and support of individuals and families, e.g. a district nursing team providing care for someone with a long-term condition and support for their carer over several years or a health visitor supporting a child and family from antenatal care to school age

Services which protect vulnerable children and adults

A focus on recovery and rehabilitation

Family-centred approaches to care and support

Enabling, empowering and supporting people to self-care so that they can live safely and independently in the environment they choose

Care for people in their own homes, adapting services to meet their needs and suit the environment.

What makes nursing in the community different?

The principles that underpin nursing practice apply to all settings, as do the skills and competencies that are required for high-quality nursing care. However, in order to provide the types of services and adopt the approaches listed above, community nurses need specific skills to work in a different way. The NMC has identified some of the key characteristics of delivering nursing care in community environments (NMC 2010):

1. *An understanding and ability to work with families, communities as well as individuals*
2. *An insight into the importance of community health profiling and patterns of health and disease across different groups, communities and populations*
3. *An appreciation of the importance of services being focused around ease of access and convenience, in meeting the needs of individuals, families, groups or communities rather than the logistics of service delivery. Nursing in the community usually means visiting people in their homes, or being available, or delivering services in the communities in which people live*

4. *Individuals and communities are empowered to take control of their health and wellbeing, emphasising choice and independence rather than conforming to imposed rules and routines*
5. *An emphasis on health promotion and prevention of ill health, either as the main objective or by finding ways to promote health and quality of life while delivering nursing care*
6. *Strong interdisciplinary networks and the ability to work with others in health and social care, as well as other statutory and voluntary agencies*
7. *A good knowledge of local services and resources to which people can go to support their health*
8. *Frequent exposure to uncertain circumstances and unplanned events with limited immediate access to resources to manage the situation*
9. *The environment, external influences, family and social factors have a major impact on nursing assessment, interventions and activities, so flexible and creative approaches to practice will be necessary*
10. *It is common for some nurses to work alone, so they must be aware of associated risks and safety issues*
11. *Nurses must be able to work without direct supervision and make judgements and decisions independently*

NMC (2010:37–38)

Activity

Perhaps not all of the characteristics identified by the NMC are unique to delivering nursing care in the community. You may feel that you have come across some of these characteristics in other practice settings. Identify three characteristics that you feel *are* unique and interest you most. Make a note of them and review your university notes related to these

Continued

topics. Discuss the three characteristics that you have chosen with your mentor and look for opportunities for learning more about them in practice. (Planning your learning experience is discussed in Chapter 4.)

Approaches to practice learning in the community

Traditional approaches to practice learning tend to rely on NHS settings with students allocated to either hospital wards or community health centres. It has not been unusual for programmes to place a greater emphasis on nursing in hospital and consequently, students have spent a greater proportion of their practice learning experience in a hospital environment. A perceived or actual shortage of placements in the community and in primary care has made this difficult to change in some areas.

With the emphasis on relevance to the programme learning outcomes, the NMC is encouraging universities to move away from traditional approaches and to develop new and creative practice learning opportunities. Newer approaches are more flexible and allow students to move between settings and experience services provided by a wider range of organisations, including social enterprises, the independent sector, schools and social services, as well as the NHS. Flexible models are more likely to give students the opportunity to gain a more holistic understanding of the patient's experience, following their journey as they move between services and different care environments.

The way in which practice learning is organised depends very much on the design of the nursing programme and the stage of implementation of new models of practice learning. It also depends on the type of practice experience that is available in the area, the range of services and how they have developed to meet the health needs of the population in that locality. Consequently, there is wide variation between universities in the length, timing and structure of periods of practice learning. However, to be approved by the NMC, all programmes must meet the NMC standards for pre-registration nursing education, and consequently, practice learning must meet the following standards:

- The programme must contain at least 2300 hours of practice learning.
- Students **must** be supervised by a mentor for 40% of the time they spend in practice but where safe and appropriate, they can be supervised indirectly, e.g. do not need to be based with their mentor for the entire practice period or may be supervised by a practitioner from another profession.
- Periods of practice learning towards the end of the first and second parts of the programme must be at least 4 weeks in length and at least 12 weeks in length towards the end of the programme.
- Reasonable adjustments must be made for students with disabilities to support achievement of the practice learning outcomes.

There are many different approaches or different ways of organising practice learning in the community. The approach may change as the student progresses through the programme, for example, beginning with observational visits or shorter periods of practice and culminating in the longer period of practice consolidation required for registration.

By providing feedback to the university on their own experience and getting involved in discussion and planning, students play an important role in helping develop the quality of practice learning. Here are some of the methods and models that support effective practice learning in the community:

- Individual or a series of focused observational visits to introduce students to clinical practice at the beginning of the programme or give insight into specialist areas of care later on
- Short practice learning opportunities or visits to a variety of areas where care is observed or where students are directly supervised in undertaking basic care
- A period of time spent with a service user, carer or family, enabling the student to work with them, observe care or self-care and discuss their experiences of health care
- A themed placement, linking each learning-in-practice experience with a particular client group, their needs and the services provided. Clark and Brown (2011) describe an effective 4-week themed placement for a 1st year nursing student focusing on understanding the needs of homeless people of all ages in the area
- A hub and spoke type arrangement where the period of practice learning is overseen by one mentor and based in a particular area or hub, and a wide range of other environments or spokes are each supervised by a named person. Overall responsibility for support and assessment remains with the mentor at the hub. This arrangement enables students to follow a patient's journey, for example across an inpatient pathway or across hospital and community settings involving a wide range of health and social care environments
- Longer periods of practice which help students consolidate their knowledge and skills, take more responsibility and develop team and leadership skills and experience
- The use of simulation to learn and practise skills in a safe environment. This may be in a clinical skills laboratory but other simulation methods such as interactive electronic learning packages, scenario building and role play are also

used to enhance practice learning. The NMC allow a maximum of 300 from the 2300 hours of practise time to be used in this way.

 Activity

Find out what your learning-in-practice journey looks like for the rest of your programme. This information will be in your programme guide or handbook. You will be able to see how the type of experience, e.g. the care of older people or surgical nursing, is aligned with the relevant theory. Some programmes are able to give students details of the student journey down to the hospital or health centre that is allocated to you and sometimes across all years from the start of the programme. In others, areas are allocated for a year at a time. Whatever the level of information, make the most of it to plan your learning and make the connections between theory modules, different types of settings and nursing practice. Some programmes also have modules which are a combination of theory and practice learning, including the assessment of learning outcomes.

What to expect in the community

Although community nurses work in teams, they spend a lot of time delivering care on their own. As a consequence, the relationship between the student and the mentor may feel different, more one-to-one than in other practice settings. However, you will not spend all of your time with your mentor; the minimum requirement is 40%. You will have a programme which will offer opportunities for learning from other members of the team. There will also be times when you will be expected to spend time on your own, and it is important that you are proactive and have already thought about the aims of this practice experience in order to make the most of this time. (There is more about how to make the most of your time in Chapter 4.)

Home visiting

Visiting people in their own homes may take a while to get used to, particularly when you do not know the person or family you are visiting and are unfamiliar with the area in which they live. It can be daunting, ringing a front door bell in a strange neighbourhood and not knowing what to expect, who else will be there, the person's condition or how they will receive you. You are unlikely to visit on your own at the beginning of your placement or to visit someone that you do not know but as you gain experience and develop competence and confidence, your mentor will give you more responsibility and may give you a small but supervised caseload. This is likely to take place towards the end of your programme when you are expected to demonstrate leadership and management skills prior to qualifying as a nurse. To give you some practise of knowing what to do and say when visiting someone in their own home, consider the following activity.

 Activity

Imagine yourself in the following situation:

Your mentor has asked you to visit Mrs Jenkins, who lives alone in a ground floor flat on a large housing estate. Mrs Jenkins has hearing impairment, difficulty with mobility since her stroke and has been having regular visits from the district nursing team to dress a

Continued

pressure ulcer on her heel. You have visited Mrs Jenkins on one occasion with the community staff nurse a few weeks ago.

What are the first three things you would do or say when Mrs Jenkins opens the front door?

You might have answered as follows:

1. Check you are in the right place and with the right person

It is not always straightforward finding the address you are looking for and the person who opens the door is not necessarily the person you are intending to visit.

So always make sure by asking them to confirm:

Hello – is it Mrs Jenkins?

2. Explain who you are and why you are visiting

Put yourself in the position of the person opening the door. Mrs Jenkins has mobility problems and getting to the door may have required some time and effort. Opening the door in an area that has problems with anti-social behaviour and finding a stranger on the doorstep may be unsettling. Mrs Jenkins does not always catch what people say, particularly if she does not know them. Mrs Jenkins may prefer not to have a student providing her care and she has a right to say No! Make your introduction very clear:

I'm here to do your dressing.

I'm Sarah Smith from the health centre.

I'm the nursing student working with District Nurse Green.

Here is my identification card.

May I come in?

Continued

3. Always be the invited guest

Wait to be invited and give Mrs Jenkins plenty of time to let you in.

Mrs Jenkins will be used to visits from the district nursing team and will know the routine for having her treatment. Ask where you can hang your coat or cardigan. If you need to put it on a surface, choose somewhere clean or put it on top of your bag.

Ask where you can wash your hands.

The community nurse enters a person's home on their invitation. Very few community practitioners have a legal right of entry, for example in certain specific circumstances a social worker can enter a house to remove a child at risk to a place of safety. Whether you are visiting someone's home with your mentor, on an observation visit with another member of the health and social care team or on your own, here are some important points to remember as an invited guest.

Always be the polite guest

To begin with, you may feel nervous or self-conscious visiting people that you do not know very well and perhaps lack confidence giving advice or performing clinical skills in unfamiliar surroundings. But remember that you are a stranger to the person or family you are visiting. Put them at their ease. You may be the only visitor they have seen all day or for days, give them time to talk and be patient.

Be self-aware and think about how the person or family sees you, your appearance and behaviour. They will notice and may be easily offended if this is not what they expect. This could have a very detrimental effect on the relationship that they have with you and their whole experience of health care. Respect people's property and take care to avoid spillages and damage. Do not touch people's possessions unless you need or are invited to do so and do not comment on things inappropriately. Always remember that you are there as an invited and professional guest.

Opportunities or challenges

Everyone has preferences for different types of nursing. Some students relish the prospect of practice learning in the community and others dread it. It makes such a positive impression on some students that they pursue a career in community nursing, while others will never choose to work there again (Box 3.1).

Expectations of practice learning in the community do not always reflect the reality. There follows an extract from a short article written by nursing student, Moyra Swan, reflecting on her experience of practice learning in the community with a district nursing team. After reading the extract, you might like to reflect on your own community experience or discuss Moyra Swan's reflection with your personal tutor prior to going out to a first placement in community.

Box 3.1 Opportunities or challenges – two sides of the same coin?
How do you see practice learning in the community?

Very wide scope for learning

New and different experiences every day – not routine

Getting to know a new area

Privilege to visit people in their own home

One-to-one attention for learning and support

OR

So much to take in that's new and different

Lots of change, unfamiliar places – out of comfort zone

Travel to community placement inconvenient and time consuming

Isolated from peers – scattered across districts

Long days away and academic work to do in the evening

Extract from reflection of practice learning: nursing student, Moyra Swan

Before I started my placement I had little idea of what to expect, having spent all my other placements on hospital wards. Some students had been dismissive: "You spend most of your time on your knees doing bandages – it's all leg ulcers".

My mentor was a district nurse – and yes, that did indeed mean leg ulcers, but this blanket term in no way did justice to the wide variety of wounds that we assessed and treated each day. I soon discovered that leg ulcers are far from being a homogenous entity, and I learnt the important differences between venous and arterial; the process of healing post-surgery; pressure sores; the organisms that can infect wounds; the complex choice of dressings and

Continued

treatments available; and the skill of bandaging. I perceived wound management as a constantly evolving and dynamic specialism.

Once I'd got the hang of it I found dressing and bandaging very satisfying. An activity that allowed me to hone my multi-tasking skills by listening and responding to the patient's news and views while assessing their wounds, choosing the relevant dressings and applying them correctly.

It was also an holistic activity; I learnt much about the patients' general state of physical and mental health while 'on my knees'. After some weeks I was allocated my own patient group and relished the responsibility and the trust that was placed in me.

During my placement, my mentor supported me in my choice to spend time with other specialists, such as the practice nurse, Macmillan nurse, health visitor and midwife. The knowledge and insight I gained was invaluable, and I can only touch on it here. I took part in clinics and visits concerned with cardiac rehabilitation, child immunisation, maternity, children at risk, diabetes, smoking cessation, asthma and wellbeing. I saw how varied people's reactions can be to discussions concerning their lifestyle. I also learnt the practical skills of venepuncture, ECG recording, immunisation and flu jab administration. How accommodating those patients were!

My placement was stimulating and thought-provoking, and the 12 weeks went far too quickly. When a placement has been as fulfilling as mine it is easy for me to feel that that's the area I want to work in, but my enthusiasm will last. I enjoyed the teamwork, the chance to follow-up patients, the autonomy and the feeling that I could really make a difference. I look forward to working in the community when I complete my training.

Swan (2006)

Specific challenges for students working within the community

Although your community learning experience is a valuable opportunity to observe and participate in the care required by clients in their own home, this particular clinical experience can present some challenges to learning. It is important to remember that you will be caring for clients from very diverse backgrounds. Some patients may require quite complex care and you may not be as involved as you would like, if you do not have the relevant expertise. You may also encounter different issues such as child protection and domestic violence, which are particularly emotionally challenging for practitioners. You also have to remember that you will be working with clients in their own environments, respecting their rights,

perspectives and views, even though they may be quite different to your own.

What is expected of students?

The NMC standards emphasise the importance of high quality nursing care; to address the challenges of an ageing population and an increasing number of people with long-term conditions; to enable children to get the best possible start in life; for people of all ages to stay well and active. Nurses are increasingly becoming the first point of contact for people and families, working flexibly across traditional boundaries such as hospital and community and health and social care and using a wider range of competencies and a greater variety of roles. Nurses will be required to have a high level of knowledge, critical thinking and autonomy at the point of registration and to develop these skills as they progress through their career. It follows that practice learning in the community will become even more important in preparing nurses to deliver safe, effective and person-centred care.

Even when you have experience of practice learning in other settings, it is not unusual for students to feel a little overwhelmed and even a little inadequate to begin with when faced with situations in the community. You will probably be struck by your mentor's knowledge of the local community, their ability to organise and co-ordinate services from numerous organisations and the range of clinical and communication skills they use in their everyday work.

Community nurses have undertaken post-registration education in preparation for their role and developed the knowledge, skills and experience to practise with competence and confidence in the community. They have well established contacts and networks and have developed, often over several years, working relationships with colleagues and therapeutic relationships with patients and families.

Nursing students are not expected to be experts in delivering nursing care in the community. However, you are expected to achieve your learning outcomes and your mentor is expected to help you to gain the experience you need to do so.

 Activity

> What support do you expect from your mentor, community practitioners, and the university during community practice learning? Identify five points. Be as honest and realistic as you can. Discuss these with your university tutor as preparation for identifying specific learning goals and then with your mentor at the start of your community placement.
>
> *Continued*

> This will be different for each field of practice learning experience or where you are expected to undertake a placement in what has been seen traditionally as a different field of practice. For example, you may be undertaking an adult nursing field of practice pathway but may have a community placement with the mental health community nursing team.

Quality Standards for Practice Placements (NES 2008) were created so that students and the individuals and organisations who support them understand their responsibilities and expectations in relation to practice learning. The extract in Table 3.3 outlines what students can expect and what they have a responsibility to do in a practice learning placement. These standards have been used widely in Scotland but would apply in any practice learning situation.

Chapter 4 describes how to make the most of your learning experience in the community. This includes further discussion of the responsibilities of students and some guidance on activities and behaviours which can have a positive influence on learning.

Professional conduct

The NMC sets out the personal and professional conduct expected of you as a nursing student in order for you to be fit to practice and to enter the professional register on successful completion of the programme (NMC 2009). The guidance is based on the Code: Standards of Conduct, Performance and Ethics for Nurses and Midwives (NMC 2008), which all unregistered nurses and midwives must uphold. It is recommended that you become familiar with the Code as you are working towards these standards while you are student.

Table 3.3 Quality standards for practice placements

Students can expect:	Students have a responsibility to:
A placement appropriate to their learning needs	Ensure they are prepared for the practice learning environment by accessing pre-practice learning environment information
Access to information about the practice area and the learning opportunities available	Contribute as a partner in the achievement of their learning outcomes
Support from a named individual who is prepared for the role of supporting students	Raise any concerns about the practice learning environment experience using the systems that exist for supporting and addressing students' concerns about the practice learning environment
An opportunity to discuss learning needs early (normally within 48 hours)	Evaluate their experience
An environment which is welcoming, supportive of their learning and in which they feel part of the team	
Access to a range of learning and teaching opportunities	
A team approach to their support	
Feedback on their performance and progress from individuals supporting their learning	
Fair, timely and objective assessment	
Access to support from their education institution when required	

NES (2008)

Universities also have guidelines regarding the conduct of students, not only while in the university but also during practice placements. Consequently, you are expected to comply with the NMC and the university guidelines regarding conduct during practice learning plus any specific guidelines relating to the organisation or setting where you are placed.

Timekeeping and attendance

Be on time. A community practitioner's day is planned ahead. If you keep them waiting they will be late for appointments, rushing to catch up and end-up shortening the time they spend with patients. This disadvantages patients, detracts from your learning experience and does nothing for your relationship with your mentor and potentially your assessment. Find out in advance exactly where you are going, confirm meeting times and places directly with the person you are meeting and get a mobile contact number just in case you are delayed or they need to inform you of a change of plan.

To get the most of your placement you must make sure you are there. Your learning experience will have been carefully planned and arrangements made for visits to and with members of the team to different services and settings. If you miss days you will miss out, as these experiences are usually difficult to rearrange. If taking time off is unavoidable, make sure you know and follow the university's notification of absence procedure and any local arrangements for informing practitioners in the placement area.

Dress code

Appearance is very important when you are in the community fulfilling a clinical role, representing the nursing profession and your university. Find out what to wear well in advance. Check the university uniform policy for practice in the community and make sure you have everything you need.

For example: Do you have suitable outdoor shoes? Does the university provide a uniform, outdoor coat? What arrangements are in place for collecting a laundered uniform (as you will need to wear a clean one every day)? You will be expected to wear a uniform when you are working with the clinical team such as the district nurse, GP or specialist nurse. You may not be expected to wear a uniform when you are visiting families with the health visitor or social worker. If a uniform is not worn, wear something clean, comfortable and smart. Knowing the correct dress code applies to all four fields of practice pathways and the placements encountered.

The care environment

There is wide variation in people's living conditions and standard of hygiene and you will encounter homes that are untidy, smelly and unclean. You may be shocked when you see the poor conditions in which some people live. Sometimes this situation has arisen because the person has been unable to cope with washing and cleaning or looking after a pet due to illness or disability. But people also choose to live in

surroundings that you would not. The health and social care visitor must assess the impact of intervening or raising their concern against the potential risks to health. They also have to consider the risk of being denied entry to the house on future occasions and the missed opportunity to help the person in need of support. It is very important that you do not express any negative feelings at the time you encounter such situations but discuss these with your mentor after the visit has taken place.

Hand hygiene facilities are not always ideal in a person's home. It is preferable to wash your hands in hot running water using pump-action liquid handwash rather than using a bar of soap. Always carry a supply of alcohol hand rub/gel. This may be used instead of handwashing if facilities are inadequate or after handwashing if hand disinfection is required. Always dry your hands thoroughly with paper towels, paper roll or a clean towel or cloth.

Hospitality and gifts

It is not unusual to be offered cups of tea when you are visiting people at home. Talking through a problem, breaking difficult news or providing social support can be more natural and effective when accompanied by a cup of tea. People sometimes offer community nurses small gifts such as biscuits to share with the team at the health centre or more personal gifts such as soap or toiletries when they are discharged from their care, as a way of thanking them. The NMC code is clear:

> You must refuse any gifts, favours or hospitality that might be interpreted as an attempt to gain preferential treatment.
>
> NMC (2008:4)

This means that you can accept that small gift or cup of tea providing you are confident that the person is not expecting preferential treatment in return. However, local policy in the area you are working in may not allow you to accept gifts or hospitality of any kind and you must check this before you consider doing so. Most community nurses do not have time for hospitality routinely but use it as a therapeutic prop, as indicated earlier.

Personal safety

Your mentor will not knowingly put you into a situation where your personal safety could be at risk. However, changes in a person's mood or the presence or arrival of friends or relatives can alter the situation and make you feel uncomfortable or even threatened. If you are visiting with your mentor, they are experienced in managing these situations, but if on your own it may be best to explain to the person that you will return at another time with your mentor. Do not take risks. It is best to leave and notify your mentor. Your mentor or named member of the healthcare team is always close at hand and it is good practice to be in mobile contact at all times.

Again, each field of practice pathway will have its own guidance for visiting patients in their own homes, and it is very important that you adhere to any local policy that is in place for any nurse, not only nursing students.

Student status

When you are a student, people often assume that you know more than you do and expect you to have the answers to their questions. On a hospital ward, if you are asked about something you do not know, there is always an experienced practitioner close by that you can refer to. If the person you are visiting at home asks you something, be honest if you do not know and there is no-one with you to ask. Do not

continue with a treatment if you are unsure or give information that may be inaccurate. Let the person know that you will discuss the issue with your mentor and that you will inform them of the outcome promptly. If it is urgent, you may be able to contact your placement and ask to speak with the mentor or leave a message for them to contact you. It is important that you reassure the person that you will do your best to find out the answer as soon as possible.

Relationships

The nature of the professional relationships that are established with people when you visit them at home feel different from the hospital environment. Trust and confidentiality are fundamental to all relationships but in the community, people can feel very vulnerable as they are exposing the way they live, aspects of their family life and personal relationships, to the home visitor.

People must feel confident in trusting the home visitor to respect their privacy and to only disclose relevant information with appropriate members of the health and social care team. The home visitor must appreciate the privilege of visiting people in their own homes and the trust which the person and family place in them. The familiarity that you may observe in the professional relationship between the person or family and the practitioner you are visiting with may have built up over successive visits or even years. McGarry (2010) studied the relationships between nurses and older people within the home and identified specific aspects, often crossing traditional nurse/patient boundaries, which enhanced the quality of care for older people.

Your experience in the community is likely to make a lasting impression on you both personally and professionally. One student reflected on her first placement in the community and summarised her feelings in the following way:

Student reflection after first community placement

I've been moved by the kindness of people and how much they appreciate even the small things we do. It's amazing how people cope with such complex problems most of the time on their own. We are only there for a tiny proportion of their day. The rest of time they cope.

I've been in situations that I've found uncomfortable, made me challenge my attitudes and beliefs. I've been shocked by the way people live, their lack of control and chaotic lifestyles. I thought I was empathetic before but I know now how important it is to see and try to understand the position of another person to be able to help them. I've learnt a lot about myself.

The privilege of being in someone's home, with them when they are at their most vulnerable, in pain, dying, upset, supporting their loved ones. I've felt so much more part of it than on the ward. I think it's the relationships, so much closer that caring with compassion is natural.

There's so much to take in that sometimes I felt a bit overwhelmed. My mentor has been a district nurse for years she knows so much about the community, who to contact, what to do when something happens. I have learnt so much from her, not just about clinical skills but about communication, management, thinking on your feet, being very flexible and of course teaching. I know I've learnt things in the community that I would never have learnt anywhere else.

Summary of learning points from this chapter

- There are distinct differences between practice learning in the community and practice learning in hospital settings.
- The potential learning opportunities available in the community reflect the unique nature of community services and the skills of community nurses.
- Students should be aware of what is expected of them to enable a successful and positive learning experience.

References

Chambers, C., Ryder, E., 2009. Compassion and care in nursing. Radcliffe, Oxford.

Clark, A., Brown, J., 2011. Partnership work in placements. Nurs. Times 107 (21), 19–21.

Holland, K., Hogg, C., 2010. Cultural awareness in nursing and healthcare: an introductory text, second ed. Hodder Arnold, London.

Innes, A., Macpherson, S., McCabe, L., 2006. Promoting person-centred care at the front line. Joseph Rowntree Foundation, York.

McGarry, J., 2010. The relationships between nurses and older people within the home: exploring the boundaries of care. International Journal of Older People Nursing 5 (4), 265–273.

NES, 2008. NHS Education for Scotland quality standards for practice placements. NES, Edinburgh.

NMC, 2008. The Code: Standards of conduct, performance and ethics for nurses. NMC, London.

NMC, 2009. Guidance on professional conduct for nursing and midwifery students. NMC, London.

NMC, 2010. Advice and supporting information for implementing NMC standards for pre-registration nursing education. NMC, London.

Swan, M., 2006. Community spirit: a student nurse's encounter. Nursing in Practice 27, 20–30.

Further reading

Brooks, N., Rojahn, R., 2011. Improving the quality of community placements for nursing students. Nurs. Stand. 25 (37), 42–47.

Chowthi-Williams, A., Woolmer, J., Harris, D., 2010. Evaluation of a primary care pre-registration programme in London. Practice Nursing 21 (6), 316–319.

Gillespie, M., McLaren, D., 2010. Student nurses' perceptions of non-traditional clinical placements. Br. J. Nurs. 19 (11), 705–708.

Hart, S. (Ed.), 2010. Nursing study and placement learning skills. Oxford University Press, Oxford.

Primary Health Care, 2011. The RCN Community Health Nursing Journal. Online. Available at: http://

primaryhealthcare.rcnpublishing.co.uk/ students/clinical-placements (accessed November 2011).

Warren, D., 2010. Facilitating pre-registration nurse learning: a mentor approach. Br. J. Nurs. 19 (21), 1364–1367.

Websites

The Equality and Diversity Forum is a national network of equality and human rights organisations. This website brings together a wide range of equality and human rights information and resources provided by EDF and other organisations: http://www.edf. org.uk/blog.

NHS Education for Scotland, Effective Practitioner Website includes learning activities for recording learning and development including a form for recording a reflective account: http://www. effectivepractitioner.nes.scot.nhs.uk/ learning-and-development/recording-learning-and-development.aspx.

Maximising the learning opportunities available in the community

CHAPTER AIMS

- To guide your preparation and organisation for practice learning in the community
- To explore the many learning opportunities available to you as a nursing student during this placement
- To examine different learning strategies which may facilitate your learning while in clinical placement

Introduction

The reasons why it is important for you to get the most from your learning experience in the community is explored in this chapter. Whether or not you plan to work in the community once you have qualified, the skills and knowledge that you have the opportunity to acquire during a community placement, have the potential to make an important impact on your beliefs and values about nursing and your approach to care in any setting.

 Activity

Look at the following two examples; one from nurse leaders and the other from a leading community nursing organisation. What message do these examples suggest to you?

Example 1

In 2006, a coalition of stakeholders from the four UK countries, led by the chief nursing officer for England, published *Modernising Nursing Careers: setting the direction* (Department of Health 2006). This report set the scene for future careers in nursing. It highlighted the importance of preparing nurses to work in a range of settings that reflected the move away from a secondary care focus to health care based in the community and primary care.

Example 2

The Queen's Nursing Institute (2009) has predicted that more nurses will need to be recruited into primary care settings on registration to cope with the shift in the balance of care. Their vision for the future is that community nurses will:

- Take on public health roles and consider community needs
- Be key workers in the care of long-term conditions

Continued

- Have the flexibility to move between roles
- Have strong leadership qualities to lead, co-ordinate and commission care
- Work across professional boundaries
- Work with families and lay carers
- Work more independently and have greater accountability
- Work with increasing advances in technology.

These examples illustrate a vision for the future of nursing roles that is very much rooted in the community. Practice learning in this environment is therefore crucial to your development as a nurse. More than ever before, nurses need to have the skills and expertise at the point of registration to work in closer partnership with service users and with other professionals and agencies. They will need to be able to deliver more care, support and treatment in polyclinics, general practice, residential care homes, walk-in centres, nursing homes and in people's homes. This reflects the rapidly changing healthcare environment where the balance of care is shifting away from a focus on inpatient and hospital services towards more services which are based in the community and closer to where people live and work.

Nurse education is becoming more focused on preparing nurses to be proactive, flexible, confident and competent to provide nursing care and support for people of all ages, wherever they use services. For many nursing programmes, this is a move away from more traditional and hospital-oriented preparation for nursing roles and is driven by the revised NMC Standards for pre-registration nursing education introduced in 2010 (NMC 2010). NMC Standard 6 for example, which focuses on the need for placement learning opportunities for students, emphasises the importance of practice learning; expecting nursing students to learn in direct contact with healthy and ill people and communities; experience 24-hour and 7-day care and learn across a range of hospital, community and other settings. The theoretical component and learning outcomes of programmes must reflect this and include more topics that support the development of skills and knowledge required for nursing in the community. These include approaches such as anticipatory care, case management, self-care and enablement, health improvement, public health and safeguarding vulnerable children and adults.

Learning outcomes

The overall aims for each module or component of your nursing programme will be described in your programme guide or handbook as general statements and overarching intentions. However, more specific statements, which describe what you should know, understand and be able to do at the end of each component are usually expressed as learning outcomes. *Learning outcomes* for nursing programmes differ between universities but all are designed to address the NMC requirements for registration; the achievement of the general and field specific competencies, the Essential Skills Clusters and demonstration of fitness to practice and fitness for an (academic) award. Practice learning gives students the experience and opportunity to demonstrate the skills, knowledge and behaviour which are required to achieve the learning outcomes associated with nursing practice. Universities work very closely with the NHS and other health and social care providers to ensure that the practice learning experience they offer involves a diversity of service users and a wide range of organisations providing services in different settings.

Make sure you are familiar with the learning outcomes for practice learning in the community and that you understand what is expected of you. The learning outcomes direct your learning experience by helping you to determine what is important for you to learn and the types of experience that would give you the opportunity. You will find this particularly helpful in the community, as there are so many learning opportunities to choose from. Of course what makes learning outcomes important, is that they are the basis of the assessment to becoming a nurse and therefore must be achieved for successful completion of specific parts of the programme.

Be prepared for practice learning before you commence your placement experience

As with all of your practice experience, it is important to do some preparation before your community placement commences. Give plenty of time for this as the information you need may not be easily accessible on the last minute. Use a checklist such as the one in Table 4.1 for ensuring that you have prepared yourself for practice.

Information that the university provides

Always check your university practice placement information site for the following information:

- Details about the practice learning setting
- Name and contact details of the mentor
- Learning outcomes to be achieved

- Paperwork associated with this part of the programme
- Assignments to be completed during practice learning
- University attendance/study days during practice learning
- Arrangements for contacting tutors
- Details of university tutor visits in practice
- Self-directed study activities.

Make sure you know where you are going and how to get there

One of the most obvious objectives before going to your community placement is to make sure you know where you are going and have planned how to get there. Within more remote areas, for example some rural areas of Scotland, it may be possible to negotiate with staff regarding your starting and finishing times, but you need to contact staff within your placement some time *before* commencing practice. You should also find out the cost of travel and how you will be reimbursed for this.

Contacting your mentor

It is important that you make the initial contact with your mentor. This is an opportunity to ensure that they are expecting you and to clarify the arrangements for your first day. You can find out what time you will be expected to arrive and leave, whether you need to wear a uniform and if not what dress code is expected. If necessary you can use this early contact to negotiate any specific requirements regarding off duty. Some areas have developed an induction or 'Welcome' pack for students and it is sometimes worthwhile visiting the area beforehand and reading this before you start.

Table 4.1 Placement checklist: Use the following as a checklist prior to starting your placement

Item	Yes	No
Checked dates of placement		
Found out location of placement		
Found out best way to get there		
What time to arrive		
What to take with me		
What to wear (see Uniform options)		
Name of mentor and base/surgery/unit/health centre		
Logged on the University Learning Resource web site and checked for any messages from programme/module leader/personal tutor		
Found the University information available on practice learning website		
Found out the University link teacher name for the placement		
Undertaken some initial reading about the community placement		
Obtained a personal file to make notes on various health problems, signs and symptoms, medications, interventions		
If time, practice some skills relevant to the placement in the clinical skills lab, with teacher agreement		
Refresh knowledge in any notes undertaken in lectures/seminars in university		
Obtain at least one book from the library or other resource, which is relevant to the clinical placement		
Ensure plenty of time to get to placement on the first day		

Relevant theory and practice

You may not have completed any specific theory relating to community nursing. However, you will have knowledge and skills which can be transferred to the community setting and it is important that you take time to explore this before commencing your placement. Nursing notes and subjects such as epidemiology, sociology and social policy are all very relevant to the community and it is worth checking reading lists for articles and text books that have been recommended. You may have already developed nursing skills in other practice learning settings or in the simulated clinical skills centre which can be transferred to the community setting. Remember that you should not take on any task that you have not been taught or that you do not feel competent in undertaking.

Personal learning objectives

Before you meet with your mentor, it is useful not only to review the specific university learning outcomes for community practice learning but also to review your personnel aims and objectives. This will help you to feel more confident when you first meet your mentor and help you to plan the learning experience more effectively.

Find out about the area before you start

The more you know about your practice learning area before you start, the more interesting and enjoyable your experience. Having an idea about the health profile of the community will give you some time to think about what you would like to see, do and learn. This will help inform discussions with your mentor when you are planning your learning experience and identify how best to achieve your learning outcomes. Ask your mentor if there is a practice profile or community profile available. Some community teams have developed these themselves and in other areas, they have been developed by the healthcare organisation. Table 4.2 gives an overview of the type of information contained within a community profile. (This is discussed in more detail later in this book.)

Table 4.2 Overview of a community profile

Community profile themes	Examples
The geographical environment	Inner city, suburban, rural or remote – the infrastructure and connections with other areas
The overall health profile of the population in the area	Information about children's and young peoples' health, adults' health and lifestyle, illness and poor health and life expectancy
The age and sex profile of the area	The number of people in each age category
Ethnic and cultural background	Different ethnic, religious and cultural backgrounds including, Black British, African Caribbean, African and Asian
Education	The provision of schools, colleges and higher education in the area
Economic	The prosperity of the area, income levels, employment/unemployment
Sociopolitical	Interaction of members of the community, community involvement in decision-making about how services are provided
Resources	Schools, shops, housing stock, health centres and hospitals, places of worship, parks and leisure facilities
The range of local service providers and access to others	Independent sector – private or voluntary, NHS, local authority

Meeting with your mentor

The learning outcomes for community practice learning will provide the focus for your initial discussion with your mentor, and should enable the development of a programme of clinical learning experiences appropriate to your specific learning needs.

Planning your learning experience

The benefits to planning your learning experience include:
- The student and the mentor are able to identify learning opportunities that match achievement of the learning outcomes and personal learning objectives and interests
- Progress can be monitored at timely intervals
- The student and mentor can be realistic about what can be achieved.

Developing a learning contract

Learning contracts or learning agreements have been used extensively in practice learning to enable the student and mentor to negotiate and agree a learning plan. They help to avoid any confusion and clarify expectations on both sides. They identify what you want to achieve personally from your practice experience and the ways in which you can achieve your learning outcomes (Hart 2010).

The following steps which can be used as a template will assist you with this:

Step 1. Identify learning needs

A learning need is the gap between where you are and where you want and need to be with regards to learning something new or extending your knowledge and skills in a previously learnt area. Discuss what you want to learn from the experience and using your mentor's guidance and knowledge, discuss clinical opportunities available which may help you to achieve your learning outcomes and personal objectives.

Step 2. Learning outcomes

The learning needs are written as outcomes or as set goals to achieve. These may often be identified as SMART goals. They must be achievable within the timeframe allowed, and they must be realistic to your needs and capabilities. Added to your programme, learning outcomes for this element of practice learning, will be any assignments or skills records that must be completed.

Step 3. Action plan

Each learning outcome is then considered and a plan constructed identifying how it will be achieved. What resources are required to help achieve the objective, such as time, visit to a Specialist Nurse, literature search. This plan describes how you propose to go about achieving each outcome.

Step 4. Evidence of achievement

For each outcome, you and your mentor can identify what evidence is required to prove that the learning has occurred and the outcome has been met.

Step 5. Evaluation

Review the outcomes as required and ensure that if objectives are not being met, then steps are taken to identify this promptly.

Developing a learning plan

Table 4.3 gives some examples that you might identify as learning needs within your learning plan. Remember to negotiate times with your mentor for regular feedback and review of your progress. To assist you and your mentor to review the learning

opportunities which exist in the community and to structure the learning plan around your learning outcomes, the key themes or components of community nursing are identified in Table 4.4.

Induction and orientation

It is always important to feel comfortable and familiar with new surroundings as soon as possible. Orientation to a new setting can enhance learning by reducing your anxiety, helping you to feel that you fit in and increase

---

Table 4.3 Developing a learning plan

Date	Brief description of learning need	Action plan
	This may include areas: in which you feel you require more practice; which are specifically related to outcomes within your university assessment documentation; where there are specific types of experience; which may only be available within this specific placement	Identify how you will achieve your learning outcomes Try to discuss specific learning opportunities which may assist you to achieve your outcomes

Examples

Understanding the main physical, social and psychological conditions common to clients using this service

Discussing referral agencies and the processes by which referrals are made

Exploring the methods for effective communication and record-keeping

Under supervision, participate in the use of health education and health promotion within the community setting

Under supervision, participate in the care of a client with a long-term condition and identify strategies used by healthcare practitioners to facilitate self-care

Demonstrate knowledge and understanding of legal and ethical aspects of care, e.g. maintaining dignity, privacy and confidentiality;

Under supervision keep accurate nursing notes

Demonstrate awareness of the need for collaboration and communication to co-ordinate care in the community

Table 4.4 Key themes for community practice learning

Themes	Indicative areas for knowledge and skills development
Community profiling	Understanding of community, concepts and definitions
Team working	Theories and concepts of team-working Multiagency working
Health promotion	Theories and concepts of health promotion Public health approaches and interventions Health promotion within specific contexts of care: sexual health, immunisation, smoking cessation, drugs and alcohol
Management	Leadership, time management, workload management, clinical governance
Communication	Communication skills, report writing and record keeping, motivational interviewing, utilisation of technology
Teaching, learning and facilitation	Mentorship, facilitation skills for teaching and health promotion Facilitation of self-care and self-management
Children, young people and family health	Working with children, young people and families, child health promotion and child protection
Long-term conditions	Management of long-term conditions, assessment, carer support, anticipatory care, medicines management
Complex needs	Identification and management of people with complex needs, co-ordination of care, needs of specific client groups, e.g. palliative and end of life care, dementia care, wound management.

your motivation to learn. As in other clinical areas, there are a number of issues which should be addressed within your orientation, which should include the following:

1. Introduction to mentor and practice staff
2. General orientation to placement
   - Layout
   - Emergency equipment
   - Emergency telephone procedures
   - Fire procedures
   - Placement phone numbers
3. Identify procedures for reporting sickness/absence, dress code
4. How to keep in contact with community staff (may be appropriate to ensure you exchange mobile phone numbers)
5. Discussion with mentor regarding philosophy of care and hours of working
6. Identify practice education facilitator and link lecturer
7. Identify and locate national and local policies/procedures/guidelines and NMC documentation.

In many areas, mentors have prepared a Welcome pack or orientation booklet for students, which also outlines specific learning opportunities available within the placement. A written orientation programme or timetable can also be very helpful. Table 4.5 is a sample timetable, for guidance only, which you and your mentor may like to discuss and adapt.

Table 4.5 Sample orientation timetable

Week 1	Morning	Afternoon
Monday	Orientation to health centre and introduction to staff Review of student learning outcomes. Identification of learning opportunities within the community placement. Discuss learning contract with mentor	Introduction to the neighbourhood and caseload Accompany mentor on home visits.
Tuesday	Day with health visitor: Home visits, attendance at clinics, health promotion/health education sessions	Continue with health visitor
Wednesday	Day with community nursing team: Accompany community staff on home visits; focus on needs of patient and family	Continue with home visits with community nursing team
Thursday	Day with community nursing team: Accompany community staff on home visits; focus on needs of patient and family.	Work-based learning activity
Friday	Day with practice nurse	Feedback with mentor/ reflection on orientation week/ finalise learning contract

You may never have been to the place where your community practice is based. It is helpful to familiarise yourself with the area as part of your orientation. Ways of doing this include: looking at maps and satellite views on the internet, visiting the area and placement itself, walking about to familiarise yourself with the area and/or taking a drive around the immediate locality. This may prove to be a great help in the future when you are trying to find an address or a meeting place. Personnel safety in the community has been discussed earlier in the book, however it is important to remember how you can reduce potential risks by developing your knowledge of the area you are to be working in. Your university and placement will have policies on health and safety and how to manage personal risk. Ensure that you are familiar with these and how to ensure your own and others' safety during your community placement.

Activities to enhance your practice learning

Remember to use your university learning resources such as the virtual learning environment (VLE) and any other online learning material which your university has recommended during community practice learning. Keep a personal learning file of notes which specifically relate to your community practice experience. These types of activity, along with many others, may be kept in your learning portfolio (Timmins 2008). You should also refer back to relevant lecture notes and read the literature related to this placement. The further reading and recommended website resources at the end of each chapter of this book are a useful starting points.

Remember that, as with other clinical placements, your contact with nursing staff, patients and other practitioners will be a major part of your learning experience; however, independent work-based activities will also enhance the achievement of your learning outcomes. For example, when community nursing staff and your mentors are involved with essential administrative duties, this is an ideal time for you to engage in some self-directed study. This may include literature searching a particular topic related to an aspect of care you have encountered or may involve specific work-based learning activities, which have been devised by the university or your mentor. Attempt to complete any work-based activities or self-directed study; they are designed to enable you to develop your knowledge and understanding. Plan regular feedback sessions with your mentor; this is an opportunity to discuss work-based learning activities and to generally reflect on your progress. This self-directed study may also be enhanced by attendance at study days for students or community staff, and regardless of the specific field of practice pathway you are pursuing, it is essential that you maximise learning about topics which can impact on the whole care experience for a patient. Study days may include learning about caring for patients with mental health problems, wound care or risk management. Find out what is planned for the time you are undertaking your placement and plan to attend if possible to gain knowledge and skills related to other fields of practice. This can contribute to your

NMC expectations with regard to, 'Exposure to other fields of practice learning' (NMC 2010).

Being an effective learner

Being a mentor is an essential part of a nurse's role. Mentors must meet the standards required by the NMC and demonstrate their continuing competence and development as a mentor (NMC 2008). Mentors guide, educate, supervise, assess, support and act as role models for students. The goal of good mentoring is also to empower students and give them confidence in taking responsibility for their own learning. This requires the students to play their part as effective learners.

 Activity

Have a look at the quotes from 2nd and 3rd year adult nursing students in Figure 4.1.

You will quickly have noticed that the quotes on the left reflect a positive experience of community practice learning and those on the right a negative one. It is likely that the learning opportunities on offer were similar for all students. Why do you think the students' comments are so different?

Mentors and students have recognised that the student's approach to learning in practice has an important effect on their personal satisfaction, learning experience and ability to achieve their learning outcomes. Teatheredge (2010) found that mentoring was more beneficial to students who were interested and willing to learn and get involved. Students preferring a participative role to a passive observation only role, appear to have a much more positive learning experience (Baillie 1993). The following are some of the behaviours which characterise willing and effective learners:

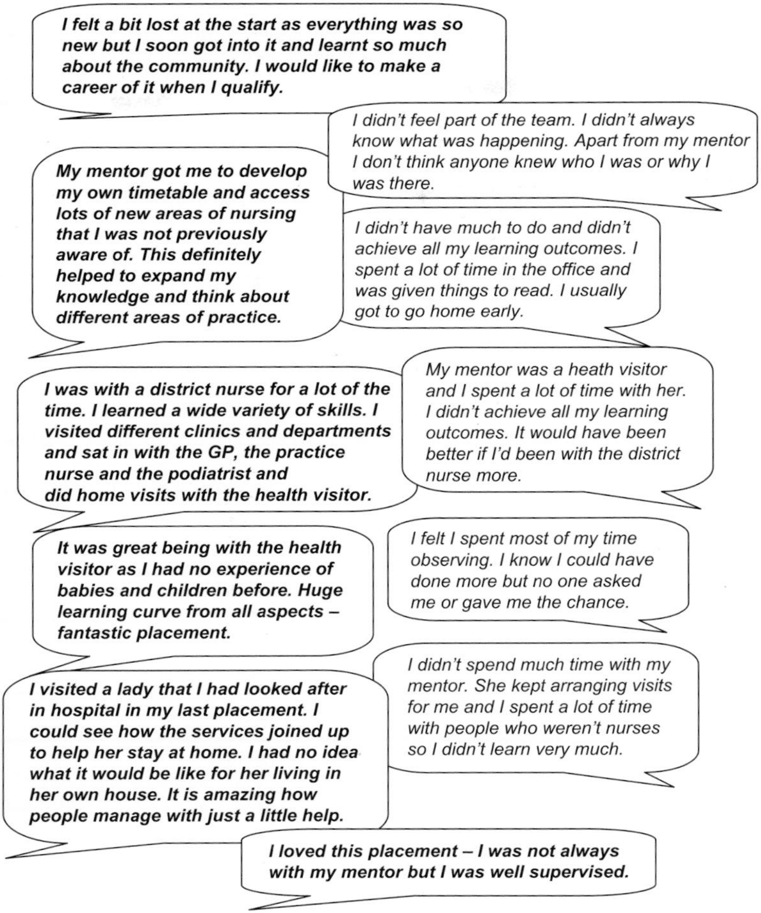

> *I felt a bit lost at the start as everything was so new but I soon got into it and learnt so much about the community. I would like to make a career of it when I qualify.*

> *I didn't feel part of the team. I didn't always know what was happening. Apart from my mentor I don't think anyone knew who I was or why I was there.*

> *My mentor got me to develop my own timetable and access lots of new areas of nursing that I was not previously aware of. This definitely helped to expand my knowledge and think about different areas of practice.*

> *I didn't have much to do and didn't achieve all my learning outcomes. I spent a lot of time in the office and was given things to read. I usually got to go home early.*

> *I was with a district nurse for a lot of the time. I learned a wide variety of skills. I visited different clinics and departments and sat in with the GP, the practice nurse and the podiatrist and did home visits with the health visitor.*

> *My mentor was a heath visitor and I spent a lot of time with her. I didn't achieve all my learning outcomes. It would have been better if I'd been with the district nurse more.*

> *It was great being with the health visitor as I had no experience of babies and children before. Huge learning curve from all aspects – fantastic placement.*

> *I felt I spent most of my time observing. I know I could have done more but no one asked me or gave me the chance.*

> *I visited a lady that I had looked after in hospital in my last placement. I could see how the services joined up to help her stay at home. I had no idea what it would be like for her living in her own house. It is amazing how people manage with just a little help.*

> *I didn't spend much time with my mentor. She kept arranging visits for me and I spent a lot of time with people who weren't nurses so I didn't learn very much.*

> *I loved this placement – I was not always with my mentor but I was well supervised.*

Figure 4.1 Adult nursing students on views community practice learning.

- Positive and personable
- Motivated and enthusiastic
- Self-directed
- Reliable and punctual
- Open to new experiences
- Conscientious
- Well prepared

- Courteous and respectful of others
- Proactive
- Ready to apply and build on learning acquired from the theoretical components of the programme and experience from other practice learning settings.

Many of the situations and events that you encounter during your community practice placement can be used as valuable learning opportunities. A positive and creative approach will greatly enhance your experience in the community and enable you to achieve your learning outcomes with ease. Table 4.6 gives some examples of how to make the most of the activities that will be included in your placement.

Reflection is therefore a very useful learning strategy, which enables you to learn about yourself and your practice. To assist you with this, you may consider keeping a reflective diary, a record of key events from your practice experience from which you can reflect. A reflective diary can be a personal record but you may consider selecting specific entries to reflect upon with your mentor or university tutor.

Student reflection

An important learning strategy for you while in your practice placement, is the ability to 'reflect' on your practical experience. A 'reflective practitioner', is someone who reflects on specific aspects of their practice and then makes changes to their future work as a result of this. Smith (1998) states that learners may find it useful to reflect on practice in the following situations:

■ When you have learned something new
■ When something within your practice experience has changed, e.g. a new practice placement, a new mentor
■ When you need to review a particular experience to learn about your strengths and weaknesses within a specific aspect of care
■ When you wish to review your personal and professional development
■ Perhaps you have made a mistake and feel unhappy about a particular outcome and so you wish to learn from this, to avoid it happening in the future.

Table 4.6 Making the most of your experience

Meetings with your mentor	Be clear about the aim of the meeting
	Have any paperwork ready, e.g. your assessment record
	Make a note of any questions you have and don't be afraid to ask
	Take a note of any actions or points of interest
Observation visits	Confirm beforehand – who you are meeting, where and at what time – *be there on time*!
	Be clear about the purpose and expectations of the visit
	Do some background reading before you go
	Clarify which learning outcomes the visit will address
	Observe the way in which practitioners work with patients and clients
	Look at the skills and unique contribution each practitioner makes to empower, support, plan and deliver care with patients and carers.

Attending team meetings	Find out about the purpose of the meeting before you attend
	Who will be there and why?
	Do you have a contribution to make?
	Be prepared to learn from all members of the nursing team, including the healthcare assistants
	Develop an understanding of the significance of working in a multidisciplinary group
	Use this experience to develop an understanding of the different roles and unique skills of different members of the multidisciplinary healthcare team
	Attending multidisciplinary team meetings and/or case conferences is another learning opportunity to develop your understanding of multidisciplinary and multiagency working.
Meeting other members of the health and care team	Your mentor will provide you with an understanding of the roles of different members of the community multidisciplinary team. Refer to the overview of roles in Chapter 2.
	Formulate questions to enhance discussions and facilitate the development of your knowledge and understanding.
Meeting up with other students in the office	Find out about each other's experience in the community
	Identify learning opportunities that you can share
Care and support in the community	The opportunities to develop your knowledge and skills regarding community profiling, team working, health promotion, management, communication, teaching learning and facilitation children, young people and family health, managing long-term conditions, and meeting complex needs are endless.
	Be an effective learner.
Travelling around the area	Use the opportunity to observe the characteristics of the neighbourhood and the types of amenities and services that are available there.
Study days at the university	Check the arrangements and make sure you give your mentor plenty of notice
	Complete any reading or preparation
	Make an effective contribution to the sessions to inform and plan further learning activities.
Reflection	Use all of these experiences as opportunities for reflection and deeper learning (reflection is covered later in this chapter).

Specific events may include any activities within your practice experience which have revealed specific strengths or weaknesses. You will find it useful to use a structured framework for reflective practice and for recording significant events. There may be a particular model that you are most familiar with or which you are encouraged to use by your university. Figure 4.2 shows an example of a reflective cycle adapted from Marks-Maran and Rose (1997).

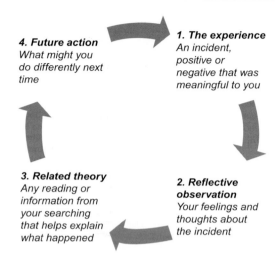

4. Future action
What might you do differently next time

1. The experience
An incident, positive or negative that was meaningful to you

3. Related theory
Any reading or information from your searching that helps explain what happened

2. Reflective observation
Your feelings and thoughts about the incident

Figure 4.2 Reflection on practice. (Adapted from Marks-Maran and Rose 1997.)

To record significant incidents accurately, you should aim to record them as soon as possible after the event. You may forget key aspects of your experience if you leave this until much later. You may find it useful to develop a daily reflective approach to your practice experience. This could include considering what went well or not so well on each shift; new skills that you have learned and plans for future work, which will enable you to develop your personal learning plan and facilitate further learning in practice.

Maslin-Prothero (2010) has identified the following self-assessment questions to assist you with reflection:

- What did I do well today?
- What could I improve on?
- What did I leave out?

Or you may prefer (Driscoll 1994):

- **What?** Returning to the situation and describing it
- **So what?** Understanding the context – feelings and effects of the different actions

- **Now what?** Modifying future outcomes – what would you change?

The reflection of significant experience is an essential learning strategy which can greatly assist you to continually question practice and enable your personnel and professional development.

The EU Directive

The EU Directive is a European law which was created to allow recognition of professional qualifications across EU countries. It stipulates, among other things, the areas of theory and practice that must be included in nursing and midwifery programmes. Students on the adult field of practice pathway are required to meet the regulations set out in European Directive 2005/36/EU (Article 31). Universities manage this in different ways, according to how the programme is structured and delivered. However, all adult field of practice students are expected to demonstrate experience in the areas of practice identified below by the end of the programme:

1.   Medical nursing
2.   Surgical nursing
3.   Care of children
4.   Maternity care
5.   Mental health
6.   Care of older people
7.   Home nursing

European Directive 2005/36/EC (Article 31): Clinical experience.

 Activity

> Think about the opportunities that could be available to you in the community for gaining nursing experience that is necessary to meet the EU directive. Could all of the clinical experience required to meet EU requirements be met? Discuss this with your mentor

Whichever branch or field of nursing practice you are studying, practice learning in the community has the potential to enable you to meet a large number and varied range of your practice learning outcomes. Read the brief overview below to see how the EU directive can be met in the community.

1. and 2. Medical and surgical nursing

Your practice learning placements will probably include medical and surgical nursing in a hospital setting. However, you are also likely to come across minor surgery in GP health centres and other outpatient settings in the community and provide care at home for people with the type of complex needs that can also be catered for in medical wards. You may have the opportunity to be involved in discharge arrangements and follow-up care at home for people who have been inpatients during your hospital experience; this is all an important part of a medical or surgical care package or pathway.

3. Care of children

You will have the opportunity to experience care of children in the broadest sense, from the interventions that promote health and wellbeing for all children, to the protection of vulnerable children and to meeting the complex care needs of children who are sick or dying. Children with complex needs and disabilities are cared for in the community by their families and supported by the primary care team including specialist nurses, community children's nurses, and in some areas, district nurses. Public health nurses, health visitors and school nurses are involved in supporting children of all ages and their families, working in partnership with other services and agencies.

It is important that any practitioner working with children and young people is aware of the rights of children so that they can be protected against harm, neglect or abuse. The United Nations Convention on the Rights of the Child (UNCRC) is an international human rights treaty that grants all children and young people (aged 17 and under) a comprehensive set of rights. The convention gives children and young people over 40 substantive rights, including the right to:

- *special protection measures and assistance*
- *access to services such as education and healthcare*
- *develop their personalities, abilities and talents to the fullest potential*
- *grow up in an environment of happiness, love and understanding*
- *be informed about and participate in achieving their rights in an accessible and active manner.*

Activity

Before or while on placement, explore the following website to increase your knowledge of the UNCRC. Online. Available at: http://www.unicef.org/crc/ (accessed November 2011).

4. Maternity care

The midwife in the community and the health visitor or public health nurse support a woman and her family from pre-birth through pregnancy, birth and the postnatal period. For some women, most or all of their maternity care is provided in the community, between the primary care team and the local midwifery-led unit or general practice health centre. Practice learning in the community should provide the ideal opportunity to gain maternity experience.

5. Mental health

For many years, the aim of mental health services has been to enable people with mental health problems to stay out of hospital and lead healthy lives in their own homes. Consequently, the community mental health nurse team, together with colleagues in other agencies, provides services to support people with long-term enduring mental health problems and provide crisis intervention for people with acute problems in the community. Other examples include the care given to people with dementia and their families by the district nursing team, the health visiting team supporting women with postnatal depression and also the role of the health visitor and school nurse in supporting children and young people with mental health problems.

6. Care of older people

The opportunities to gain experience and learn about nursing care for older people are many and varied in the community. As our population ages and more people seek to lead healthier lives for longer, services for older people have become more oriented towards health improvement, enablement, rehabilitation and self-care. Assessing risk for the most vulnerable and anticipating problems has been a positive move in reducing hospital admission and helping people stay in their own homes for longer. Nursing care and support in residential and nursing homes is another aspect of caring for older people in the community.

7. Home nursing

Home nursing is a key function of district nursing care and in many areas, the district nursing teams provide a generic service, which includes surgical and medical nursing, care of sick children, people with mental health problems and care of older people. However, a variety of nurses care for people at home, including community mental health nurses, community children's nurses and specialist nurses, e.g. tissue viability, palliative care, respiratory nurses.

Summary of learning points from this chapter

- Preparation and organisation are important aspects of effective practice learning in any placement
- A positive and proactive approach to learning not only enhances learning opportunities but motivates and encourages both the student and mentor to engage in collaborative learning experiences
- Learning strategies such as reflection facilitate learning and promote achievement of personal objectives and learning outcomes.

References

Baillie, L., 1993. Factors affecting student nurses' learning in community placements: a phenomenological study. Journal of Advanced Nursing 18 (7), 1043–1053.

Department of Health, 2006. Modernising nursing careers; setting the direction. DH, London.

Driscoll, J., 1994. Reflective practise for practise. Senior Nurse 13 (Jan/Feb), 47–50.

EC Directive 2005/36/EC of the European parliament and of the council. Recognition of professional qualifications. Updated 19 May 2010.

Hart, S. (Ed.), 2010. Nursing: study and placement learning skills. Oxford University Press, Oxford.

Marks-Maran, D., Rose, P (Eds.), 1997. Thinking and caring: new perspectives on reflection. In: Reconstructing nursing: beyond art and science. Bailliere Tindall, London.

Maslin-Prothero, S. (Ed.), 2010. Bailliere's study skills for nurses and midwives. 4th ed. Bailliere Tindall, London.

NMC, 2008. Standards to support learning and assessment in practice. NMC standards for mentors, practice teachers and teachers. NMC, London.

NMC, 2010. Standards for pre-registration nursing education. NMC, London.

Queen's Nursing Institute, 2009. 2020 Vision: Focusing on the future of district nursing. QNI, London.

Smith, A., 1998. Learning about reflection. Journal of Advanced Nursing 28 (4), 891–898.

Teatheredge, J., 2010. Interviewing students and qualified nurses to find out what makes an effective mentor. Nursing Times 106 (48), 19–21.

Timmins, F., 2008. Making sense of portfolios: a guide for nursing students. Open University Press.

Further reading

Holland, K., Roxburgh, C.M., 2012. Preparation for learning in practice. In: Placement learning in surgical nursing. A guide for students in practice, Bailliere Tindall, London.

Jasper, M., 2006. Professional development, reflection and decision-making. Blackwell, Oxford.

NHS Education for Scotland, 2008. Quality standards for practice placements, 2nd ed. NES, Edinburgh.

Nursing and Midwifery Council, 2009. Guidance on professional conduct for nursing and midwifery students. NMC, London.

Sharples, K., 2010. Learning to learn in nursing practice: a guide for student nurses. Learning Matters, Exeter.

Websites

There are a number of helpful publications for student nurses at the RCN website, which would be helpful to read prior to any clinical placement experience. For example, 'Helping students get the best from their practice placements' (RCN 2002, reprinted with amendments in 2006). Please keep in mind when reading it that the NMC have now amended their Standards for pre registration nursing education (NMC 2010): http://www.rcn.org.uk/ development/publications.

NHS Education for Scotland (NES) is NHS Scotland's education and training body. The website contains a wide range of educational materials: www.nes.scot.nhs.uk/.

Nursing and Midwifery Council, http://www. nmc-uk.org/.

United Nations Convention on the Rights of the Child (UNCRC 2011), http://www. education.gov.uk/ childrenandyoungpeople/ healthandwellbeing/b0074766/uncrc.

Section 2. Practice learning opportunities

5 Assessing and addressing need in the community

CHAPTER AIMS

- To examine how 'need' is assessed within the community and to explore the concept of 'health needs assessment'
- To explore the different issues to be addressed in the individual assessment of care including the use of a person-centred approach
- To discuss the role of the nurse in promoting health and wellbeing and what students can learn in a community placement

Health needs assessment: getting to know your community

To enable primary care staff to understand and plan appropriate services to meet the healthcare needs of the practice population, several sources of data are gathered. Data related to health needs normally includes aspects of the community which can affect health such as housing, education, socioeconomic status and unemployment/ employment statistics. Associations have been identified between deprivation and behavioural factors which affect health, for example people who are economically inactive and in lower socioeconomic groups are more likely to be cigarette smokers and live in areas of deprivation (Robinson & Harris 2011). Deprived areas also have higher levels of death due to coronary heart disease (Naylor et al 2012). The term 'community profile' is sometimes used to describe specific aspects of the practice locality and normally includes issues related to the specific characteristics of the population (the demography), local amenities and public services, employment, transport. Data related to the specific incidence and pattern of disease which relates to the local pattern of need is also significant when planning appropriate services.

Activity

In discussion with your mentor, select one specific health issue which is significant within your specific practice placement population and compile information from different sources on this topic, which would help a new community nurse coming to work within the locality.

Continued

You may wish to refer to:

- Resources on topics that previous students may have considered during their placement
- Information on the locality held at the nursing department and the health centre
- Local NHS computerised data available (ask your mentor about this as you may not be permitted to access it yourself)
- Local information sources such as libraries, employment agencies, Citizens Advice Bureaux, local practitioners (e.g. practice nurse, practice manager, community mentor).

You may also like to use the links below, to see how comprehensive and easily accessible information about the community can be. Both are excellent resources for finding out about public health and needs of populations.

Look at 'The Network of Public Health Observatories' website, which produces information, data and intelligence on people' health and healthcare practitioners across the UK and has expertise in utilising data and information into meaningful health intelligence: www.apho.org.uk.

There is also a European Public Health Observatory which has information on European Health Care systems and other countries worldwide: http://www. euro.who.int/en/who-we-are/partners/ observatory.

an evidence-based reference list. It may be that some of you are required to compile a community profile for an assignment or for meeting your personal and professional development goals. The health issue identified for the community profile can also be used to look at how that health need is managed in the community.

Assessing 'need' in the community

Health needs assessment could be considered equivalent to a clinical consultation when the doctor will take a medical history from the patient, collecting information that assists with a diagnosis of the person's problems, which then helps to identify solutions. The health needs assessment process takes a medical history at a population level, collecting data, which helps to diagnose the population's health problems and assist in the planning and implementation of services, which will help to meet the population's problems.

 Activity

Discuss with your mentor the advantages of using a health needs assessment approach and how this will enable the health and social care team to plan an integrated approach to meeting the health needs of the community population.

Once you have gathered the information it is important that you then compile them into a folder, ensuring that sections are organised in a way that the information is easily accessible for you and others reading it. It is important to ensure that whatever you gather, there is a clear contents list and

Health needs assessment provides an opportunity to evaluate the population's health status, in order to understand the needs and priorities of the practice and local population (NICE 2009). This should assist in developing clear aims and objectives to design and develop services to meet the population's needs. Ultimately, this process aims to improve the health of the practice and local population, targeting groups and specific population needs.

 Activity

- Ask your community mentor about the health needs assessment in your specific practice placement; this may involve spending some time with the health centre practice manager who will normally manage some of the data involved, such as the epidemiology of the practice population, including data related to the prevalence and incidence of disease, morbidity and mortality statistics, age/sex ratio.

- Consider the social determinants of health within your practice population such as housing type, socioeconomic status of the practice population, ethnicity, single parent families, age profile and disability.

- Discuss with your mentor the local healthcare services, which have been developed to meet the local community needs.

This type of information will be invaluable if you are undertaking a health profile project of the community where your practice placement is to be found. This can build onto the information already collected on the profile of the community.

Including service users in the assessment of health needs

Health needs assessment should also involve the gathering of data from a wide range of sources, which should also include service users, their families and carers.

Depending on where you are in your programme of study, you will have varied interaction with families and carers of service users. It is important to remember that if a person (service user) in the community has a long-term health problem, that they probably know more about this and its management than the main healthcare professional. They are living with the health problem – an example of this is someone who has had diabetes (mellitus) since they were 8 years old and who is now 48 years old! Determining their health needs as they get older however, may involve their family and/or carer.

 Activity

Try to find out the different ways in which healthcare practitioners within your community practice placement consult their practice population; you might like to ask your mentor and other members of the community team.

In some health centres, for example there is a patient/healthcare professional forum which meets every 2–3 months to discuss a range of matters, from resources available in the health centre, to access to GP appointments. Patient satisfaction surveys, focus groups, one-to-one interviews, public meetings and interviews with key leaders of specific services, are additional ways in which user involvement can be integrated within service development. Some of these local questionnaires can be linked to the work of the general practice nurse for example, such as managing smoking behaviour or alcohol reduction. This is an excellent meeting to attend with permission from the person leading such a forum, and can also be an opportunity to meet members of the community and their families and carers.

When exploring the concept of needs assessment within your university lectures, a reference may have been made to Bradshaw's Taxonomy of Need (1972), which describes different types of need. These are:

1. 'Normative' need, which is a need defined by professionals
2. 'Felt' need, which is a need defined by the population
3. 'Expressed' need, which is a demand for a felt need to be met by health professionals and others.

For appropriate services to be developed, healthcare practitioners need to take account of all 'types' of need. An example which illustrates these three different needs could be:

1. Normative need: the practice team may decide that there is a definite need to introduce a smoking cessation programme in the health centre
2. Felt need: the patient forum at the health centre has undertaken to talk to members at the local community centre where there are a number of clubs for all ages, and they have been asked by a number of young and older people if there is anything at the health centre for helping them give up smoking, and they think there is a need for support and help to stop smoking group
3. Expressed need: The patient forum have discussed the need for a smoking cessation support and 'help give up smoking' group and have requested that this need be met by the health centre staff.

National targets for improving health

National targets often underpin government health policy and may be enacted through legislation, for example the ban on smoking in any public place in the UK, such as

cinemas, restaurants, university campuses and pubs, with many places not even having a dedicated space for smoking and smokers. They clearly impact on healthcare delivery within local communities. These targets for health improvement are normally identified because they constitute a major public health issue, which has not been resolved through existing interventions. Smoking prevention and cessation is one of these.

Activity

Identify the key national targets for improving the health of the population in the part of the UK that you are based. You will find it helpful to access the government websites referred to in Chapter 1.

Discuss with your mentor how these targets are addressed locally and the services that are in place to meet them. The practice manager at the health centre may also be able to give you information.

Identify a learning action for yourself to discuss with your mentor and how this knowledge can help you achieve your programme and NMC learning outcomes with regards to public health and wellbeing.

The Scottish Government (2007) has developed a set of core objectives and measures for the NHS known as HEAT targets, which include work within areas such as mental health, focusing on decreasing the use of antidepressants utilisation, reducing suicide rates and improvements in the earlier diagnosis and management of clients with dementia.

A health needs assessment approach enables practitioners to critically examine current provision of services and how this addresses local healthcare needs. It is also an opportunity to review the contributions of all healthcare professionals in that particular aspect of care.

Activity

With guidance from your mentor, look at how a health needs assessment approach could be used for a specific client group. This could be looking at services to prevent or treat disease or services to promote health. An example could be women aged over 60 years (at risk of osteoporosis) or men over 50 (at risk of prostatic cancer).

- Consider the contributions of different healthcare practitioners in meeting the needs of this specific client group.
- You should try to include an examination of current services for this specific client group and all the best practice, newly published guidelines, which should be referred to in the future development of services. Remember you are looking at what 'is happening' and what 'should be happening', in terms of service provision, resulting in the identification of clear objectives of what changes are required and how these changes can be achieved. Try to identify what an action plan might entail for the specific client group you have chosen.
- Refer to the National Institute for Clinical Excellence's (NICE 2005) Health needs assessment: A practical guide, at: www.nice.org.uk will assist you with this activity.
- A report of your findings could be used in your portfolio to evidence the achievement of learning outcomes relating to public health, health needs assessment and health improvement.

Meeting the needs of individual patients and their carers

In this chapter so far, you have explored assessing the needs of the community but you must also consider meeting the needs of the individual and their carers, all of whom are part of your mentor's caseload of patients/clients. It is helpful to use the stages of the nursing process, in particular the first stage of assessment.

Assessment

Assessment is the first stage in the process of planning individualised care for the client; it requires gathering information, which can significantly influence the plan of care and assist the client to retain their independence (Holland and Whittam 2008). Approaches to assessment differ according to the clinical setting. Assessing the needs of the client within the home environment, for example may help them and their carers to feel more at ease and therefore more comfortable in giving an honest expression of their concerns and needs. However, the home environment can also pose significant challenges such as an untidy, smelly or unclean environment, as referred to in Chapter 3. The distractions within the 'business' of a clinic or surgery, however, may also pose difficulties in the facilitation of a therapeutic relationship.

During your community experience, you will be aware that some individuals and their families have been known to the community nurse and to the general practice over a long period of time. The longer the duration of the nurse–patient relationship, the more conducive to developing a more holistic perspective of the person's actual and potential needs. For example, although the district nurse may have an initial request to visit an older person to dress a venous ulcer, over a number of visits the person may disclose issues such as loneliness, difficulty with medication and mobility problems. The first visit to a client's home can present the community nurse with an overwhelming amount of information and great skill is required to be able to identify the client's key issues and concerns and plan care which addresses their specific needs.

 Activity

Try to use some agreed time during your community placement to review the different ways in which client's needs are assessed. Discuss with your mentor how you might practise assessment skills, as this will contribute to achieving your learning outcomes associated with NMC competencies in the domain: Nursing practice and decision-making (NMC 2010). Ensure that you observe your mentor or member of the team undertake an assessment first and when you are undertaking one yourself under supervision, do not forget to ask the patient/client for permission to do so, explaining that you are a student nurse and also that you would value very much their feedback on how you undertook the assessment, as well as how effective your communication skills were. This inclusion of service users and carers in the assessment of student nurses is also to be encouraged as part of the assessment of skills and knowledge within the NMC 2010 standards (NMC 2010).

Similar to patient assessment within the hospital setting, the focus of the first visit to the client at home is normally to identify the client's concerns, identify actual and potential healthcare needs/problems and in collaboration with the client and if appropriate their carer, plan an appropriate

programme of care. This assessment approach will be different, depending on the initial needs of the client/patient, and if undertaking the mental health nursing pathway, the community nurse may be identified as a community psychiatric nurse or CPN. (See Felton et al 2012 for additional information on specific roles and assessment approaches within mental health nursing in the community placements.)

Good communication skills, regardless of the client/patient group, are vital in the facilitation of a good assessment and can:

- create rapport
- facilitate thorough collection of all information which can assist in the development of an appropriate plan of care which meets the approval and needs of the client
- facilitate invitation to the client and family to give an honest perspective of their wishes and needs.

 Activity

You will probably have lots of opportunity to observe the communication skills of the different healthcare practitioners you encounter during your community learning experience. Try to identify some of the key communication skills you have observed when you have accompanied the community nurse/community psychiatric nurse/children's nurse on home visits. Discuss with your mentor why certain communication techniques were used in some situations and not others.

Reflect on how you communicated with the client and their family or carer in the home.

Learning to communicate effectively is an essential skill required for registration (NMC 2010). Chapter 9 looks in more detail at communication in community practice.

Your list of communication skills should include the ability to initiate discussion; to listen to the client's 'narrative' or story on their perspective of their current health problem and be able to respond in a way which demonstrates to the client that you understand the problem from their perspective. You will probably have also included the skill of questioning; the ability to find out the 'what, where, when, how, who and why' in assessment, this can greatly assist in the identification of specific needs and problems. However, it is important to remember to avoid extensive questioning, which could be considered as intrusive. The skill is to initiate general conversation, which elicits relevant information and enables the client to feel comfortable in discussing their health problems. Remember also that when visiting a client within their own home, the practitioner has the responsibility to pick up on cues which may influence the care plan such as hazards in the home environment, which may increase the risk of falls.

 Activity

Imagine you are at home and you are expecting a visit by the district nurse. How would you like the nurse to approach you? In Chapter 3, reference was made to the student being an invited guest in the client's home.

What impact do you think it will have on the visit by a nurse if the person has dementia and is unable to communicate very well because of memory problems, or if the person has a mental health problem? Visiting a mother who has young children will also make a difference in how the nurse approaches them in the home. Often a discussion takes place, which ensures inclusion of family members or carers and thus helps the communication between nurse and patient/client.

Most of us would like to feel that we have been given opportunity to participate and be involved in the decisions about our care; that the healthcare practitioner demonstrated understanding of our problems/needs and that we had time to ask questions.

The initial visit to a client's home is a significant time to collect information, which can help facilitate the development of an appropriate individualised plan of care and includes:

- Confirmation of general data, name, date of birth, source and reason for referral
- Details regarding present complaint/ needs and potential problems
- How the present complaint has interfered with daily life
- The identification of underlying concerns the client has about the current situation
- Details regarding family and carer support, the potential for self-care
- Assessment of the home environment for any adaptation which may assist daily living.

During your placement experience, you will have opportunities to assist both your mentor and the client to create an individualised care plan using a framework for the assessment.

Assessment frameworks and models of nursing

Within any previous clinical placements, you will have encountered different models of nursing to assist in the process of assessment and planning of appropriate care. You may have also had lectures in the university as well as directed study looking at various models in the literature and have had the opportunity to discuss these in the classroom.

Activity

In discussion with your mentor, identify models of nursing, assessment frameworks or assessment tools used within the community setting. Use what you know already to consider the possible nursing models/frameworks that would be appropriate for assessment of clients in the community. You should already have accessed information prior to the placement, as to possible models of care planning that they use in the placement you are experiencing.

 Activity

You may find it useful to refer to the text by Holland et al (2008), which uses a case study approach to examine the application of the Roper–Logan–Tierney model. Access other literature to find out about other models and compare them with each other in terms of how valuable they are in helping you to identify a patient/client's care needs and to undertake a health assessment with regards to lifestyle and quality of life. Health promotion models are often used for this latter exercise.

It is not the purpose of this book to review nursing models in detail but it is important that you identify the nursing models being used in each area in which you work and also become acquainted with any other assessment frameworks or tools which assist in the assessment process. You may find that your practice learning area has developed its own model of nursing from a range of different models. Roper et al's (2000) activities of the 'living model' is widely used in nursing, both in the acute and community area and guides nurses to assess, plan, deliver and evaluate care in relation to 12 key activities of living. Macduff and Sinclair (2008) identify Orem's (1971) self-care deficit model as being particularly applicable in the care of clients with long term conditions, assisting nurses to identify gaps in self-care and resulting in the planning of care which optimises the individual patient's behaviour. Orem's model of care has also been considered particularly relevant to rehabilitation and community care. Roy's (1976) adaptation model has been used to effectively support people with mental health problems and Casey's (1988) partnership model has been utilised in the caring of children and families.

A variety of different assessment tools help with specific aspects of care such as wound care, nutritional status, oral health, pain relief and pressure area risk assessment. (Assessment tools are discussed in Chapter 6, in relation to the management of long-term conditions.)

 Activity

Refer to the Royal College of Nursing publication regarding the nursing assessment of older people (RCN 2008): www.rcn.org.uk.

This assessment tool is designed to assist anyone who is involved in the care of an older person and includes 25 categories of ability or need that can be used to assess an individual's complex health status. You may wish to use this as an example of using an assessment tool in practice. Discuss with your mentor the possibility of using it with a person on the caseload, ensuring that any information is anonymised.

SIGN and NICE guidelines

A set of frameworks available to practitioners to assist in planning appropriate care, are the NICE clinical guidelines, which have been developed by the UK National Institute for Health and Clinical Excellence (NICE): www.nice.org.uk. Similar to this, in Scotland, are the SIGN guidelines by the Scottish Intercollegiate Guidelines Network: www.sign.ac.uk. These guidelines outline specific plans of action for specific conditions, from the onset of illness to the client's rehabilitation. (Details of how to access these resources are included at the end of this chapter and they are discussed in more detail in Chapter 11.)

Integrated care pathways

Many clinical settings use integrated care pathways based on evidence and best practice, which outline the most appropriate care for a variety of different conditions. These pathways can be used by different members of the multidisciplinary team and assist in comprehensively addressing the treatment of many conditions. Other names for 'integrated care pathways' include: 'clinical pathways', 'clinical care pathways' and 'care pathways'. Examples of palliative care pathways, such as the Liverpool Care Pathway (Marie Curie Palliative Care Institute 2010) and the Gold Standards Framework (Thomas 2005) are included in Chapter 6. You can access examples of a variety of different care pathways, by accessing: www.library.nhs.uk.

Person-centred care

We have given a brief overview of the different tools and frameworks which can assist with comprehensive assessment of the client's needs, however it is essential to look at the approach healthcare practitioners

should adopt in trying to assess and plan care *with* the client. Person-centred care is a partnership way of working with clients and their families to plan, implement and evaluate health care. This approach to care is referred to throughout the book with specific reference to care of the client with dementia in Chapter 6. Table 5.1 includes the components of a person-centred approach to care (DH 2003).

Components of person-centred care

The following characteristics of a therapeutic relationship are also essential in developing person-centred care:

- *Clear professional boundaries are maintained*: it is essential that the patient, family, carer and nurse are all fully aware of each other's roles and expectations
- *Satisfies the needs of the patient*: it is important that the nurse collaborates with the patient, carer and family to identify nursing needs and plan appropriate and realistic goals of care
- *Facilitates patient autonomy*: Effective communication skills are essential to respect and maintain the patient's autonomy
- *Is a positive experience for the patient*: the nurse-patient relationship should focus on meeting the patient's needs and facilitate patient empowerment.

 Activity

Read the Guidance on professional conduct for nursing and midwifery students (NMC 2009) and consider the importance of accountability, maintaining confidentiality and maintaining clear professional boundaries and treating people as individuals in the context of person-centred care.

Table 5.1 Components of person-centred care	
Dignity and respect	To provide appropriate health care and to meet the individual needs of the client, healthcare practitioners must listen and respect client's perspectives and choices. Patient-centred care includes giving respect and consideration to client's cultural traditions, personal preferences and values, family situations, special circumstances and lifestyle.
Information sharing and communicating effectively	To make informed choices and to be able to self-care, clients and carers need accurate comprehensive information. Clients are more likely to adapt their behaviour and adhere to treatment if they receive information which helps them understand their health problems.
Participation and empowerment	Healthcare practitioners encourage and support in care and empower clients to make their own decisions.
Collaboration	The views of service users are considered in planning services, this necessitate the need for healthcare practitioners to establish what the client wants, to negotiate what is possible and to deliver an agreed plan of action.

Dignity in care

Providing dignity in care means respecting diversity, respecting the individuality of clients, their beliefs and values. Values-based practice is part of providing dignity in care. The National Service Framework for Mental Health (DH 2004) refers to the principles of values-based practice for mental health, which includes:

• Working positively with a diversity of values
• Making the inclusion of the views of service users as essential in the development of services
• Understanding personal values and beliefs and utilising this in a positive way
• Respecting the values of our colleagues.

These principles are relevant to nurses working in all areas of practice.

Tackling inequality

Reference has been made to protocols, guidelines and policies; although necessary to ensure standards, they cannot meet the specific individual needs of the client. The Equality Act (2010) guides and supports staff to tackle discrimination and promote equality. It includes factors such as disability, gender, age, race, sexual orientation. The act can be accessed on: www.equalities.gov.uk

Promoting health

Your community practice experience can provide you with a valuable opportunity to develop your knowledge and understanding of health promotion and to develop an awareness of the competencies required to promote health. Health promotion is the process of enabling clients to adopt lifestyles which are conducive to improving health and wellbeing.

 Activity

From your practice experience, identify a number of health promotion activities undertaken by different practitioners you have spent some time with, e.g. the health visitor, the district nurse, the general practice nurse, the community psychiatric nurse (community mental health nurse), the school nurse or the GP. Identify the different approaches and strategies that aim to promote health for different client groups and see what you can find out about their effectiveness. (Also access the Nursing and Midwifery Council Standards for entry to the register: www.nmc-uk.org, Domain 2 Communication and Interpersonal Skills, competency 6.)

From your list, you have probably included a number of very varied activities, which may include the community staff nurse engaging in one-to-one discussion with a patient on healthy lifestyle changes such as smoking cessation, controlling alcohol use, improving diet and encouraging exercise, school nurses promoting health with school children and public health nurses/health visitors planning and initiating health promotion awareness on a variety of issues such as smoking cessation or healthy eating. What is important from this activity, is to recognise that health promotion consists of a variety of activities which include health education, preventive health services, e.g. screening, immunisation, community-based work, environmental health measures and healthy public policies.

Communicating effectively is an essential skill for all healthcare practitioners and is particularly significant in health promotion practice. There are many ways to communicate health promoting messages but the skill of the healthcare professional is being able to select the most effective method of health promotion for that particular client or client group. For example methods appropriate for adult health care may differ from mental health requirements, which again may differ greatly from the promotion of health in children.

 Activity

Using your community experience, identify some of the different forms of communicating health promotion messages, e.g. posters/leaflets within the health centre, text, health fairs, magazines, newspapers, health awareness days, internet communication, group teaching by public health nurses or school nurses. Consider some of the skills required by the healthcare practitioner to promote health effectively. Discuss with your mentor ways in which you can develop your skills in this area, e.g. plan and deliver a health promotion talk or awareness session in the local health centre, school or day care centre.

You will probably have identified a number of health promoting activities within your practice placement, promoting 'healthy eating' is just one example of health promotion delivered by community practitioners who have direct contact with families. Weight and obesity are linked to many illnesses such as childhood diabetes, cardiovascular disease, cancer and osteoporosis. Poor diet is a significant contributor to ill health. The promotion of healthy eating is therefore a significant health promotion issue for all healthcare professionals.

Activity

Access some of the following government policies and initiatives that help to inform and advise practitioners of the possible issues to examine when promoting healthier eating:

■ The promotion of breast-feeding is included within employer occupational health and safety advice (www.healthyworkinglives. com) and encourages companies to support breast-feeding mothers to continue with breast-feeding for the first 6 months of life.

■ 'Healthy Start' (www.healthystart. nhs.uk) includes advice regarding the application of free vouchers to spend on milk, plain fresh and frozen fruit and vegetables, infant formula milk and free vitamins. Advice is also give regarding breast-feeding and recipe ideas to promote a healthy diet.

■ The National Healthy Schools Programme (www.healthyschools.gov. uk) is a joint Department of Health and Department for Children, Schools and Families project intended to improve the health of pupils and includes themes such as personal, social and health education, including sex and relationships, including bullying.

It is important for students following all the fields of practice pathways to learn about these studies and government initiatives, because the people they meet in the community are members of a wider community. They may be parents or grandparents who have a significant influence in shaping the future of children's and their own eating and lifestyle habits.

Within this chapter, you have reviewed the process of assessment from the health needs in the community to individual patient need, using a patient-centred approach. Communication skills are referred to here but are discussed in further detail in Chapter 9. Health promotion activities have also been touched upon, as they impact on health needs assessment at both community and individual level.

Summary of learning points from this chapter

- There are different ways to assess 'need' within the community from both an individual and community perspective
- The use of a person-centred approach to care
- The variety of health promotion activities within the context of community care.

References

Bradshaw, J.R., 1972. The concept of social need. New Society 19, 640–643.

Casey, A., 1988. A partnership with child and family. Sr. Nurse 8, 8–9.

Department of Health, 2003. The essence of care: patient-focused benchmarks for clinical governance. Online. Available at: http://www.dh.gov.uk.

Department of Health, 2004. The ten essential shared capabilities – a framework for the whole of the mental health workforce. DH, London.

Equality Act. 2010. Online. Available at: www.legislation.gov.uk (accessed November 2011).

Felton, A., Sheppard, F., Stacey, G., 2012. Exposing the tensions of implementing supervision in pre-registration nurse education. Nurse Education in Practice 12 (1), 36–40.

Holland, K., Whittam, S., 2008. Applying the Roper-Logan-Tierney Model in practice, second ed. Churchill Livingstone, Edinburgh.

Macduff, C., Sinclair, J., 2008. Evidence on self-care support within community nursing. Nurs. Times 104 (14), 32–33.

Marie Curie Palliative Care Institute, 2010. The Liverpool care pathway for the dying patient. Marie Curie, Liverpool. Online. Available at: http://www.mcpcil.org.uk/.

National Institute for Clinical Excellence, NICE, 2005. Health needs assessment: a practical guide. Online. Available at: www.nice.org.uk.

Naylor, C., Parsonage, M., McDaid, D., et al., 2012. Long term conditions and mental health: the cost of co-morbidities. The Kings Fund Centre for Mental Health, London.

Nursing and Midwifery Council, 2009. Guidance on professional conduct for nursing and midwifery students. NMC, London.

Nursing and Midwifery Council, 2010. Standards for proficiency for pre-registration nursing education. NMC, London.

Orem, D., 1971. Nursing concepts of practice. McGraw-Hill, New York.

Robinson, S., Harris, H., 2011. Smoking and drinking among adults, 2009. A report on the 2009 General Lifestyle Survey. Office for National Statistics, London.

Roper, N., Logan, W., Tierney, A., 2000. The Roper-Logan-Tierney model of nursing. Churchill Livingstone, London.

Roy, C., 1976. Introduction to nursing: an adaptive model. Prentice Hall, New Jersey.

Royal College of Nursing, 2008. Defending dignity – Challenges and opportunities for nursing. RCN, London.

Scottish Government, 2007. NHS Scotland performance HEAT-Targets. Online. Available at: www.scotland.gov.uk.

Thomas, K., Department of Health, 2005. The gold standard framework: A programme for community palliative care. Online. Available at: www.goldstandardsframework.nhs.uk.

Further Reading

Department of Health, 2004. The NHS improvement plan: putting people at the heart of public services. DH, London.

Department of Health, 2007. Policy and guidance: health and social care topics: long term conditions. DH, London.

Ewles, L., Simnett, I., 2005. Promoting health: A practical guide, fifth ed. Elsevier, London.

Naidoo, J., Wills, J., 2009. Foundations for health promotion, third ed. Bailliere Tindall, London.

Royal College of Nursing, 2007. Nurses as partners in delivering public health. RCN, London.

Scottish Executive, 2006. Visible, accessible & integrated care: Report of the review of nursing in the community. Scottish Executive, Edinburgh.

Scottish Executive, 2007. Better health, better care. A discussion document. Scottish Executive, Edinburgh.

Watkins, D., 2010. Public health and community nursing: frameworks for practice, third ed. Bailliere Tindall, London.

Websites

The National Institute for Clinical Excellence, A practical guide to health needs assessment. www.nice.org.uk (updated 2009).

Department for children, schools and families, 2010. Early intervention: securing good outcomes for all children and young people. Office of Public Sector Information. www.dcsf.gov.uk/evrychildmatters

Department of Health, www.dh.gov.uk.

Department of Health, 2006. Dignity in care. www.dh.gov.uk

Department of Health, 2009. NHS 2010–2015. From good to great, preventative, people-centred, productive. www.dh.gov.uk/qualityaccounts

Equality Act, 2010. www.equalities.gov.uk.

European Public Health Observatory, www.euro.who.int/en/who-we-are/partners/observatory.

Healthy Start, www.healthystart.nhs.uk.

Healthy Working Lives, www.healthyworkinglives.com.

Help the Aged/Picker Institute, 2008. On our own terms: the challenge of assessing dignity in care. www.helptheaged.org.uk/policy

Mental Welfare Commission, 2010. Decisions for dignity. www.mwcscot.org.uk

Modernising nursing in the community, www.mnic.nes.scot.nhs.uk.

National Healthy Schools Programme, www.healthyschools.gov.uk.

Network of Public Health Observatories produces information and data on health and has expertise in analysing data into meaningful health information: www.apho.org.uk.

Nursing and Midwifery Council, www.nmc-uk.org.

Parliamentary Office of Science and Technology, www.rsc.org/scienceandtechnology.

Royal College of Nursing publication regarding the assessment of older people: www.rcn.org.uk.

Scottish Government, www.scotland.gov.uk.

Scottish Government, 2011. Getting it right for every child (GIRFEC). www.scotland.gov.uk/Topics/People/Young-People/gettingitright.

Scottish Household Survey, www.scotland.gov.uk.

Scottish Intercollegiate Guidelines Network, SIGN guidelines. www.sign.ac.uk.

UK National Institute for Health and Clinical Excellence (NICE), www.nice.org.uk.

6

Managing long-term conditions in the community

CHAPTER AIMS

- To introduce the student to the principles of the management of long term conditions within the community, including assessing and anticipating individual and carer need and promoting self-care
- To examine the principles of palliative care referring specifically to the end-of-life care for the person with dementia
- To explore the care of the older adult within the community setting in particular with regards to rehabilitation

Introduction

Nurses who work in the community have the challenge of planning care for a variety of different health needs within a person's home and other community settings such as the health centre or care home. Care can range from helping people to manage their medication at home, providing long-term condition management services at nurse-led clinics, dressing acute and chronic wounds, to providing specialist palliative care at home. Your community practice experience can provide you with a valuable opportunity to see some of the challenging roles community nurses undertake in order to benefit their local practice population. This chapter does not attempt to refer to every role the community nurse may fulfill but does make reference to some contemporary aspects of care which will enable you to understand and appreciate the variety of care which can be delivered by the community nursing service.

Caring for patients with long-term health conditions

A long-term condition can be defined as an illness of prolonged duration which affects the individual physically, mentally and emotionally and may require ongoing or intermittent support from healthcare services. Such conditions include: diabetes, epilepsy, some mental health problems such as schizophrenia, heart disease, cancer, arthritis, eczema, chronic obstructive pulmonary disease (COPD), asthma and inflammatory bowel disease. The World Health Organization (WHO 2005) defines chronic conditions (long-term conditions) as the healthcare challenge of this century.

Within the UK, it is estimated that clients suffering from a long-term condition account for 80% of all general practice consultations and have an increased risk of being admitted to hospital (DH 2007). Research has also suggested that on-going support to prevent complications or acute exacerbations of illness is limited, care being more 'reactive' rather than 'proactive'.

To facilitate better management of long-term conditions, numerous government policy documents have been published. The Department of Health (DH 2005a) published the National Service Framework (NSF) for long-term conditions and, although this outline focuses on individuals with long-term neurological conditions, much of the advice is applicable to all long-term conditions. In addition to this framework, the Department of Health (DH 2005b) also published a strategy for the management of people with long-term conditions which included guidelines regarding the stratification of treatment into one of three levels according to need:

- Level 1. The majority of patients within this level are able to self-manage their condition with support and advice.
- Level 2. Clients within level 2 require more professional input to manage their condition.
- Level 3. Clients within level 3 have more complex needs, often requiring intensive co-ordinated care from a variety of different services. The role of the case manager within level 3 is discussed later in this chapter.

Using the above categorisation, clients can therefore be assessed for the complexity of their needs and then allocated to the level of care they require. The model provides a framework to assist health and social services to deliver an integrated and co-ordinated approach to the management of long-term conditions.

In summary, effective management of long-term conditions aims to give support and advice to minimise the effects of disease and reduce complications, resulting in a better quality of life for the client. A number

of the components for improving care for people with a long-term condition are discussed here and include the holistic assessment of clients, the role of the community matron and case manager in promoting independence in long-term illness, including the promotion of self-care and self-management and the promotion of anticipatory care.

Activity

Reference was made earlier to the assessment of client's needs. Discuss the possible issues to be addressed in the assessment of a client who is suffering from a long-term condition, with your mentor. Plan a learning goal to achieve with regards to the care of a patient with a long-term health problem and the steps your mentor can take to help you to achieve this.

You may have the opportunity to accompany the district nurse on the first home visit to a client or to observe the practice nurse's assessment of a client during their first clinic appointment at the health centre. Try to identify with your mentor, your perceptions of the person's needs and if possible, those of the family members and discuss the plan for care at this stage of their health problem.

You will probably find that the assessment includes such factors as:

- The patient's physical/medical status, the stage of illness, current issues that affect the patient's day-to-day living
- Medication usage and adherence
- Psychological status, current functional abilities and activity
- A review of all the current services provided
- The patient, carer and families coping abilities, family support, carer dynamics
- The patient's willingness to 'self-care'.

You may also have observed how the client's needs may vary depending on the stage of illness, for example the physical and psychological needs of the client will change over time from diagnosis, returning to stability after an acute exacerbation or adapting to disability.

have a responsibility to ensure that that they are also maintaining a healthy lifestyle. Completing these tools yourself can also give you an insight into how the patient/client can be encouraged to do so and you will be able to help them to understand their meaning in a supportive way.

Assessment to facilitate the management of long-term conditions

To facilitate a holistic assessment of the client with a long-term condition, a variety of different assessment tools may be used such as:

- Nutritional assessment: Eberhardie (2004) makes reference to the utilisation of a Mini Nutritional Assessment Tool for use with older people
- Quality of life assessment tools: referred to by Chamanga (2010) for use by community nurses improving quality of life for patients with chronic leg ulcers.

🔖 Activity

Identify, with your mentor, some of the different assessment tools which are utilised in your placement for the management of patients with long-term conditions. Access NICE (www.nice.org.uk), to look at the assessment of depression in adults with a chronic physical health problem or to review long-term conditions self-assessment tools.

Complete some of these available tools yourself – such as the healthy eating assessment tool and fitness test assessment. All health professionals are prone to the same potential long-term health problems such as obesity, heart problems and depression and

The following case study is given to demonstrate how more effective management of a client's long-term condition can facilitate a better quality of life.

▮ Case study

A patient with chronic obstructive pulmonary disease (COPD)

Mr King is an 88-year-old man who lives alone with support from his daughter, who lives nearby. He has chronic obstructive pulmonary disease (COPD) and is partially sighted. He manages to mobilise slowly around the house and a carer visits him in the morning and at night but he has not been out for several years. Over the past 2 years, he has had multiple admissions to hospital often through the local A&E department.

A visit by the district nurse to assess Mr King noticed that he appeared to have developed a pattern of going into hospital; this appeared to happen when his condition worsened, frequently when he experienced episodes of increasing breathlessness and, increasingly, his daughter was away on business. He was encouraged to contact the district nurse when he recognised the early symptoms of not feeling well, instead of ringing for an

Continued

ambulance. When he did this the next time, he was found to be having a mild exacerbation of his COPD worsened by a chest infection and anxiety, however hospital admission was avoided. He has been instructed to recognise the early symptoms of a worsening of his condition, which includes early identification of possible infection by regular observation of his sputum. He now has a store of antibiotics which he can commence as early as possible, after telephone consultation with the relevant staff within the health centre. He now also attends a day centre 2 days a week, where he enjoys the company and can be regularly assessed to enable early identification of any problems.

This case study demonstrates a move away from a reactive service towards a more proactive one; monitoring patients with a long-term condition even in a 'well' phase to identify any early signs of changes which may require treatment.

Activity

With your mentor, identify a patient suffering from a long-term condition who receives regular visits from the community nursing service and, with reference to the proactive measures within the above case study, consider how such actions can be applied to your chosen patient.

So who takes overall responsibility for the management of the team caring for patients such as Mr King? We have considered the immediate professional carer as the district nurse but in many community teams, there are now roles called community matrons, who take on more holistic overarching care roles.

The role of the community matron and case manager in the management of long-term conditions

The district nurse will often be the 'key worker' within the management of long-term illness, using her skills of communication, co-ordinating and collaborating with colleagues to draw health and social care together to provide an appropriate holistic programme of care for the patient and family. However, the role of the community matron (referred to in Chapter 2) has also been referred to in the management of patients with long-term conditions.

The community matron has developed skills and competence within the following areas:

- Advanced clinical nursing skills related to management of specific long-term illnesses including the management of care at the 'end-of-life'
- Leading and co-ordinating interagency and partnership working
- Proactive management of long-term conditions, including health promotion
- Supporting self-care and self-management
- Identifying high-risk patients.

Within some community settings, reference will also be made to a case manager who may also be a district nurse or community matron, the case manager specifically manages a caseload of clients with long-term conditions The main responsibilities for this practitioner include identification of 'high-risk' clients to proactively manage personalised care for patients and carers. *Case management* is a method of enabling practitioners to achieve this, identifying those at risk and co-ordinating and collaborating with different care services to enhance the quality of life for patients living with a long-term condition within the community.

Activity

Find out from your mentor if there is a practitioner who is also a case manager for long-term conditions and organise to spend some time with this person to gain further understanding of this role. This can be taken as a Spoke placement or insight visit for those of you undertaking a long placement for the adult nursing field of practice pathway or as an exposure to other fields of practice for those of you pursuing the mental health, learning disability of children's nursing pathways. Understanding how long-term conditions can impact on families and especially children, who may end-up being the main carer, is important for all students.

An excellent website for considering mental health and wellbeing across all ages can be found at: http://www.nhs.uk/livewell/mentalhealth/pages/mentalhealthhome.aspx.

Promoting independence in long-term illness

The increase in incidence of long-term conditions has resulted in an increase in focus by healthcare practitioners to encourage patients to self-manage their own condition. 'The expert patient: a new approach to chronic disease management for the 21st century' (DH 2001b) is a programme to empower people with a long-term condition such as diabetes, to develop their knowledge and skills of their condition to enable effective, appropriate, daily management, prevent complications and generally enhance quality of life. The main objective of this self-management approach is to increase the number of patients with a long-term condition whose condition is improved, remains stable or deteriorates more slowly and who:

- *are able to manage specific aspects of their condition*
- *experience less symptoms of their condition such as sleep deprivation, low levels of energy and depressing emotional consequences of illness*
- *are more effective in accessing health and social services appropriately and gaining and retaining employment*
- *are well informed about their condition and medication, feel empowered in their relationships with healthcare professionals and have higher self-esteem.*
  Department of Health (2001b)

 Activity

Access the NHS Choices homepage regarding long-term conditions management to gain a further understanding of the advice and support available for patients to self-care. There is a short questionnaire that you can access which tells you if you are receiving the right kind of care and support along with a printed out checklist, available at: http://www.nhs.uk/planners/yourhealth/pages/yourhealth.aspx

Self-care

Facilitating self-care and self-management for the client suffering from a long-term condition is significant and can increase confidence to manage their illness and enable better day-to-day coping. This may result in fewer symptoms or complications of the condition, which results in a generally better quality of life for the patient and their family. With greater confidence in managing their condition, patients are also less likely to require consultations with their GP and are also less likely to require hospital admission, resulting in more efficient use of NHS resources.

A self-management approach involves establishing a relationship with patients based on their health being their responsibility; the healthcare practitioner is supporting and empowering them in their choices, rather than being paternalistic, prescribing solutions to symptoms. This empowering approach necessitates motivating the patient to make lifestyle changes, developing an understanding of their condition and complying with care and treatment.

 Activity

The following case studies demonstrate the significance of self-management. Consider these in the context of patients that you have come across during your clinical placement. How typical are they from your experience of caring for patients with similar situations?

Consider their impact on their families and their own health and wellbeing.

Case study

Sarah's story: Living with an acquired brain injury

Sarah is 35 years old and lives with acquired brain injury and epilepsy as a result of a road traffic accident 5 years ago. She is no longer in paid employment but works part time as a volunteer in the local charity shop. She lives with her husband and her 7-year-old son and with daily help from her mother who lives nearby, she manages to attend to most of the household chores, except for the weekly supermarket shopping, which her husband does with her on a Saturday morning. Her husband takes their son to school every day in the car, however Sarah enjoys walking to the school at the end of the day to meet the other Mums and to collect David.

Sarah's short-term memory was damaged by her brain injury. However, she has 'self-managed' since her accident, which has meant she has been able to 'get on' with life and has continued to find ways of living with her short-term memory problems, receiving support from others when required. She has developed techniques to deal with her memory difficulties such as the use of a Google calendar. She takes anticonvulsant medication and has not had a seizure for the last 2 years.

With reference to her condition Sarah says:

I think it's really important to be in control, and get on with life despite your difficulties, the doctors, nurse and everyone are really kind but they don't understand all the everyday challenges you have to face when you have a brain injury. You only start learning about how to manage when you get home, accept that you have a long-term condition and start to understand what you need to do to manage normal day to day living; you need to identify all kinds of help and support. I think my ability to manage has been helped by being aware of my condition, knowing what kind of help I need, this has helped me to plan for the future.

Case study

Iain's story: Living with insulin dependent diabetes

Iain is a 21-year-old, third-year student studying history and politics at university. He lives with insulin dependent diabetes (type 1), which was diagnosed when he was very young, it has always been hard to bring his diabetes into control and as a result has presented him with many challenges; he needs to monitor his blood sugar levels and his insulin requirements on a regular basis. In his first year of study, Iain became very depressed, due to his condition, and his attendance at lectures suffered and may have contributed to his failure to achieve pass grades from his end of semester examinations. He has also felt that his condition interfered with his social life and this resulted in a year out of university to recover from severe depression. He then returned and, with support, continued his studies.

For Iain self-management means being able to control his diabetes, monitoring his blood glucose levels and adjusting his insulin requirements accordingly. He now works part time in the student's union which he enjoys and he says makes him feel better. He knows what to do now when he feels 'low', arranging to meet with friends or family and going out for walks. Iain has also become a 'buddy' for new students in their first year of study, helping them to settle into university life.

Self-management

Self-management is empowering, helping put people at the centre of services and in control, providing an opportunity to develop a partnership relationship with different services, to enable quality of life. Sarah refers to the importance of developing knowledge and understanding of your long-term condition which enables you to understand your symptoms and experiences which increases your confidence and ability to manage your condition. David refers to the importance of being able to manage his diabetes and recognising what to do when he feels 'low.'

Support for self-management involves collaboration between the client and a range of different services. Figure 6.1 identifies some of the support services, initiatives and skills which may be required by the client to facilitate self-management.

Activity

Try to find out what support activities exist to enable patients, with a variety of long-term health problems, to self-care. This may include looking at information given by healthcare practitioners to patients but may also include 'lay, self-led' management programmes that the patient may be referred to.

Access the NHS Choices video library on: http://www.nhs.uk/Video/Pages/ for videos on self-care and patients and professionals talking about self-care experiences and management.

Some of you may be fortunate enough to be studying at a university where there has been a significant involvement with both local service user/carer groups and where they also contribute to the delivery of teaching sessions as 'expert patients' or 'carers'. These can make a significant impact in

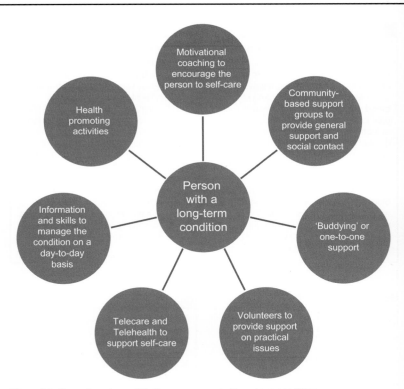

Figure 6.1 Support services within the management of long-term conditions.

understanding patient's health and social care experiences, as well as their 'expert' view of their own health problem.

The 'expert patient'

Campling and Sharpe (2006) define the 'expert patient' as the patient who is suffering from a long-term illness, who has become quite knowledgeable about the management of their condition. This knowledge is normally the result of

gathering information about the causes and possible progression of their illness and by developing an individualised regime of care which has developed from what has worked within their experience of illness. They are therefore 'empowered patients' who feel generally in control over living well with their illness and adapting positively to their condition. Healthcare practitioners can assist patients to become 'experts' by addressing their information needs as discussed earlier and by giving advice on the possible range of sources of information which may assist in the development of their knowledge regarding their specific condition. Self-management courses provide tools and techniques to assist clients to 'take control' of their health and manage their condition on a daily basis. Such courses are designed to develop the client's confidence, skills and knowledge.

 Activity

Try to find out about the provision of local self-management courses within your community practice learning area and the topics which are covered within such courses.

You could also access: http://www. expertpatients.co.uk

Find out from your university the extent to which service users are involved in the programme to share their experiences of living with long-term illness; listening to the patient's perspective is a very valuable learning opportunity for students.

Many expert patient programme courses are delivered by trained tutors who have also had experience of living with a long-term condition. Courses can include subjects such as managing pain and tiredness, coping with depression, learning to relax, adopting a healthy lifestyle, dietary advice. The expert patient website: http://www.expertpatients.co.uk, offers advice on a range of chronic health conditions such as asthma, arthritis and diabetes.

Anticipatory care

There is now substantial evidence which indicates that many crises situations within long-term illness can be prevented.

Anticipatory care focuses not only on the client's current health status but, also on proactive management, considering the avoidance of problems and emergency situations in the future. This requires contingency planning, making a plan to facilitate the future management of a possible complication and individual plans of care for acute episodes of illness. Although the term 'anticipatory care' is currently mostly associated with long-term conditions and contingency planning, there are a variety of proactive and preventative actions taken by healthcare professionals within different aspects of care and include activities such as:

- Child health surveillance, immunisation, lifestyle advice, contraception
- Health needs assessment
- Screening for asymptomatic disease
- Reversing risk, smoking, blood pressure, cholesterol
- Postnatal depression screening
- Respite care.

Anticipatory care within the management of long-term illness is carried out during routine consultations and deals with 'today's' problems but also assesses potential problems. This can result in a number of benefits for the patient and healthcare provider and include:

- Avoidance or reduction of negative effects of illness
- Reduced number of admissions to hospital
- Reduced length of stay in hospital
- Improved use of intermediate care
- Improved patient outcomes
- Improved patient satisfaction.

 Activity

Find out more about the national anticipatory care programme from NHS Health Scotland: www.healthscotland. com/anticipatory-care.aspx

Kennedy et al (2011) argue that community nurses are appropriately placed and have the relevant competencies and skills to anticipate care needs which help the patient to self-care and prevent or detect potential problems at an early stage. Patient assessment by community nurses often include anticipating care needs, which enables the patient to remain well at home. Community nurses often work with frail patients who are suffering from a variety of health problems and within the holistic assessment of such a patient, potential care needs can be identified. Practice nurses managing clinics for specific medical conditions are also involved with patient education which enables anticipating care needs. Anticipatory care interventions can include simple measures such as giving the patient with chronic obstructive pulmonary disease specific instructions to be able to identify the early stages of chest infection to initiate early treatment.

 Activity

Using the definition above of anticipatory care, reflect with your mentor on the anticipatory needs of a number of patients with a long-term condition who you have encountered while in your community practice placement.

On the next visit to a client, where you can undertake their first assessment, identify and discuss their possible anticipatory needs and the appropriate interventions to meet these. Make a plan of action to meet these needs and discuss them with your mentor. This will enable you to develop the problem-solving and critical thinking skills essential for a graduate nurse (NMC 2010).

Different nursing services in the management of long-term conditions

The different roles of community staff are discussed within Chapter 2 of this book, however it is useful to consider these roles with specific reference to the management of long-term conditions.

 Activity

Before continuing with reading this chapter, re-visit Chapter 2 and read about the different roles in practice.

The district nursing team

District nurses play a significant role in the care of patients and families within their own home or in residential care homes. Their role includes planning and managing care, supporting, advising and assisting the patient to self-care or supporting the carer to 'care'.

District nursing responsibilities also include liaison with hospital staff to ensure continuity of care for patients being admitted or discharged from hospital. The district nurse will often work with different healthcare services such as social services, voluntary agencies and other NHS organisations, particularly when assisting clients with a long-term condition.

The out-of-hours nursing service

The 'twilight nursing service' and 'over night nursing service' enables continuation of care. Similar to the day district nursing service, work within this service includes planning, managing and delivering direct nursing care in the patient's own home or in residential homes.

The practice nurse

The practice nurse may be involved with the running of nurse-led clinics for long-term conditions, monitoring symptoms and providing general advice and support and assisting in the management of acute exacerbations of the condition.

The occupational health nurse

The occupational health nurse can be included within the care of a client with a long-term condition who wishes to remain at work and requires specific changes to his work environment or hours to enable this. They may also assist carers who wish to retain some part-time work commitment. Their role in giving general counselling and support can also be invaluable.

NHS Direct

NHS Direct is a NHS telephone service led by qualified nurses which aims to provide the public with advice on various health issues. The utilisation of computer-based guidelines support and assist the nursing staff to give appropriate advice to address a variety of health-related inquiries. In relation to long-term conditions, advice can range from self-care to emergency service referrals for a sudden acute exacerbation of the condition.

The role of the community pharmacist

Many patients with a long-term condition may require quite complex medication regimes, which should be reviewed regularly to assess drug effectiveness, adverse side-effects and patients' medication regimes;

ensuring they receive the maximum benefit from their medication. The GP plays a key role in regularly reviewing any non-compliance issues, while at the same time, ensuring the minimum of side-effects. To assist with this, clients can review their medications with the community pharmacists; a medication use review (MUR) consultation with the pharmacist can provide the client with the opportunity to further their knowledge about their medication regime and ask any questions in relation to this. Chapter 11 provides a comprehensive introduction to all aspects of medication review.

Carers

Within your community learning experience, you will meet a number of informal carers; this could be someone caring for an elderly relative, looking after a child with a disability or supporting a partner who is ill or suffers from a mental health problem. Every year many family members and friends become carers; informal caregivers generally have received no formal training and normally receive no significant financial reward for this difficult and demanding job. Many informal carers provide care on a full-time basis, some carers are very young, i.e. children looking after parents, and some carers are caring for more than one person.

 Activity

Access the following website to read some of the stories of how young carers can be supported: www.barnardos.org.uk. The Macmillan website: www.macmillan.org.uk also provides support and advice for young carers caring for someone with cancer.

It may be possible for you to visit one of these organisations to find out how

Continued

they link with young carers and those that they care for. Some of you may meet young carers as part of your curriculum timetable involving engagement with service users and carers.

Being in the community and engaging in visiting people's home will also bring you into direct contact with carers of all ages. The carer's role is often demanding and meets numerous challenging demands. Carers carry out a number of responsibilities, which will often include giving, at times, quite complex daily physical care and emotional support; their role, however, differs from the role of the professional carer in a number of ways. Normally, family carers receive no financial payment for their services; it is difficult to take any leave away from their responsibilities and it may be that they were never really consulted about their wish to care but it has been assumed that this is their role as partner, parent, daughter or son. Care giving may have to be balanced with work and other family responsibilities and is further complicated by the unique, special relationship that care giving takes place within. Carers may also feel socially isolated, never getting any break from caring.

◥ Activity

- Consider the changes in a family's lifestyle as a result of a family member requiring continual care.
- How might the carer feel about this?
- Do you think the change in situation might change the carer's feelings towards the person needing care?
- What do you think might be the best/worst aspects of the carer's role?

The following case study demonstrates the possible experiences of carers:

▉ Case study

Christine and Tom (a patient who suffered from multiple sclerosis)

Christine cared for her husband Tom who suffered from multiple sclerosis (MS) until his death last year. They were married in 1984 and 2 years later Tom was diagnosed with MS at only 29 years old. Over the next few years, Tom experienced several relapses, which resulted in early retirement from work. Tom and Christine moved to a bungalow with a purpose built extension and tried to live a normal married life. Christine attended to most of Tom's everyday needs such washing, dressing, toileting, lifting him, with the help of a hoist into his wheelchair; this was all on top of the general housekeeping duties such as cooking and shopping. As Tom found it increasingly difficult to move, Christine got up four to six times during the night to help change his position and make him more comfortable. During this time, Christine could not go out very much, which frequently made her feel quite depressed and the demands of care made her feel permanently exhausted. She also worried a great deal about the future; what would happen to Tom if she became ill or her ability to cope when he died. It was also difficult to be unable to make any future plans, not knowing how Tom was going to be and wondering if his condition would change. She also at times grieved for the lost opportunity to have children; they decided not to have children at the time of his diagnosis.

Activity

The above case study identifies a number of stressors experienced by the carer. With your mentor, discuss the challenges and concerns faced by some of the carers you have visited while in your community practice placement and explore some of the ways in which carers may be supported.

Access: www.communitycare.co.uk to read the case study of a young carer of just 13 years of age, who cares for her mother who suffers from mental health problems.

Discuss with some of your student colleagues, during a reflection session, what you have learnt or when you have a session on the role of the carer. Take the opportunity to learn more about the way in which social policies influence the role of the carer in the community setting.

Carers often suffer ill health due to the demanding nature of their caring role. To continue caring and to preserve their own physical and mental health, carers need support, information and recognition from the professionals with whom they are in contact. Care for carers should be proactive and should therefore consider respite care, emotional support, employment, education and information. Carers' needs should be assessed independently but along with the patient being cared for.

The information needs of carers

The specific areas of information needs which may be required by carers include:
- Information needs
- Skills needs
- Emotional support needs.

The diagnosis of chronic illness often takes place in hospital, surgery or clinic, when time is unfortunately limited and it may not be until the patient and carer returns home that they may begin to think of questions related to the significance of their recent diagnosis. Questions may relate to many different issues such as specific progression of the condition or what help may be available, to assist with planning for the future patients need the opportunity to discuss their concerns with healthcare staff. Carers also need to have access to information about services, which may be specifically relevant to their need.

 Activity

Access the following websites to examine the range of support and advice which is available to carers:

Carers UK: www.carersuk.org

Carers Direct: www.nhs.uk

Carers Trust: www.carers.org

Make brief notes about each site to add to others you may have come across. One idea would be to keep a notebook of all the websites you have been recommended in this book, in the university or that you yourself have found and make notes about what each contains in terms of information and links etc. This will be an invaluable resource for you when undertaking assignment work or if your computer malfunctions and all your 'Favourite' sites have disappeared!

Skills needs of family caregivers

Informal carers are often involved with giving personal care which, if the patient was in hospital, would be carried out by registered nursing staff. Such care may include washing, bathing, managing incontinence, urinary catheter care and giving injections. The case study of a child carer identified earlier makes reference to the carer's ability and skill in discussing and distracting her mother when she heard voices in her head. She had also developed extensive knowledge regarding her mother's medication. Qualified community practitioners have developed their competency with such skills from their educational preparation, however informal carers may have received little preparation or training to carry out such clinical tasks. Community practitioners have an important role in teaching carers who have demonstrated a willingness to take part in carrying out care, to enable them to implement care safely, reducing risk for the carer and the person receiving care.

 Activity

When you are visiting clients in the community, reflect on the daily tasks carried out by some of the carers you meet and consider how the community nurse can support carers to fulfil their role. Discuss with your mentor or a member of the team when you return to the main health centre after a morning or afternoon visiting and caring for patients/clients.

Emotional needs of carers

Carers' emotions may swing dramatically from feeling rewarded to feeling physically and emotionally exhausted and overwhelmed. Informal carers are also normally in a situation where they deliver care continuously, with very little time off from their responsibilities and this can lead to feelings of frustration and depression. Complete focus on the needs of the patient can be at the expense of

the needs of the carer, this may result in the carer's failure to recognise their own physical, mental and social health needs. Caregivers who have information about the availability of support and help which specifically relates to their situation can feel more empowered and in control of their situation.

 Activity

Identify local carer support groups within your community practice placement locality and discuss with your community nursing mentor how they may assist in raising the self-esteem of carers. This could be linked to any field of practice placement.

Access some of the carer's websites referred to earlier in this chapter to review some of the advice and support given to carers to relieve stress and facilitate wellbeing. Make yourself some key notes on these sites and identify some that may help some of the carers you have met. Discuss with your mentor their value and ensure that the sites are evaluated by the professional team prior to telling carers about them. It may not be possible, however, for some carers to access them due to not having a computer or direct access in the home, but they may already make use of the computer in the local library or community centre. Please remember to make sure that carer websites are culturally appropriate whenever possible, and many now offer options to read the material in different languages.

See: http://www.nhs.uk/carersdirect/Pages/CarersDirectHome.aspx.

This website has a 'Translate' button linking to Google Translate for many different languages such as Hindi and Italian.

It is important to remember that with an ageing population, healthcare practitioners will increasingly encounter families and friends who have become carers therefore carers' support is an essential aspect of their work.

Summary

Thus far, we have explored, as an integral and considerable part of the NHS remit, the management of long-term conditions, including: assessment; the facilitation of self-care and self-management; the concept of anticipatory care and the expert patient; the different services and roles required to address this agenda. The carer's role is integral to these issues.

A key aspect of the work of health and social care professionals in the community in relation to both long-term conditions and other care needs is in the role of rehabilitation (see below).

Rehabilitation and caring for patients with complex care needs

Rehabilitation in the community

Appropriate rehabilitation care within the community is vital to promote independence, support timely discharge from hospital and also prevent unnecessary hospital admission. For some clients, rehabilitation is a process which has a defined 'end point'. However for others, e.g. clients suffering from a long-term condition, their needs normally change over time, therefore regular review is required. Rehabilitation for older people includes proactively supporting people living at home and providing appropriate rehabilitation prior to returning home from hospital and being supported on their return to home.

Rehabilitation involves assisting the client to regain some or all of the skills they had before they were ill or injured, to enable them to live as independently as possible. Within primary care, the community nurse will assist clients with a variety of rehabilitation needs, caring for clients who may have needs relating to:
- Complex or chronic disease
- Disability
- Stroke
- Brain injury
- A fall
- Severe mental illness (rehabilitation from severe mental illness is discussed in more detail in Chapter 8).

The King's Fund (2010) refers to rehabilitation as a journey in which the individual progresses to achieve independence. However, Wade and de Jong (2000) provides a more detailed examination of rehabilitation which is divided into the following components:
- **Structure** refers to the multidisciplinary team who work together to involve and educate the family and have the relevant skills and knowledge to them in this process.
- **Process** refers to the assessment and identification of the patient's problems and how they could be resolved; this includes goal setting and planning interventions with the patient and family.
- **Outcomes** refers to the outcomes of the rehabilitation process maximising the participation of the client in his social setting while minimising pain and distress experienced by the patient and family and carers.

Most definitions of rehabilitation include reference to the importance of enabling maximum physical, psychological, emotional, social and occupational potential of the individual and improving quality of life. Social engagement and purposeful occupation are significant components in people's lives; to give self-worth and wellbeing, therefore rehabilitation teams often include a wide range of services and agencies to enable this.

Activity

Clients requiring rehabilitation frequently need on-going access to a variety of different services and support to meet their changing needs and to maintain their independence. Identify with your mentor a client requiring rehabilitation, who has experience of different services and (after your mentor has asked permission) discuss with the client the different services they require to maintain their independence. Find out what they know about their health problems and how to manage their wellbeing as well as health in order to manage their independence.

The community rehabilitation team often consists of a number of different healthcare professionals, which will differ according to the specific needs of the client. For example the following range of health and social service staff are identified in relation to the rehabilitation of a client after a stroke:

- Physiotherapists: to help with walking, balance, general strength and mobility
- Occupational therapists: to help with skills which need to be 're-learnt' and to identify possible adaptation in the home to enable the client's independence
- Psychologist: to give emotional support and help with difficulties such as memory loss
- Social worker
- Speech and language therapist
- Nursing staff
- General practitioner (GP)
- Dietitian.

Figure 6.2 outlines the many different services and personnel who can be part of the rehabilitation team.

Intermediate care

Intermediate care has been developed to assist clients to stay at home, to prevent admission to hospital or to enable early discharge from hospital, assisting the client to maintain or regain their independence. To enable clients to remain in their own home intermediate care services can provide support during an acute illness or initiate extra support to help carers or relatives. To enable discharge from hospital, intermediate care can provide 'supported discharge' home services to initially support the client or can provide a short stay in a residential rehabilitation unit. Care often involves multi-agency working and to differentiate from mainstream services intermediate care is often time limited, maximising client independence to remain in your own home or in a setting such as local community hospital or care home.

 Activity

Access the following websites to develop your knowledge and understanding of intermediate care:

This website defines intermediate care and also outlines the different intermediate care services available in Scotland: http://www.jitscotland.org. uk/action-areas/intermediate-care

This website examines intermediate care for older people: http://www.dh. gov.uk/prod_consum_dh/groups/dh_ digitalassets/@dh/@en/documents/ digitalasset/dh_4065694.pdf

A range of intermediate care examples are discussed here: http://www.bgs. org.uk/index.php?option=com_ content&view=article&id=363: intermediatecare&catid=12: goodpractice&Itemid=106

As before, make notes about each of these websites and their content. Evaluate them for usefulness of information for a multicultural community.

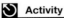

Activity

Many services which contribute to intermediate care have been developed in response to local need. Try to find out what intermediate care services have been developed within your community area. Ask your mentor if it is possible for you to visit one of these as a planned professional development opportunity or an insight day.

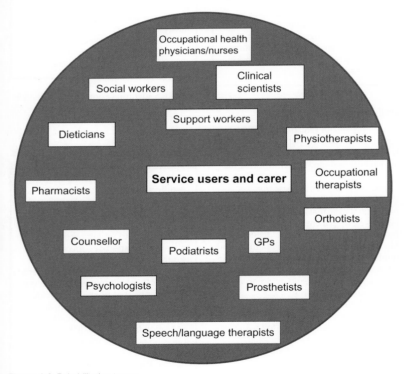

Figure 6.2 Rehabilitation teams.

A number of initiatives have been developed to support intermediate care. Chapter 2 discusses some of the following initiatives in more detail:

- Rapid response teams
- Community rehabilitation teams
- Residential re-ablement units
- Hospital at home schemes
- Hospital supported discharge teams
- Community assessment and rehabilitation schemes

- Private/voluntary/social services sector nursing
- Stroke rehabilitation outreach teams
- Nurse-led units
- Day hospitals
- The role of the community hospital has also been re-examined and developed.

 Activity

Consider services identified above and consider how you can learn more about these from a visit or talking to different healthcare professionals working in these teams.

Palliative care

The World Health Organization (WHO 2009), when defining palliative care, highlights the importance of quality of life for patients and families confronting life-threatening illness.

Lawton (2000) emphasise the significance of palliative care for community nurses by stating that approximately 90% of palliative care patients are cared for within the primary care setting. The district nurse often plays a key role in the planning and implementation of care to control and alleviate symptoms, co-ordinates care and gives general support and advice to the client, carer and family.

The World Health Organization at: http://www.who.int/cancer/palliative/definition/en/ identifies the following as key aspects of palliative care:

- Providing the relief of pain and other distressing symptoms
- Enabling the patient and family to regard dying as a normal process
- Neither hastening nor postponing death
- Offering support to enable patients to live as actively as possible until death
- Offering support to the family during the patient's illness and to cope with bereavement

- Utilising a team approach to care to enable the utilisation of appropriate expertise to support the patient and family.

 Activity

Discuss with your mentor the WHO's aims of palliative care and if possible, focus your discussion on a patient and family who you may have both visited who requires this type of care. Identify the range of expertise involved with care to support the patient and family.

Figure 6.3 identifies some of the palliative care services which you may have included in your discussions in the above activity.

 Activity

In discussion with your mentor, identify and contact some of the different palliative services and agencies and arrange a clinical visit to enable you to develop your knowledge and understanding of this area of expertise, you may also like to try to arrange a visit to the local hospice. You may like to refer to Chapter 2, which makes reference to the services that hospices provide. Some of you may have an opportunity to undertake a clinical placement in a hospice (see below). If you do, then consider how the nurses in the hospice work with the palliative care team in the community and/or how the hospice teams are also involved in such work as 'hospice at home' services: see http://www.hospiceathome.org.uk/ for the national organisation which links on a local community hospice level.

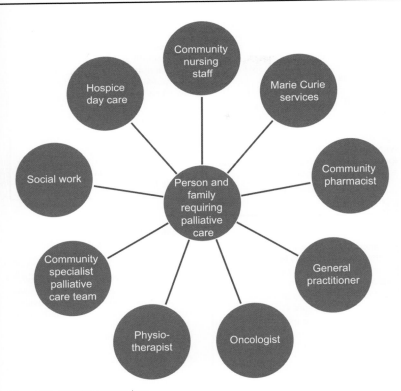

Figure 6.3 Palliative care services.

Supportive agencies

Many different supportive agencies contribute to care within the arena of palliative care. Their role is to assist in the general support of the client, carer and family to promote quality of life. You may have encountered the Marie Curie nursing service during your community practice placement. This service provides nursing care within the home, supporting clients with terminal cancer and other illnesses who wish to die at home. Marie Curie nurses can be with the client for several hours, frequently overnight, providing the family with the opportunity to rest (Marie Curie Palliative Care Institute 2010).

Macmillan nurses are registered nurses who have normally completed specialist training in the psychological support and the management of pain and other symptoms related to cancer and palliative care. Their role is primarily supportive, giving advice and guidance to clients and their families and other colleagues. Some Macmillan nurses specialise in specific types of cancer such as breast cancer, giving advice and support at the time of diagnosis and during treatment. There are also paediatric Macmillan nurses who work with children with cancer and their families. The Macmillan Website can be accessed at: www.macmillan.org.uk.

Hospices

Hospices provide expertise in the care of clients with terminal illness, offering respite care, day services and treatment to alleviate symptoms. Some hospices also employ specialist nurses who provide support and advice for clients at home.

Activity

In discussion with your mentor, try to find out if it would be possible to arrange a visit to the local hospice within your community learning placement, this could be a very valuable opportunity to:

- Understand the role of the hospice within the community
- Identify resources that may assist practitioners in caring for people with life-limiting illness
- Have the opportunity to ask questions about the hospice services.

Within your university placement learning time, it may be possible to request an elective placement at the local hospice; this is a valuable opportunity to develop your knowledge and skills in palliative care. Find out about this when you visit.

A significant aspect of palliative care is the respect given to patients and carers to enable them to make choices over their care at the end of their lives. To address this important issue, the Department of Health End of Life Health Care Strategy (2008a) was

published. Access this paper at: http://www.dh.gov.uk/prod_consum_dh/groups/dh_digitalassets/@dh/@en/documents/digitalasset/dh_086437.pdf to develop your understanding of how healthcare professionals can enhance end-of-life care, regardless of disease.

Activity

Referring to the above Department of Health Strategy, consider the main objectives of this and discuss with your mentor how they can be achieved in practice.

Good multidisciplinary communication and co-ordination is essential within this specific aspect of care and the Gold Standards Framework assists in the achievement of this. The Gold Standards Framework (Thomas 2005), found at www.goldstandardsframework.nhs.uk, provides general practitioners and community staff with advice and guidance to enhance their care and hopefully to enable the patient to stay at home. The document provides guidance and advice within the following specific aspects of care:

- Communication
- Co-ordination
- Control of symptoms
- Continuity
- Continued learning
- Carer support
- Care in the dying phase.

Activity

Access The Gold Standards Framework on www.goldstandardsframework.nhs.uk, which aims to improve cancer and palliative care in the community and review some of the practical tools,

Continued

guidance and examples of good practice contained within this document. Discuss with your mentor how this is integrated in practice.
If you are a student nurse in another country, find out what standards are available for palliative care in the community.
Compare these with those in the UK.

The Liverpool Care Pathway for the dying patient is another significant document that you should refer to, see: http://www.mcpcil.org.uk/liverpool-care-pathway. This pathway of care is implemented in the last hours and days of life and aims to advise the multidisciplinary team on aspects such as the continuation of medical treatment, discontinuation of treatment and the implementation of comfort measures during the last stages of illness. It is essential that practitioners using the pathway ensure that the patient and family are aware that the structure and focus of care has now changed and that focus of care is now on comfort and the alleviation of symptoms during the end stages of life.

Support for carers in palliative care

Reference has been made earlier to the needs of carers; the role of carers is essential if a patient wishes to die at home.

Understandably, this can be a particularly challenging, stressful, emotional and fearful time for the carer. Newbury (2011) refers to the experiences of carers within this specific aspect of care:
- Financial strain due to disruption at work
- Social dysfunction and relationship challenges
- Difficulties in providing care and trying to achieve normal household tasks and activities

- Dealing with future loss of the loved one.

Clayton et al (2005) emphasise that, in order to support carers, an understanding of their unique experience is required. Carers within this situation have taken an overwhelming dramatic responsibility with very little preparation and the community nurse plays a crucial role in assisting carers with this.

Community nurses access different resources and expertise within the field of palliative care, as this is often a challenging experience and requires a range of specific skills and expertise to deliver high-quality care. Poorly informed but kind care is not enough; what is required is the delivery of evidence-based care that follows the most current guidance.

The health and social care needs of the older adult in the community

You will probably find that a great deal of the community nursing caseload includes patients who are over 65 years of age. This is because this sector of the UK population is large and is expected to increase. The Office for National Statistics states that life expectancy in the UK has reached its highest level on record for both males and females: 78.1 years at birth for males and 82.1 years at birth for females. By 2035, 23% of the UK population is projected to be over 65 years of age, compared with 18% aged under 16. Unfortunately, the increase in life expectancy results in the increasing likelihood of more years spent in ill health. Approximately 700 000 people in the UK suffer from dementia; Alzheimer's Scotland (http://www.alzscot.org/pages/info/whatis.htm) predicts that this figure will increase to 940 000 by 2021 and 1.7 million by 2051.

Activity

In discussion with your mentor, identify the number of older people within the practice population and within the community nursing caseload. Consider the reasons for the substantial current and future increase in the number of elderly people in the population.

 Activity

What do you think are the possible positive and negative experiences of growing older in society today? Determine the health profile of the local community around your placement area and identify the health problems prevalent in this older age group. These profiles are available from the health organisations. Discuss with your mentor how to obtain the latest data to read and consider possible impacts in the future on meeting the long-term needs of the older adult with long-term and complex health needs.

Your discussions may have identified some of the following issues:

• Life expectancy is increasing. In 2003/2004, life expectancy at birth in Scotland was 73.8 years for men and 80.7 years for women. It is predicted to increase over the next few years, with life expectancy for women rising to 83.6 years and men to 78.9 years by 2031 (Age Concern 2007)
• There was a very significant surge in the birth rate in the UK in the late 1950s and 1960s and these people will start to retire over the next few years
• Health care has improved
• Living conditions have improved.

The increase of an ageing population may result in an increasing health burden; age is often associated with increased morbidity. Half of those over 70 years of age report health problems (Scottish Household Survey 2003). An estimated 61% of people in Scotland have dementia: 3% are under 65; 21% are between 65 and 74; 40% are 74–84; 37% are 85 or older (Alzheimer Scotland 2006). Older people can also have problems with common mental health problems such as anxiety, depression, schizophrenia, bipolar disorder and substance misuse. However, older people also continue to contribute to society by taking an active role in areas such as voluntary work, caring for a partner, relative or neighbour and providing a regular baby-sitting service for grandchildren.

Growing older may be perceived as having more time to be with a partner, family and grandchildren, to pursue hobbies, travel, to undertake further education opportunities or to undertake other responsibilities such as voluntary work. The more negative perceptions of growing old may include the increased risk of ill health; the risks of chronic disease such as heart disease, stroke, osteoarthritis and respiratory disease are higher in older people, this can then result in increased dependency on family and friends. Other health concerns for the elderly may include vision problems such as cataracts and hearing loss. Normal life changes at this stage such as loneliness, bereavement, retirement, inadequate income, poor health and functional capacity can lead to depression.

 Activity

Access the Joseph Rowntree Foundation at: www.jrf.org.uk, which examines the experiences of older people living in residential and nursing care homes. It is a useful study to help develop your understanding of the older

Continued

126

person's aspirations regarding their care and what might need to change so that older people have a 'better life'.

Also access the RCN website on caring for the older person, at: http://www.rcn.org.uk/development/practice/older_people, in order to review the resources, support and advice for practitioners caring for this specific client group.

There are several issues which are identified within this work and are particularly significant to healthcare professionals working within this specific client group. Developing our understanding of old age is relevant to all of us; this includes an understanding of both the losses and the more positive experiences of ageing. To enable us to do this, we need to support older clients to voice their concerns; this is particularly significant when attempting to provide individualised person-centred care. These issues must be considered in relation to living in a multicultural community and that management of health and wellbeing, as well as caring for those with long-term conditions and complex care needs, is influenced by the cultural background of the individual and the local communities in which they live.

Care, compassion and dignity

The results of the investigations of complaints made in 2009 and 2010 are included within the Parliamentary and Health Service Ombudsman report: Care and Compassion (2011). Many of the complaints are related to the care of older people. There are 10 case histories which all reveal unnecessary suffering and include difficulties with basic aspects of care such as pain relief, indignity, distress, lack of personal care, badly managed medication and lack of discharge planning.

 Activity

Access the report: Care and Compassion (2011), at: www.ombudsman.org.uk and read or listen to the case histories. In discussion with your mentor, identify the issues which could have been prevented. Although many of the case histories took place within the hospital environment, there are many issues which are relevant to all healthcare practitioners, regardless of the workplace setting and include lack of discharge planning and medication review within primary care, lack of attention to the client's and families wishes and general lack of attention to personal care and nutrition and hydration needs. The stories related to 'Mrs Y', 'Mr D' and 'Mrs G' specifically relate to community care. You will also find that the case studies demonstrate failure of staff to meet the Nursing and Midwifery Council (NMC) five essential skills clusters of:

- *Care, compassion and communication*
- *Organisational aspects of care*
- *Infection prevention and control*
- *Nutrition and fluid management*
- *Medicines management*

NMC (2010)

Ask your tutors in the university if this report and case studies can be accessed during an appropriate session or use them when presenting directed study opportunities on caring for patients in hospital and community. Opportunity can also be taken to consider the professional and ethical aspects, which will help you with meeting the requirements of the NMC competencies. Discuss with your mentor how the placement team are ensuring care and compassion in their community nursing activities.

Falls in older people

Falls among older people in the UK are an increasing cause of injury, treatment cost and death, and in many cases, these falls occur in the client's own home and are preventable.

The consequences of a fall for an older person are considerable and can result in severe injury and resulting disability, long hospital stays and long rehabilitation periods. NICE (2004) recommends that comprehensive risk assessment and multi-agency intervention represent the most effective strategy to reduce the incidence and impact of falls.

Falls result in approximately 400 000 presentations to emergency departments each year in the UK. Falls are a major cause of disability and the leading cause of mortality due to injury in older people aged over 75 in the UK (DH 2006). It is therefore particularly significant that attention is given to this when looking at care of the older adult within the home setting. Standard 6 of the National Service Framework for the Elderly aims to decrease the incidence of falls which result in serious injury, and to plan and organise effective treatment and rehabilitation for those who have fallen.

Falls for the older adult can result in:
- Loss of confidence
- Loss of mobility, social isolation and depression
- Increase in dependency and disability
- Hypothermia
- Pressure-related injury
- Infection.

Activity

There is a wealth of material available on the topic of falls in older people. However, you could start by accessing Standard 6 of the National Service Framework for Older People (DH 2008b), which specifically deals with the management and prevention of falls. This can help you develop your understanding of this problem and should help develop your insight into:

■ The reasons why falls prevention is seen as a priority

■ Different approaches taken to prevent falls

■ Local and national policy relating to falls prevention.

If you are undertaking an international placement in another country, e.g. Australia – consider the differences between community experience and care in the UK and that in rural Australia, where distances are vast in comparison and the services very different.

Access the following report on Primary Health Care in Australia, published in 2009, for an insight into some of the issues managed by primary care nurses and colleagues:

http://www.rcna.org.au/WCM/Images/RCNA_website/Files%20for%20upload% 20and%20link/policy/documentation/position/consensus_statements_PHC_ Australia.pdf (accessed July 2012)

and for Caring for Older People in Rural Australia:

http://www.agedcareaustralia.gov.au/internet/agedcare/publishing.nsf/content/ Living+in+a+rural+area (accessed July 2012).

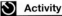 **Activity**

While visiting older adults with the district nurse, observe some of the factors within the home environment which might put the client at risk of falling.

Access the National Service Framework for Older People on the Department of Health website, at: www.dh.gov.uk to review Standard 6, which specifically focuses on the prevention of falls.

Your observations made may have included some of the following issues:
- Stairs
- Inappropriate footwear
- Inadequate lighting
- Uneven surfaces
- Slippery surfaces
- Low chairs
- Outside steps to the front or back door.

You may have also considered physical health factors such as:
- Effects of medication
- Altered gait from, e.g. Parkinson's disease
- Cerebral-vascular disease, dementia
- Cognitive impairment
- Communication difficulties
- Exacerbation of chronic disorder
- Muscle weakness
- Pain/disability
- Poor diet
- Poor eyesight
- Restricted movement
- Orthostatic hypertension
- Diabetes.

Within the home setting, there are a number of issues that the district nurse may take into account when assessing the older person's risk of falling, which may include taking a history of falls, what appears to have contributed to the fall, reviewing the client's current prescribed and over-the-counter medication, assessing any problems with balance and mobility, impaired vision or urinary incontinence. Consideration should also be given to any environmental factors within the home which may pose a risk and details regarding social support, mobility problems, smoking and cognitive ability are also significant. Remember also that even modest alcohol consumption may compound or exacerbate other risk factors for falls.

Key interventions to prevent falls include:
- **Prevention**, including the prevention and treatment of osteoporosis
- **Improving the diagnosis, care and treatment** of those who have fallen
- **Rehabilitation and long-term support**

There are a number of public health strategies regarding falls prevention, which include:
- Encouraging physical activity
- Promoting healthy eating, adequate intake of calcium
- Keeping pavements clear and in good repair and making property safer
- providing information, addressing ways to prevent falling such as 'avoiding slips, trips and broken hips' (National Patient Safety Agency 2007).

The role of a 'falls co-ordinator'

Within the National Service Framework, reference is made to a 'falls specialist'. Within some areas, the appointment of a falls co-ordinator assists in the achievement of reducing emergency admissions and re-admissions of people aged 65 and over due to falls. A falls co-ordinator can:
- Review the use of risk assessment tools
- Disseminate and recommend the use of falls risk assessment tools across all agencies who are involved with the care of older people
- Provide training regarding risk assessment and patient safety
- Develop an integrated care strategy.

Primary care has a responsibility to assess older people at risk of falling, however this can only be achieved through a well thought out falls strategy, which outlines a multidisciplinary service, where patients are assessed appropriately and referred if they are at risk or have sustained a fall. A falls strategy can contribute to a reduction in fragility fractures and a reduction in emergency admissions and readmissions to hospital.

Living with dementia

Throughout the UK, there are increasing numbers of people who have dementia; community nurses can play a significant part in caring for them and their families. In 2007, Dementia UK estimated that there were 683 597 people in the UK with dementia and by 2021, it is stated that this number will have increased to 940 110 and by 2051, to 1 735 087. This increase is linked to the increasing number of elderly people in the UK, specifically those over 85 years.

Dementia is a chronic condition, which results in the patient becoming increasingly forgetful and unable to cope with activities of daily living; it is an illness which not only affects memory but has a significant affect on all aspects of a patient's life and that of their family.

 Activity

Early interventions such as memory clinics and information giving, regarding community services are advocated as good practice within the arena of dementia care. Try to find out the early intervention services which exist within your practice placement to help support service users and carers within this specific area of care. Access the UK Alzheimer's Society website at www.alzheimer's.org.uk to help you to understand this debilitating condition from the person suffering with it and also for their carers and families.

In the early and middle stages of dementia, clients and their families may receive help and support from a variety of community services, which may include day hospital care, respite care and carer support groups. Throughout each stage of dementia, care is based on developing the physical, psychological and social wellbeing of the patient and family.

 Activity

Depending on your field of practice pathway, and your learning objectives, discuss with your mentor the possibility of spending some time with the community mental health nurse who may have a significant role to play in supporting patients and families within this specific area of care. For some of you, your whole placement will be with the Community mental health nursing team who are employed by the primary healthcare provider and who are actually based in the local health centres. For others, this could be an excellent opportunity to negotiate a longer Spoke placement to gain a more in depth insight into the management and support for the service user with dementia and their carers.

Please take time to read the NMC Report on the experience and views of people with dementia and carers by the Alzheimer's Society as part of the review of

Continued

pre-registration nursing education. Here are some examples of patients/carers narratives from the paper:

NMC Report

Recommendation: *Dignity and respect: despite the growing dignity and respect agenda, this is not being reflected in the care of people with dementia. It must become a priority.*

"Give dignity priority, because with that comes a lot of other things".

"In this particular home, they change their pads at certain times of day, i.e. morning, lunchtime, afternoon 4 pm and eve. But not everyone needs to be changed at the same time. I got shouted at by one of carers, 'she was changed at lunchtime'. May well have been, but she's dirty now. These people are not in care homes for a week, but have often been in there 12 or 15 years. So, surely they should be changed not by the clock but by need. But you can't keep going to the nurses as they don't listen".

"Going to the toilet used to upset me, I think . . . she used to be changed by a man. Why couldn't she have a lady to take her in? That used to upset me more than her. I couldn't see why that had to happen".

And here is one of the questions to carers and patients:

How do you think that nurses can best be helped to understand what dementia is?

People with dementia and their carers strongly assert that nurses must understand the experience of dementia if they are to truly provide compassionate and respectful care that acknowledges the person behind the dementia and their needs and wishes. This can come from visiting someone with dementia in different care settings, or from a person with dementia or a carer speaking to student nurses about their experiences.

"A lot of people think, 'just pull yourself together' and things like that . . . they've got to experience it".

"If nurses go to someone's house where there is a personal carer and see the experiences the carer is going through to fulfil their duties . . . would be learning curve . . . see problems that arise, behaviour etc . . . grass roots experience is better than all the books . . . . People with dementia, their attitude can change from hour to hour".

"Spend some time in a care home, to just be in there for a morning and note some of the things . . . . the deal should be 24 hours!".

"Personal contact is needed . . . it may jolt them, because we are hard work to care for . . . we keep saying the same thing over and over again, we keep asking, 'what am I doing today?' We need to make them aware".

"First hand experience is the only way to learn . . . . And not a flying visit, because what happened at 9 o'clock yesterday morning will not happen at 9 o'clock today".

See: http://www.nmc-uk.org/Documents/Consultations/RPNE/Report-on-the-experiences-and-views-of-people-with-dementia-and-carers.pdf (accessed July 2012).

All student nurses in all fields of practice pathways should gain some placement learning experience in caring for patients with dementia, as it impacts on the whole family. This holistic impact will require a patient-centred care approach by the health and social care team.

Patient-centered care for the client with dementia

Earlier discussions here made reference to a person-centered approach to care. With this in mind, it is important to remember to focus on the individuality of the client with dementia; this can be achieved by taking a comprehensive history of the client's past interests, hobbies and work; this information may be gathered from the client and family. Awareness of the 'whole person' enables a more individualised person-centred approach to care.

 Activity

During your community learning experience you may encounter clients who are about to be admitted or who have been admitted to residential care. Some of you may have a specific community placement in this environment. Consider how person-centeredness can be maintained within this setting. The NMC document above, as well as the narratives highlighted, give some indication of how their needs need to be accounted for and managed.

Access it and other documents such as the RCN website for student nurses and gain a further insight into student nurses' experiences in caring for patients with dementia in a variety of settings, see: http://nursingstandard. rcnpublishing.co.uk/students/clinical-placements/community-placements/nursing-patients-with-dementia/ (accessed July 2012).

There are a variety of ways in which person-centeredness can be maintained:

- A comprehensive history taken from the client, carer and family to ascertain client's past interests, hobbies, likes and dislikes and their normal pattern of daily activities
- Observing the client in their new environment to observe their likes and dislikes, what seems to create problems and distress?
- Providing material such as television, clock, reading, photographs and other things which the client appears to like and results in an improvement in the quality of life
- If possible, making modifications to the surrounding environment to make life easier
- Finding out about food preferences and dietary needs
- Addressing cultural needs.

Access the article, 'Changing the Culture of Residential Care' at: http://www. alzheimerbc.org/getdoc/a4351fef-546b-44d1-90d5-19604ca8cd90/Changing-the-Culture-of-Residential-Care-for-web-p.aspx for a further understanding of the implementation of person-centeredness.

Although some clients with dementia may often be unable to recall recent events, they often remember how events have made them feel. It is therefore essential that the informal and professional carer adopt a person-centered approach to enable individualised care based on the needs and wishes of that particular client.

 Activity

To further develop your knowledge and understanding of the needs and support of the patient and family with dementia, read the following case study (Mr Smith) and consider the implications of dementia for Susan, and issues such as human rights, ethical issues, safety, privacy, dignity and respect.

Case study

Mr Smith and his family – caring for a person with dementia

Mr Smith is an 89-year-old widower of 16 years, who lives in a large isolated house in a pleasant area of town. He spent most of his working career as a very successful businessman. Susan his daughter lives nearby but works away from home a great deal; she also has a teenage son who has recently commenced university.

Mr Smith suffers from increasingly severe dementia, leading to neglect of himself and his property. He is reluctant to accept help, allowing only his daughter and grandson into the house at weekends. The house has recently been burgled three times and this has resulted in his anxiety about anyone entering the house in case they are 'casing the joint'. Susan tries to do a weekly shop and takes this to her father every Saturday but she does not know what he really eats.

Recently, crisis point was reached when a small fire broke out in Mr Smith's house, caused by a tea towel which had fallen onto a lit gas cooker ring, which he had left on. Although Mr Smith is not safe on his own, he does not wish to leave.

The following reading may help you with this:

Dalton JM (2005) Client-caregiver-nurse formation in decision making situations during home visits. Journal of Advanced Nursing 41(1):22–33

Department of Health (2001) National Service Framework for Older People. Standards 2, 7 and 8.

Nolan MR, Davies S, Brown J et al (2004) 'Beyond person-centred' care: a new vision for gerontological nursing. Journal of Clinical Nursing 13(S1):45–53.

Nolan M, Dellasega C (2000) 'I really feel I've let him down'; supporting family carers during long-term care placement for elders. Journal of Advanced Nursing 31 (4):759–767

Taylor P (1987) A living bereavement. Nursing Times 83(30):27–30

Wilson HS (1989) Family care giving for a relative with Alzheimer's dementia: coping with negative choices. Nursing Research 38(2):94–98.

These articles were published over a number of years. In reading them, consider the social and political issues arising at the time of their publication and determine if there are any differences with current narratives and examples from the RCN Website in terms of understanding of dementia by nurses and the care given to individuals experiencing this long-term health condition.

Palliative care for people with dementia

Earlier discussions here referred to palliative care, however it is important to refer to this again to develop your awareness of the specific challenges of palliative care for this specific client group. Read the text again and then consider some of the following issues.

Earlier in this chapter, reference was given to anticipatory care, specifically in relation to the management of long-term conditions, however anticipatory care planning is also recommended in palliative care to meet patient's wishes for end-of-life

Activity

Examine some of the issues included in the document: 'Exploring Palliative Care for People with Dementia' (NCPC/Alzheimer's Society 2006). This document emphasises the significance of palliative care for this specific client group and also refers to the importance of collaborative working between mental health services and palliative care services to facilitate the development of good end-of-life care. Discuss the possible care pathways involved with a hospice nurse and a community mental health nurse. Identify how they collaborate to ensure good and appropriate end-of-life care.

care, including preferred place of care. This is particularly significant in the care of clients suffering from dementia, when loss of capacity and communication problems are frequently experienced. However, in the early stages of dementia, when the client is able to make informed choices and decisions, an anticipatory care plan can provide the client with the opportunity to indicate the services and care they wish to receive later in illness, when they no longer have the capacity to decide for themselves. An anticipatory care approach should therefore assist in the achievement of person-centred care, dignity, choice and control. The approach can also facilitate communication between the client, the family, health and social care services.

Summary of learning points from this chapter

- There are different ways to assess 'need' within the community from both an individual and community perspective, as well as the role of the community nursing teams in achieving this
- The use of a person-centred approach to care is essential to the care of any individual requiring care in the community and which takes into account the increasing life expectancy of individuals and the health problems that they might experience long term

- It is important for all students to learn about the principles of management of long-term illness within the community, including assessment of individual and carer need, promoting patient self-care and self-management, anticipatory care and medication management
- Caring for someone with dementia requires specific knowledge as well as development of specific skills, which student nurses need to acquire during a community clinical placement.

References

Campling, F., Sharpe, M., 2006. Living with a long-term illness: the facts. Oxford University Press, Oxford.

Chamanga, E.T., 2010. How can community nurses improve quality of life for patents with leg ulcers? Nurs. Times 106, 10.

Clayton, J.M., Butow, P.N., Arnold, R.M., et al., 2005. Discussing end of life issues with terminally ill cancer patients and their carers: a qualitative study. Support. Care Cancer 13, 8.

Department of Health, 2001a. National Service Framework for Older People. DH, London.

Department of Health, 2001b. The expert patient: a new approach to chronic disease management for the 21st century. Online. Available at: www.dh.gov.uk.

Department of Health, 2005a. National Service Framework for long-term conditions. DH, London.

Department of Health, 2005b. Supporting people with long-term conditions: An NHS and Social Care Model to support local innovation and integration. DH, London.

Department of Health, 2006. National Service Framework for older people, Standard Framework (Standard 6). DH, London.

Department of Health, 2007. Policy and guidance: health and social care topics: long-term conditions. DH, London.

Department of Health, 2008a. End of Life Care Strategy: promoting high quality care for adults at the end of life. Online. Available at: www.dh.gov.uk (accessed May 2012).

Department of Health, 2008b. National Service Framework: Falls, No. 6. DH, London.

Eberhardie, 2004. Assessment and management of eating skills in the older adult. Online. Available at: http://www.nursingtimes.net/nursing-practice-clinical-research/assessment-and-management-of-eating-skills-in-the-older-adult/199540.article.

Kennedy, C., Harbison, J., Mahoney, C., et al., 2011. Investigating the contribution of community nurses to anticipatory care: a qualitative exploratory study. J. Adv. Nurs. 67 (7), 1558–1567.

King's Fund, 2010. How to deliver high-quality, patient-centred, cost-effective care. Consensus solutions from the voluntary sector. Kings Fund, London.

Lawton, J., 2000. The dying process: patient's experiences of palliative care. Routledge, London.

Marie Curie Palliative Care Institute, 2010. The Liverpool care pathway for the dying patient. Online. Available at: www.mcpcil.org.uk (accessed April 2012).

National Patient Safety Agency, 2007. Slips, trips and falls in hospital. NHS, London.

NCPC/Alzheimer's Society, 2006. Exploring palliative care for people with dementia. Online. Available at: ncpc.org.uk.

NICE, 2004. Clinical Practice Guideline for the assessment and prevention of falls in older people. NICE, London.

Newbury, J., 2011. Support for home carers dealing with the drama of death. Nurs. Times, 21 March.

Nursing and Midwifery Council, 2010. Essential skills clusters and guidance for their use. Online. Available at: www.nmc-uk.org.

Parliamentary and Health Service Ombudsman, 2011. Report of the Health Service Ombudsman on ten investigations into NHS care of older people. Parliamentary and Health Service Ombudsman, London.

Scottish Household Survey, 2003. Online. Available at: www.scotland.gov.uk.

Thomas, K., Department of Health, 2005. The Gold Standard Framework: A Programme for Community Palliative Care. Online. Available at: www.goldstandardsframework.nhs.uk.

Wade, D.T., De Jong, B.A., 2000. Recent advances in rehabilitation. Br. Med. J. 320, 1385–1388.

World Health Organization, 2005. Caring for people with chronic conditions, a health systems perspective. Online. Available at: http://www.euro.who.int/__data/assets/pdf_file/0006/96468/E91878.pdf.

World Health Organization, 2009. Definition of palliative care. Online. Available at: www.whoint/cancer/palliative/definition.

Further reading

Clayton, J.M., Butow, P.N., Arnold, R.M., et al., 2005. Discussing end of life issues with terminally ill cancer patients and their carers: a qualitative study. Support. Care Cancer 13 (8), 589–599.

Department of Health, 2008a. End of life care strategy: promoting high quality care for all adults at the end of life. DH, London.

Department of Health, 2009. Your health, your way: a guide to long-term conditions and self care. DH, London.

Donnelly, S.M., Michael, N., Donnelly, C., 2006. Experience of the moment of death at home. CMRT Mortality 11 (4), 352–367.

Funk, L., Stajduhar, K., Toye, C., et al., 2010. Part 2: Home based family caregiving at the end of life: a comprehensive review of published qualitative research (1998–2008). Palliat. Med. 24 (6), 594–607.

Hunter, S., 2009. Distinguishing between acute and chronic elements of ill health when assessing patients. Nurs. Times 105 (37), 20–23.

National Council for Hospice and Specialist Palliative Care Service, 2002. Definitions of supportive and palliative care. NCPC, London.

National Collaborating Centre for Chronic Conditions, 2006. Parkinson's disease: National Clinical Guideline for diagnosis and management in primary and secondary care. Royal College of Physicians, London.

Naylor, C., Parsonage, M., McDaid, D., et al., 2012. Long-term conditions and mental health: the cost of co-morbidities. The Kings Fund Centre for Mental Health, London.

Parkinson's UK, 2008. Life with Parkinson's today – room for improvement. Parkinsons' UK, London.

Payne, S., 2010. White paper on improving support for family carers in palliative care. European Journal of Palliative Care 17 (5), 238–245.

Roe, B., Howell, F., Riniotis, K., et al., 2009. Older people and falls; health status, quality of life, lifestyle, care networks. J. Clin. Nurs. 18 (16), 2261–2272.

Royal College of Nursing, 2004. Nursing assessment and older people. A Royal College of Nursing toolkit. RCN, London.

Royal College of Nursing, 2008. Defending dignity – challenges and opportunities for nursing. Royal College of Nursing, London.

Rubenstin, L.Z., 2006. Falls in older people; epidemiology, risk factors and strategies for prevention. Age Ageing 35 (Suppl. 2), 37–41.

Scottish Executive, 2006. Rights, relationships and recovery: The Report of the National Review of Mental Health. Scottish Government, Edinburgh.

University of Stirling, Final report on the Hub & Spoke Model for Clinical Practice Placement. Online. Available at: dspace. stir.ac.uk/bitstream/1893/3574/1/MRoxburgh-HS-FinalReport-13Sept 2011.pdf.

Wong, W.K.T., Ussher, J., 2009. Bereaved informal cancer carers making sense of their palliative care experiences at home. Health Soc. Care Community 17 (3), 274–282.

Websites

Alzheimer's Scotland, www.alzscot.org/pages/info/whatis.htm.

Barnardos, www.barnardos.org.uk regarding the stories and support of young carers.

Carers UK, www.carersuk.org.

Carers Direct, www.nhs.uk.

arers Trust, www.carers.org.

Community care, www.communitycare.co.uk.

Macmillan, regarding the support and advice for young carers caring for someone with cancer: www.macmillan.org.uk.

Marie Curie Website, www.mariecurie.org.uk.

Websites relating to intermediate care

Age UK, www.ageuk.org.uk. Information about aids and benefits for the elderly.

Alzheimerâs Society, 2006. www.alzheimers. org.uk provides a network of support for patient, families and carers living with Alzheimer's disease.

British Geriatrics Society, http://www.bgs.org. uk/index.php?option=com_content& view=article&id=363:intermediatecare& catid=12:goodpractice&ltemid=106.

Department for children, schools and families, 2010. Early intervention: securing good outcomes for all children and young people. Office of Public Sector Information.www. dcsf.gov.uk/everychildmatters.

Department of Health, www.dh.giv.uk. Information regarding many health issues such as long-term conditions.

Department of Health, www.endoflifecare.nhs. uk. NHS National End of Life Care Programme which works with health and social care across England to improve end-of-life care for adults and implements the End of Life Care Strategy.

The Equality Act. 2010. www.equalities.gov.uk.

Expert Patients, www.expertpatients.co.uk. A variety of patient self-management courses for a different of long-term conditions.

Health Service Ombudsman, www. ombudsman.org.uk. To read the case histories within the Care and Compassion Report of the Health Service Ombudsman on 10 investigations into NHS care of older people (2011). There are many care issues which are identified within each case study and important lessons to be learned for all healthcare practitioners.

Healthy Working Lives, www. healthyworkinglives.com.

Healthy Start, www.healthystart.nhs.uk.

Help the Aged/Picker Institute, 2008. www. helptheaged.org.uk/policy. On our own terms: The challenge of assessing dignity in care.

JIT Scotland, http://www.jitscotland.org.uk/ action-areas/intermediate-care/.

Joseph Rowntree Foundation, www.jrf.org.uk. Examines the experiences of older people living in residential and nursing care homes; the study enables you to develop your understanding of quality care through the perspective of the older adult.

National Healthy School Programme, www. healthyschools.gov.uk.

National Institute for Clinical Excellence, www. nice.org.uk gives a practical guide to Health Needs Assessment.

National Service Framework for Older People, http://www.dh.gov.uk/prod_consum_dh/ groups/dh_digitalassets/@dh/@en/ documents/digitalasset/dh_4065694.pdf.

Network of Public Health Observatories, www. apho.org.uk produces information and data on health and has expertise in analysing data into meaningful health information.

NHS Choices, www.nhs.uk/planners/ yourhealth/pages/yourhealth.aspx.

NHS Gold Standards Framework, www. goldstandardsframework.nhs.uk. The Gold Standards Framework which aims to improve cancer and palliative care in the community.

NHS Staff, http://nhslocal.nhs.uk/story/ national-links-staff. This Website is for staff working in the NHS to access the many links to resources available for them to help their patients and clients. It also shows you how to make your information more accessible to those it is aimed at.

Royal College Nursing, www.rcn.org.uk. A publication regarding the assessment of older people.

Scottish Government, 2011. Getting it right for every child.http://www.scotland.gov. uk/Topics/People/Young-People/ gettingitright.

7

Infection prevention and control in the community

CHAPTER AIMS

- To enable the student to gain an understanding of infection control measures as they apply within the community placement environment
- To enable the student to gain an understanding of the principles of infection prevention
- To enable the student to use their developing knowledge and skills of infection control in the community through focusing on the specific prevention and control of infection in wound care

Introduction

This chapter begins by focusing on prevention and control of infection and then elaborates on the prevention and control of infection in wound care.

Healthcare-associated infections (HCAIs or HAIs) are infections that are acquired in a hospital or other healthcare setting, such as a hospice or care home, or as a result of a healthcare intervention or procedure (Turner 2008). They pose a significant threat to the safety of patients and the public. Consequently, policies and procedures for the control of infection are a major concern to the NHS and a particular area of responsibility for all practitioners within all aspects of care. It is important to note here that this does not only apply to what may be called adult nursing placements, but those related to children's nursing, where more children are also being cared for in the home. Patients suffering from mental health can also be at risk of infection from issues such as self harm. Students who are learning in mental health nursing placements (Stacey et al 2012) may also be called upon to administer care with their mentors for patients with mental health problems who have been discharged home following surgery. Collaborative working with the district nurse in such situations is essential to ensure holistic care of the patient.

The community nurse is responsible for the holistic care of the person at home and this includes helping to prevent and control infection. More people of all ages are discharged home earlier from hospital, many on the day of surgery and an increasing number of procedures and treatments are offered at the local health centre by their doctor (GP) and specialist nurses such as practice nurses and advanced nurse practitioners. It is now commonplace for people to receive care at home such as intravenous medication, urinary catheterisation and enteral feeding.

These various procedures emphasise the importance of the prevention and control of infection within a variety of settings in the community, including nurseries, schools, residential and nursing homes, health centres and the person's home. The physical environment within the home can also vary markedly, resulting in the community nurse requiring considerable adaptation skills to prevent or maintain control of infection: changing a dressing in a person's home where space is at a minimum might for example entail kneeling on the carpet or even on the bed and the community nurse must make the environment as safe as possible by implementing the same principles of infection control that would be adopted in hospital.

The Nursing and Midwifery Council (NMC) require all student nurses to demonstrate essential skills in infection prevention and control. The 'Essential Skills Cluster: Infection Prevention and Control', states that people can trust the newly registered graduate nurse to:

- *identify and take effective measures to prevent and control infection in accordance with local and national policy*
- *maintain effective standard control of infection precautions and apply and adapt these to needs and limitations in all environments*
- *provide effective nursing interventions when someone has an infectious disease including the use of standard isolation techniques*
- *fully comply with hygiene, uniform and dress codes in order to limit, prevent and control infection*

- *safely apply the principles of asepsis when performing invasive procedures and be competent in aseptic technique in a variety of settings*
- *act, in a variety of environments including the home care setting, to reduce risk when handling waste, including sharps, contaminated linen and when dealing with spillages of blood and other body fluids.*

NMC (2010: 124)

 Activity

Some of the skills in this essential skills cluster will be more applicable in your community placement than others, depending on the specific learning outcomes which you are expected to achieve and the scope of the learning experience that is available. However, most skills are fundamental to community nursing practice. Following discussion with your mentor, identify examples within the community placement, which might demonstrate your progress in developing these skills and evidencing achievement in your portfolio. With their support, gain experience according to your development needs in these areas, ensuring that you gain permission from patients/clients in doing so. Your mentor should be prepared to explain to the patient/client that you are a student nurse learning to gain knowledge and skills to become a qualified nurse.

A variety of key personnel are specifically involved with infection prevention and control. For example, infection control nurses are specialists in infection prevention and control and provide advice on infection prevention and control in hospital and in the community.

Hospital infection control teams provide an infection control service for the hospital, which can also include community hospitals. These teams are often led by a nurse consultant in this field and a lead consultant microbiologist. Infection control link personnel are normally employees working in a surgery or care home who have completed additional training in infection control and act as a link between the workplace and the infection control nurse. Environmental health officers work for local authorities and advise on food safety, pest control and waste disposal. The Public Health departments in many community health organisations play a key role in the prevention and control of infection across the community as a whole, including areas such as child care centres (Health Protection Scotland 2012: http://www.documents.hps.scot.nhs.uk/hai/infection-control/guidelines/infection-prevention-control-childcare.pdf – accessed July 2012.)

 Activity

In discussion with your mentor, plan to spend some time with one of the control of infection specialist advisers within your community practice placement. Find out their specific responsibilities and when you would refer to them on behalf of a patient/client, including children and their parents. When a student nurse is undertaking a children's nursing pathway, a period of time should be spent focusing on the special infection and prevention needs of children in a variety of care and education settings.

 Activity

Find out about the infection prevention control policy and procedure for the community in which you are based and make yourself familiar with it. Ask members of the community nursing team how the procedures work in practice. This may well be one of the key learning experiences that you will need to comply with on your first clinical placement in any setting, and will often be linked to the clinical skills learning of hand washing and good practice in personal hygiene and infection prevention.

Lawrence and May (2003) outline a checklist of questions which can help the nurse with control of infection in the home; this includes the following:

- Has the client been discharged from hospital recently and if so, did they have any infections during their stay?
- Is there a history of known infections/antibiotic treatment?
- What other services are involved with care?
- What procedures need to be carried out in the home?
- Can hands be washed in the home?
- Is a sharps box required?
- Is there adequate storage space in the home for necessary equipment?
- Are there any other family members ill or immunocompromised?

Normally, discharge from hospital will be planned and the community nurse will have been given sufficient time to make appropriate arrangements to enable continuity of care; in some cases, a home visit may have been organised for example before surgery, enabling the above questions to be addressed.

Activity

In discussion with your mentor (this applies to all field of practice pathways – adult, mental health, learning disability and children's nursing), select a patient from their allocated caseload and with their agreement, use Lawrence and May's (2003) checklist (or an assessment template used locally) to assess their infection prevention and control status. You should be able to follow this through by mapping your assessment against local infection prevention and control policy and discussing with your mentor where action is required to manage risk. This exercise could be used to evidence learning about infection prevention and control in the community in your portfolio and contribute to meeting the requirements of the NMC Essential Skills Cluster outcomes as well.

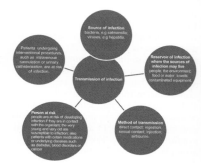

Figure 7.1 Transmission of infection.

same high standard and in some community contexts, the risks are very different. For example, risks such as cross-infection between people in close proximity as in a hospital ward are significantly reduced in the home but it is also more difficult to control the environment when it is a person's home. The elements of standard infection control precautions are listed in Table 7.1. It is

Standard infection control precautions

The practice of standard infection control precautions aims to prevent the transmission of infection. Potential sources of infection include blood and body fluids or excretions and any equipment in the care environment that could become contaminated. Figure 7.1 outlines the ways in which infection can spread. It is important that you learn about this process and most importantly, the physiological aspects of infection and its causes and outcomes.

It is essential that all practitioners carry out standard infection control precautions at all times, irrespective of whether infection is present or not and irrespective of the setting in which they are caring for their patients. However, compared with the hospital setting, it can be challenging to practise all standard infection control precautions to the

Table 7.1 Elements of standard infection control precautions

Patient positioning

Hand hygiene

Respiratory hygiene

Personal protective equipment

Occupational exposure management including sharps

Management of care equipment

Safe care of linen including uniforms

Control of environment

Management of blood and body spillages

Safe waste disposal

HPS (2012).

also important to include the patient's family and/or immediate carer in any risk assessment of infection and how to prevent it happening. Patient education will often include the family member or carer, especially when the patient is unable to undertake any procedure necessary.

Lectures covering standard infection control precautions such as hand decontamination, personal protective clothing and safe handling of sharps will have been included in your preparation for practice learning and will also form an essential part of your practice assessment (formative or summative) in many placements.

Hand hygiene

Handwashing is an essential component in the prevention and control of infection and regular careful handwashing is vital when you are looking after someone at home. However, within someone's home, hot and cold running water might not always be readily available. Community nurses therefore carry alcohol hand rubs/alcohol hand gel and tissues to address this problem but it must be remembered that this must be accompanied by an appropriate hand decontamination technique. (See an online example of this technique at the CETL website: http://www.cetl.org.uk/learning/hands/hand-washing/data/downloads/print-sheet.pdf – accessed October 2012.)

In your initial preparation for clinical practice, you will have received specific instructions on how to wash your hands, covering all the surfaces of your hands including the tips of your fingers, your thumbs and the areas between the fingers. It is essential to explain the risks associated with poor hand hygiene to service users and carers and educate them to undertake effective hand hygiene, particularly within the home setting, when an informal carer may be delivering the majority of nursing care. (See an example of information for patients and carers to use in the home at the Stroke4Carers website: http://www.stroke4carers.org/?p=5086 – accessed October 2013)

 Activity

We all have a responsibility to ensure that colleagues and all members of staff who are involved in delivering care comply with hand hygiene. However, people can be careless or forgetful. How would you approach a situation where you witnessed another member of the healthcare team not washing their hands before or after performing a procedure for a person in their care?

Discuss with your mentor how to manage this situation and work together to identify a decision-making plan according to your own NMC Student Code and that of your mentor's qualified nurse NMC Code.

Personal protective equipment

The main purpose of protective clothing is to prevent the spread of potentially pathogenic micro-organisms to another client, preventing contamination of the nurse's uniform or clothing (NICE 2003). It is important that you adhere to the local policy and protocols regarding protective clothing such as gloves and aprons.

Gloves

Staff should wear seamless, non-sterile disposable gloves when in direct contact with blood or body fluids. Sterile gloves will normally be worn when asepsis is required. Cuts and abrasions on exposed skin should always be covered with an appropriate waterproof dressing and the wearing of disposable gloves is also recommended to reduce the risk of infection. Gloves should not be worn as an alternative to hand hygiene

Aprons

Plastic disposable aprons will normally be worn when direct contact with blood or body fluids is anticipated. They are for single use only and should be changed between tasks.

Uniforms should not be considered as protective clothing and you should not wear your uniform to and from work. However, if you find that this is unavoidable when undertaking patient care in your community placement, such as visits to patients/clients, then your uniform should be covered with an outer layer when travelling. Please refer to the university policy on wearing uniform during your community placement.

Sharps management

One of the potential hazards facing nursing staff is the potential risk of needle stick injury. Safe practice should be maintained at all times, as it is not always possible to know who is infected by bacteria or viruses. Within the community setting, it may be difficult to reach local occupational health or accident and emergency departments if needle stick injury occurs, therefore you should always check local policy regarding the procedure if this occurs. Practices to prevent injury are similar to hospital practice and include:

- Never re-sheathing needles after use
- Disposing of syringes and needles as one complete unit immediately after use
- Never leaving sharps lying a round
- Ensuring secure closure of sharps boxes after three quarters full
- Storing sharps container in a secure place out of the reach of others.

Remember also that inoculation can also occur if abrasions, cuts or scratches are exposed to blood or body fluids. Within their everyday work, nurses risk exposure to dangerous viruses such as hepatitis as a result of needle stuck injury (RCN 2009).

You must become acquainted with the local guidelines and policies in relation to

needle stick injury and sharps management. However, most protocols regarding needle stick injury will follow the same general guidelines which include:

- Encourage bleeding from the inoculation site and wash under running water
- Cover with a waterproof dressing and report to a senior member of staff on duty
- Record the incident
- Inform occupational health, GP (or visit accident or emergency) and client's carer
- Assess risk of hepatitis B and C or HIV
- Obtain relevant blood samples from source and recipient with informed consent
- Seek specialist advice if there a need for post-exposure prophylaxis or follow-up for Hepatitis B and C or HIV?

Activity

Read the policy and procedure for the safe disposal of sharps in your community placement area. Although practice may be very different in the community, for example district nurses may carry sharps boxes in the boot of the car, you will see that the principles of safety and risk management are the same.

Access the CELT website: www.cetl.org.uk/learning/tutorials, where you can access a number of videoclips on different clinical skills such as hand-washing, handling and disposal of sharps, dealing with sharps injury. This is a useful learning resource to revise your control of infection skills.

Clinical waste management

Clinical waste is any waste such as swabs, dressings, syringes, needles, which have been in contact with tissue, blood or body fluids. The increasing number of complex treatments being delivered within the home and other community settings has increased the amount of clinical waste requiring safe disposal. Local policies and guidelines must be adhered to by community staff and collaborative working may be required with the local infection control nurse and local council to arrange appropriate disposal and removal of clinical waste from people's homes.

 Activity

> Find out the local arrangements for the safe disposal of clinical waste within your community practice placement.

Contaminated linen

Within the client's own home, linen is normally laundered in a domestic washing machine. Thorough washing at temperatures of 65–70° centigrade for at least 3 minutes, will remove most organisms (Infection Control Services 2007). Linen which is heavily contaminated should be dealt with by a hot wash cycle of 80°. However, in homes where this is not possible, it may be necessary to make arrangements with social services for linen to be laundered.

Blood and body fluid spillage

All spillages must be dealt with immediately to prevent contamination and also to prevent damage to client's furniture. If any abrasion, cuts or eczematous lesions become contaminated, then the local policy regarding this must be followed.

Aseptic technique

You will have covered the theory of aseptic technique to prevent microbial contamination of tissue and either practised this in a previous placement or in a simulated clinical skills environment in preparation for practice learning. However,

within the client's home, nursing staff do not have specific equipment such as dressing trolleys to assist them with this and consequently, they adapt their skills based on the principles of asepsis. There are times when the standards of hygiene and cleanliness in the home environment are far from conducive to aseptic practice, but the nurse must respect how people wish to live and use professional judgement to provide the most appropriate care. This does not mean however, that their own practice with cleanliness and asepsis should be compromised in any way. It is essential that all possible activities requiring infection prevention and control to be carried out in the patient's home must be risk assessed and all risks to patient and nurse safety minimised.

We can consider some of these issues by considering many of the procedures that you might be involved in undertaking under the supervision of your mentors.

Examples of procedures frequently undertaken in the community

Urinary catheter care

Catheter care within the home setting is usually associated with long-term or permanent catheters and an essential part of this care is to prevent infection. Similar to hospital practice, the principles of asepsis must be adhered to with catheter insertion, drainage bag changes, bladder installations, urinary sampling and catheter removal, and must be carried out using an aseptic technique (NICE 2003).

Intravenous therapy

Increasingly, intravenous therapy is delivered to clients within the home environment for a variety of treatments. Normally a comprehensive risk assessment will be carried out to see if the person's home circumstances are suitable for this. Many people with conditions such as cystic fibrosis, renal conditions and human immunodeficiency virus (HIV) will manage their own therapy. Patient-controlled analgesia using an infusion device will also be self-managed. Intravenous therapy is often delivered at home for clients receiving chemotherapy, total parental nutrition and haemodialysis. With intravenous therapy, the cannula site should be observed regularly for the early identification of infection (Lavery 2010).

A number of different intravenous catheters can be used, some of which you will have already encountered in your earlier clinical learning experiences, such as Hickman lines or peripherally inserted central catheters (PICC lines). Catheters for long-term vascular access are normally inserted in the hospital setting. All community nursing staff caring for patients with intravenous devices receive specific training and education to enable them to deliver this care safely. Intravenous catheter care includes daily inspection of the site to identify any infection, pain, inflammation or swelling, as early as possible. Local guidelines and protocols should be adhered to regarding dressings and dressing changes for intravenous catheter sites and an aseptic technique should be applied when dressings are changed. Any intravenous tubing should be replaced on a regular basis and reference to local protocols will give advice regarding this.

Enteral feeding

Enteral feeding is a way of giving nutritional support. However, there are possible infection risks associated with this and so the community nurse must consider the prevention of infection as an important part of the care for clients receiving this kind of therapy. To facilitate this, the nurse must consider the type of delivery system, the procedure for preparing and administering feed and the care of the gastrostomy site. The gastrostomy site must be kept clean and dry; a dressing may not be required. Regular

monitoring of this is essential to enable early identification of infection. Normally, food for this particular form of administration is already prepared and pre-packed in a sterile container. When administering feed, a strict aseptic routine adhering to local protocol should be established.

When using equipment related to the above procedures, it is important to use a system with few connections to reduce the potential for infection. To prevent transmission of infection, decontamination of equipment must be carried out between uses; local guidelines should be referred to regarding this.

Activity

During your home visits with the community nurse, observe and discuss with your mentor how asepsis is maintained when completing different procedures such as wound cleansing and urinary catheterisation. Although this type of experience will most often be undertaken by students undertaking the adult nursing pathway, other students on different pathways will also be exposed to similar procedures. Make a note in your portfolio of all the clinical procedures that you are exposed to/or undertake during each placement.

Notifiable diseases

A significant aspect of control and prevention of infection is to be aware of specific infectious diseases which can be easily transmitted among people. Under the Public Health (Control of Diseases) Act 1984, some diseases such as tuberculosis or food poisoning must be notified to the local authority. Normally, the medical practitioner who makes the diagnosis would notify the relevant individual. (See Table 7.2 for a list of notifiable infectious diseases.)

Activity

In discussion with your mentor, identify a particular infectious disease which has occurred within your community placement area and access the Health Protection Agency at: http://www.hpa. or.uk to further develop your knowledge and understanding about this infection and its management. Consider how the infection is spread; is anyone at particular risk? How is the spread of infection avoided? Those of you undertaking the children's nursing pathway can focus on the specific ones that can affect children and young people.

Table 7.2 Diseases notifiable to local authority under the Health Protection Regulations (2010)

Acute encephalitis	Acute meningitis
Acute infectious hepatitis	Measles
Acute poliomyelitis	Meningococcal septicaemia (without meningitis)
Anthrax	
Botulism	Mumps
Brucellosis	Plague
Cholera	Rabies
Diphtheria	Rubella
Enteric fever (typhoid or paratyphoid)	Scarlet fever
	Smallpox
	Tetanus
Food poisoning	Tuberculosis
Haemolytic uraemic syndrome	Typhoid fever
	Typhus
Infectious bloody diarrhoea	Viral haemorrhagic fevers (Lassa fever and Marburg disease)
Invasive group A streptococcal disease	
	Viral hepatitis
Legionnaires	Whooping cough
Leprosy	Yellow fever
Leptospirosis	
Malaria	

Prevention and control of infection in wound care

It is not the purpose of this portion of the chapter to examine wound care in depth but to focus on the implications of infection for delayed wound healing and the importance of the implementation of standard infection control precautions to prevent infection. All wounds increase the risk of infection and chronic wounds such as pressure ulcers are at increased risk of becoming colonised with, e.g. MRSA. Infected wounds take longer to heal and are uncomfortable and frustrating for the patient and costly in terms of nursing interventions (Gethin 2009). Patients with infected wounds suffer greater pain than those with uninfected wounds (White 2009). It is therefore crucial that control of infection measures are taken to prevent wounds such as pressure ulcers and to prevent infection in existing wounds (Lawrence and May 2003, DH 2006).

Identification of wound infection

Early identification of infection is vital in the avoidance of delayed wound healing and potential complications. Infected wounds often have an increase in exudate and the immediate skin around the wound is often inflamed. Gray (2011) outlines the following characteristics of inflammation which include: erythema, heat, oedema, pain and functional disturbance. Increased pain or unpredicted pain and wound breakdown can indicate infection. The infection and subsequent inflammation not only delays wound healing, but can result in systemic disease and potentially life-threatening sepsis (DH 2006).

To add to the above symptoms of inflammation and infection, the person's quality of life can be adversely affected. (See later in the chapter for further discussion.)

Normally a wound-swab is taken when infection is suspected, however this, although identifying some or all of the bacteria in a wound, is not a guarantee of the identification of specific, clinically significant bacteria (European Wound Management Association, EWMA 2006, Best Practice Statement, BPS 2011).

It is important to continue regular assessment and documentation of a patient's wound to help identify early signs of infection. However, in some situations infection can be present even where there is a lack of symptoms; infection in chronic wounds may manifest itself with delayed healing only, with other signs of infection absent. Gray (2011) refers to this as 'critical colonisation'. Patients with nerve damage, for example a patient with burns or suffering from neuropathy due to diabetes, may not experience pain where infection is present. Patients who are immunocompromised may present with discreet and few signs and symptoms of infection, or indeed present none at all. These instances highlight the importance of regular assessment of a variety of symptoms to ensure early identification of wound infection.

The following activities are essential to help prevent wound infection and contain an infected wound to the host patient:
- Hand hygiene before changing the wound dressing
- Wearing gloves when handling wounds
- Using an appropriate wound dressing and changing the dressing when indicated.

Aseptic dressing technique should be employed when dressing surgical wounds, recent trauma, burns and scalds and for chronic wounds, particularly when patients are at increased risk of infection due to other disease conditions such as circulatory problems, diabetes or cancer.

The basic principles of caring for a client with a wound remain the same whatever the care setting and include:
- Removing the cause of the wound
- Local wound debridement
- The application of an appropriate dressing

- Developing a good nutritional plan
- Treating any underlying disease and psychological support.

Activity

Reflect on the care of a client, with a wound, you have visited during your community practice experience and consider the initial assessment and how this contributed to a holistic plan of care to facilitate wound healing and prevent the occurrence of wound infection.

You may find that you can divide the assessment into the following components:
- If appropriate, remove the immediate cause of the wound to prevent complications and recurrence; this might include addressing any underlying pathology that may impair wound healing or alleviating factors which may delay wound healing; this also includes determining if a wound is infected. When dealing with surgical wounds, although it is not possible to eliminate the cause of the wound, care should be focused on regular observation to enable the early identification of infection.
- Improve the quality of life by exploring various issues such as alleviating mobility restrictions, pain, loss of socialisation, emotional wellbeing.
- Explore ways in which the client and carer can be involved in care to empower them, facilitate motivation for self-help and to promote wellbeing and hence facilitate wound healing. Patient and carer wound care education may include advice regarding good nutritional intake. If required, educate in the importance of the regular administration of pain relief, the avoidance of undue trauma and information regarding wound observation and education, to enable the early identification of any complication which may impede wound healing such as infection.

Wound assessment charts and wound measuring

The use of wound assessment charts contributes greatly to the assessment process and you may have completed such documentation within other learning practice experiences. They can be used in the treatment of all wounds including chronic open wounds such as pressure ulcers, leg ulcers and surgical wounds.

Most wound assessment charts include information about the size and location of the wound; within leg ulcer treatment, the size of the ulcer should be measured and documented, also the depth, any bone or necrotic tissue should be noted, as this will aid the choice of dressing. Langemo et al (2008) states that the measuring of the wound can be used as an indicator to assess wound healing progress; this can be achieved by tracing. Details regarding any exudates should be noted – factors which may lead you to the diagnosis of wound infection include pyrexia, increasing exudates, odour and increasing pain. If infection is suspected, a wound swab should be taken for bacteriological analysis.

Earlier reference has been made to the range of wounds you may encounter in practice, unfortunately this may include wounds as a result of cutting and self-harm. This is normally representative of someone who is suffering from severe distress, and specialist advice should be sought for this particular aspect of care.

 Activity

Discuss this specific aspect of care with your mentor and if possible, arrange to spend time with the community mental health team to gain further knowledge and understanding regarding the signs of self-harm and the specialist help available for patients facing this.

Malnutrition and wound care

It is important to always consider the nutritional status of the client receiving wound care. Stignant (2009) stated suggesting that weight loss may reduce swelling can be used as a significant motivating factor for clients. Nutritional screening is an important aspect of the initial assessment of the client requiring wound care to identify malnutrition or to identify clients at high risk of becoming malnourished, and should be carried out during the initial assessment and throughout the client's duration of care. Nutritional assessment is normally carried out by a healthcare professional with specific expertise regarding nutrition requirements such as a dietitian and includes dietary history, physical assessment and anthropometry, with biochemical analysis.

 Activity

There are various assessment tools and guidelines that can assist with the above responsibility. Consider the nutritional assessment tools that you have encountered during your practice learning experiences. You may find it useful to refer to the Department of Health (2001) publication: 'Essence of Care', which includes a toolkit to develop the quality of care in eight fundamental areas, one of which is food and nutrition. You may also find it useful to access The National Institute for Health and Clinical Excellence (NICE 2006): www.nice.org to read Clinical Guideline No. 32 on nutrition support in adults.

Psychosocial issues and quality of life

Morison et al (2004) discussed the social conditions which can play a role in delaying wound healing, many clients with leg ulcers for example are older, poor and live alone. King et al (2007) referred to the inability of such patients to wear their normal footwear while receiving treatment can result in inadequate ankle flexibility, which may increase risk of falls and social isolation if they cannot go out. Chronic wounds such as leg ulcers can result in the client experiencing changes in body image and loss of self-esteem. Hareendran et al (2007) discussed the restrictions that can result in activities of daily living and role performance, along with the experiences of pain and anxiety, which can then result in depression and perhaps further isolation. With a holistic assessment, the nurse should be able to view the experience of wound care from the client's perspective; this should enable the appropriate strategies to facilitate quality of life. Listening to clients and providing psychological support is an essential component to the healing process. Quality of life in patients with chronic wounds can be severely compromised. Posnett and Franks (2008) declare that in the next 20 years, there will be a significant rise in the number of patients with chronic wounds. It is suggested that this may be related to the increase in people living longer and the increase in incidence of type 2 diabetes. It is therefore imperative that quality of life becomes a set aspect of wound care.

 Activity

Consider the holistic approach to wound care for the following patient:

Mr Jones is a 75-year-old man who lives with his wife who suffers from dementia. Mr Jones suffers from pulmonary disease and has a very painful chronic leg ulcer over the posterior-lateral malleolus. The tissue surrounding the ulcer is very inflamed and the ulcer is producing a yellowish discharge.

Points to consider from Mr Jones' case study

The discomfort, inflammation and discharge that Mr Jones is experiencing indicates possible infection and a wound swab should be taken – although this must not delay initial treatment of the wound when awaiting results. O'Meara et al (2010) make reference to UK prescribing guidelines, which indicate that systemic and topical antibiotics should be avoided with chronic wounds to prevent antibiotic-resistant strains of bacteria from developing and that antibacterial preparations should only be used to treat clinical infection in leg ulcers, not for bacterial colonisation. An appropriate dressing should be applied to absorb exudate and to protect the wound bed.

Mr Jones suffers from chronic obstructive pulmonary disease, which compromises his respiratory function and which could be a significant factor in delaying wound healing. It is important therefore to proactively manage this, trying to prevent episodes of respiratory distress and initiating early treatment of any chest infections. Mr Jones also takes prednisolone for his respiratory condition. This is increased during acute exacerbations and steroid therapy can compromise healing. Mr Jones becomes extremely anxious at times; this anxiety is predominantly related to the difficulties in caring for his wife. The occurrence of stress in carers can affect cytokine activity, which can also result in delayed wound healing. Care should therefore consider ways in which Mr Jones could be assisted with his wife's care to help alleviate this anxiety.

General aspects of wound care within the home environment

Wound cleansing
The main aim of wound cleansing is to remove foreign materials; to prevent or treat

infection; to prepare the wound for grafting or to reduce odour or exudates. Antiseptics, antibiotics, saline and water are all commonly used for cleansing wounds. However, a recent Cochrane update (Fernandez & Griffiths 2010) concluded that using tap water to cleanse acute and chronic wounds in adults did not increase infection and that there was some evidence to suggest that it reduced infection. In the community, people with leg ulcers routinely have their legs washed with tap water in a lined container to avoid contamination and find this benefits skin care, comfort and general wellbeing.

 Activity

During your community learning experience, observe and take note of the solutions used for cleansing wounds; how they are stored in the client's home and also the way in which wound cleansing is delivered. Also observe how the community nurse maintains aseptic technique within the client's home environment.

The temperature of the solution and the method of its delivery are also important components to the cleansing of wounds. Solutions that have been refrigerated or sometimes even kept at room temperature can reduce the surface temperature of the wound, resulting in local hypothermia. Gannon (2007) reports that it can take the wound several minutes to return to its original temperature and several hours to resume cellular activity.

Cleansing agents must be delivered in such a way as to effectively wash away debris but avoid excessive force, which might only displace debris within the wound; irrigation with a syringe is often effective in achieving effective cleansing but preventing displacement of debris.

Selecting the appropriate dressing

Selecting the appropriate dressing can be a challenging task for the nurse. Within your community placement, you will encounter a wide variety of different dressings, including materials such as transparent films, alginate fibres, hydrocolloid wafers and collagen sheets. An important component of selecting a dressing is to consider the function and performance of the dressing. Morison et al (2004) promotes the utilisation of the following questions to assist the practitioner with the selection process:

- What does the wound need?
- What does the product do?
- What does the patient need?
- What is available?
- What is practical?

By addressing the above questions, the practitioner is adopting a performance-based approach, assisting in the matching of available dressings and their functions to wound needs. Note the earlier reference made to O'Meara et al (2010) in the discussion of the UK prescribing guidelines that advise the cautious use of systemic and topical antibiotics with chronic wounds to prevent the development of antibiotic-resistant strains of bacteria. When there is wound exudate, an appropriate dressing should be applied to absorb this and to protect the wound bed.

 Activity

Identify the different dressings that you have encountered during your clinical practice experience and with your mentor, discuss the rationale for the dressing choice. Consider how the situation of the patient affected the choice of dressing used, e.g. for some patients a re-usable type dressing would be more practical, as in the case of a patient who would constantly rip away any dressing applied.

Your identification of different dressings may have included some of the following:
- Foams/alginates to absorb excess exudates
- Films/hydrocolloids to promote tissue hydration
- Products containing activated charcoal to absorb wound odour.

 Activity

There are numerous antimicrobial products for wound infections. Access the Tissue Viability Society Website at: www.tvs.org.uk to gain an understanding of the utilisation of this treatment.

As discussed earlier, it is not the purpose of this chapter to examine wound care in depth but to include this area of care within the control and prevention of infection as they are unquestionably intertwined. It is also important for you to appreciate that your community learning experience can provide you with a valuable opportunity to review and develop your knowledge of wound care. You may encounter a variety of different wounds such as, burns, surgical wounds, malignant fungating lesions, pressure ulcers, self-harm wounds, diabetic foot ulceration and radiotherapy skin reactions.

It is important to utilise the opportunity of dealing with a variety of different wound care activities to further develop your wound care knowledge and skills.

 Activity

To assist your professional development within this aspect of care, you might like to refer to the following websites: www.tissuevaibilityonline. org and the European Pressure Ulcer Advisory Panel: www.epuap.org

Practitioners must remain aware of the signs and symptoms of wound infection and also, where symptoms are more discreet or indeed absent, be mindful of the potential presence of infection. Early identification, management and treatment of infection is essential to avoid deterioration, complication or any preventable suffering of the patient. Ultimately however, the prevention of infection is the best approach, achieved through the effective implementation of standard control of infection measures.

Summary of learning points from this chapter

After reading this chapter and completing the learning activities, you should be able to achieve the following actions which will support your achievement of the NMC Standards (NMC 2010):
- Knowledge and understanding regarding the principles of infection prevention and control as an essential part of the holistic care of patients
- Knowledge and understanding of local and national prevention and control of infection policy
- Knowledge and understanding of the principles of infection prevention and the skills required in the implementation of infection control measures within the patient's own home
- The skills required to safely deliver the principles of asepsis when performing invasive procedures
- The principles of infection control and prevention in the management of wound care.

References

Best Practice Statement (BPS), 2011. The use of topical antiseptic/antimicrobial agents in wound management, second ed. Wounds UK, London.

Department of Health (DH), 2001. The essence of care: patient-focused benchmarking for health care practitioners. DH, London.

Department of Health (DH), 2006. The Health Act 2006; Code of Practice for the prevention and control of healthcare-associated infections. DH, London.

Department of Health (DH), 2006. Revised essential steps to safe, clean care: introduction and guidance. DH, London.

European Wound Management Association (EWMA), 2006. Position document: identifying criteria for wound infection. MEP, London.

Fernandez, R., Griffiths, R., 2010. Water for wound cleansing (Review) 1. The Cochrane Collaboration. John Wiley & Sons, London.

Gannon, R., 2007. Fact file: wound cleansing; sterile water or saline? Nurs. Times 103 (9), 44.

Gethin, G., 2009. Role of topical anti-microbials in wound management. Journal of Wound Care/Activa Supplement S4–S8.

Gray, D., 2011. Assessment diagnosis and treatment of infection. Wounds UK 7 (2 Suppl.), 4–22.

Hareendran, A., Doll, H., Wild, D.J., et al., 2007. The venous leg ulcer quality of life (VLU-QoL) questionnaire: development and psychometric validation. Wound Repair Regen. 15 (4), 465–473.

Health Protection Scotland (HPS), 2012. National infection prevention and control manual. HPS, Glasgow. Online. Available at: http://www.documents.hps.scot.nhs.uk/hai/infection-control/ic-manual/ipcm-p-v1.0.pdf (accessed May 2012).

Infection Control Services, 2007. Primary care policies. Online. Available at: http://www.infectioncontrolservices.co.uk/

primary_care_disinfection_and_decontamination_linen.htm.

King, B., Wesley, V., Smith, R., Smith, R., 2007. An audit of footwear for patients with leg bandages. Nurs. Times 103 (9), 40, 42–43.

Langemo, D., Anderson, J., Hanson, D., et al., 2008. Measuring wound length, width and area; which technique? Adv. Skin Wound Care 21 (1), 42–45.

Lavery, I., 2010. Infection control in IV therapy: a review of the chain of infection. Br. J. Nurs. 19 (19), S6–S14.

Lawrence, J., May, D., 2003. Infection control in the community. Churchill Livingstone, London.

Morison, M.J., Ovington, L.G., Wilkie, K., 2004. Chronic wound care: a problem-based learning approach. Mosby, Edinburgh.

National Institute for Clinical Excellence (NICE), 2003. Infection control: prevention of healthcare-associated infection in primary and community care. NICE, London.

National Institute for Clinical Excellence (NICE), 2006. Clinical Guidelines, No. 32. Nutrition support for adults: oral nutrition support, enteral tube feeding and parenteral nutrition. National Collaborating Centre for Acute Care (UK), London.

Nursing and Midwifery Council (NMC), 2010. Standards for pre-registration nursing education. Online. Available at: http://standards.nmc-uk.org, Annexe 3, Essential Skill Cluster. Infection Prevention and Control. NMC, London.

O'Meara, S., Al-Kurdi, D., Ologun, Y., et al., 2010. Antibiotics and antiseptics for venous leg ulcers. Cochrane Database Syst. Rev. (1), CD003557.

Posnett, J., Franks, P.J., 2008. The burden of chronic wounds in the UK. Nurs. Times 104 (3), 44–45.

Royal College of Nursing (RCN), 2009. Needlestick injuries: the point of prevention. RCN, London.

Stacey, G., Felton, A., Bonham, P., 2012. Placement learning in mental health nursing. Bailliere Tindall, London.

Stignant, A., 2009. Tackling obesity as part of a lymphedema management programme. Br. J. Community Nurs. 14 (10), s9–s14.

Turner, R., 2008. Healthcare associated infections. Kings Fund, London.

White, R., 2009. Wound infection – associated pain. J. Wound Care 18 (6), 245–249.

Further reading

Benbow, M., 2008. Exploring wound management and measuring quality of life. Journal of Community Nursing 22 (6), 14–18.

Bryant, R., 2010. Acute and chronic wounds. Elsevier, Edinburgh.

Burnett, E., 2009. Innovative infection prevention and control teaching for nursing students: a personal reflection. Journal of Infection Prevention 10, 204–210.

Moore, M., 2008. Mosby's pocket guide to nutritional assessment and care. Elsevier, Edinburgh.

Pellowe, C.M., Pratt, R.J., Loveday, H.P., et al., 2003. Infection control: prevention of healthcare-associated infection in primary and community care. British Journal of Infection Control 4 (Suppl.), 1–100.

Pratt, R.J., Pellowe, C.M., Wilson, J.A., et al., 2007. Epic 2: National evidence based guidelines for preventing hospital acquired infection in England. J. Hosp. Infect. 65 (Suppl. 1), S1–S64.

Smith, B., 2010. Student nurse infection control survival guide. Pearson, Harlow.

Ward, D., 2010. Infection control in clinical placements: experiences of nursing and midwifery students. J. Adv. Nurs. 66 (7), 1533–1542.

Websites

The following organisations protect the population by giving support and advice to the NHS, the government, local authorities and other organisations that play a part in protecting health. An important part of their role includes infection prevention and control.

Health Protection Agency (England), http://www.hpa.org.uk.

Public Health Agency (Northern Ireland), http://www.publichealth.hscni.net.

Health Protection Scotland, http://www.hps.scot.nhs.uk.

Public Health Wales, http://www.wales.nhs.uk/sites3/home.cfm?orgid=457.

The Compendium of Healthcare Associated Infection Guidance

The purpose of the HAI compendium is to provide NHS Scotland staff with all current HAI guidance, as well as the key messages from the guidance and all the associated supporting materials e.g. checklists, care bundles, patient information leaflets and training scenarios. This can be accessed on: http://www.documents.hps.scot.nhs.uk/hai/hai-compendium/hai-compendium.pdf.

The Infection Control Nurses Association can be accessed on www.icna.co.uk and deals with a variety of issues related to infection control including a framework of competencies for practitioners in working in infection control and prevention.

National Patient Safety Agency informs and supports all healthcare practitioners on an array of healthcare practices which facilitate safer care for patients: www.npsa.nhs.uk.

Evidence-based practice in the prevention of healthcare associated infections can be accessed on: www.epic.TVu.ac.uk.

The National Institute for Clinical Excellence (NICE) Guidelines, www.nice.org.uk.

Tissue Viability Society (TVS), which aims to provide expertise in wound management to all healthcare professionals: www.tvs.org.uk.

The latest news regarding wound care practice and research for nurses can be accessed on: www.nursingtimes.net/section2.

The *Journal of Tissue Viability*, which can be accessed on www.journaloftissuevaibility.com deals with all aspects of the occurrence and treatment of wound including patient assessment, managing pain and nutrition and refers to the most recent wound healing research.Information regarding best practice in tissue viability can be accessed on the Institute for Health Care Improvement website: www.ihi.org.

The City University London and Barts and The London Hospitals – Centre for Excellence in Teaching and Learning (CETL) – Clinical and Communication Skills learning resources Centre: see a range of resources regarding infection control and risk management at: http://www.cetl.org.uk/learning/downloads.php and http://www.cetl.org.uk/learning/tutorials.html.

Royal College of Nursing, 2012. Essential practice for infection prevention and control: Guidance for nursing staff. RCN publication.http://www.rcn.org.uk/__data/assets/pdf_file/0008/427832/004166.pdf (accessed July 2012).

Mental health and care in the community

Iain Murray

Iain Murray

CHAPTER AIMS

- To examine a range of mental health problems which may affect people living in the community
- To explore the role of the community mental health nurse and other members of the team
- To discuss treatment options for patients/clients within a community care context
- To reflect on how the knowledge and experience gained in mental health services in a community placement can be applied across a range of other placement settings

Introduction

This chapter will help you to prepare for a placement within the community where you may gain experience working with nurses who care for people with mental health problems. It is a chapter for all student nurses pursuing all fields of practice pathways, as mental health and wellbeing and managing to care for patients with diagnosed mental health problems will be essential skills at exposure level for all. It is an introduction to the mental health issues to which a student may be exposed in many placements. (To focus in more detail on mental health-specific placements and learning, see Stacey et al 2012).

Major mental health problems are relatively uncommon in comparison with minor or common mental health disorders. In the 2007 household survey of adult psychiatric morbidity in England (NHS 2009), the level of common mental health disorder in the population requiring some form of treatment, was identified as 7.5% of the population. In the same publication, the prevalence of 'psychoses', a term which captures the majority of major mental health disorders, is 0.5%. When you compare these two percentages and given that people with major mental health problems are more likely to be admitted to hospital, it is clear that nurses working in the community are more likely to encounter people with minor, less severe mental health problems, albeit these can be quite disabling and impact significantly on the life of sufferers and their families. Table 8.1 shows common mental health and major mental health disorders.

On placement you may be able, if the patient consents, to observe basic

Table 8.1 Common mental health and major mental health disorders

Common mental health disorders	Major mental health disorders
Generalised anxiety disorder (GAD)	Psychoses
Mixed anxiety and depressive disorder	Schizophrenia
Depressive episode (including mild, moderate)	Bipolar disorder
Phobias	Manic depressive illness
Obsessive-compulsive disorder (OCD)	Unipolar disorder
Panic disorder	Severe depression

The NHS (2009).

 Activity

At times, people with mental health problems are misunderstood; occasionally negative attitudes expressed towards such people and their behaviour, often borne out of ignorance and prejudice, can have a detrimental effect on an individual's wellbeing.

The terminology used by mental health practitioners is often not fully understood; derogatory and stigmatising terms such as 'crazy', 'mad' or 'having a screw loose' are commonly used by the public to describe people with mental health problems.

Research common mental health terminology through websites such as:

■ http://www.open.ac.uk/inclusiveteaching/pages/understanding-and-awareness/ common-terms-in-mental-health.php

■ http://www.mentalhealth.org.uk/help-information/mental-health-a-z/T/ terminology/

or

■ from a textbook such as *Mental Health Nursing* (Videbeck 2009).

Discuss your findings with your mentor and reflect on how your understanding of mental health terminology varies from that used by professionals, carers and service users.

counselling, relaxation therapy, sleep hygiene counselling, etc. (People with mental health problems such as mild depression and anxiety-related problems are covered in more detail later in this chapter.)

Mental health nursing in the community is often seen to be the domain of the Community Psychiatric Nurse/Community Mental Health Nurse (CPN/CMHN). While many people with a mental health problem, particularly long standing conditions such as schizophrenia or bipolar disorder, are supported by CPNs, there are a wide range of conditions, often referred to as minor

mental health problems, and those who experience them are occasionally cared for and supported by other community nurses such as general practice nurses, district nurses and health visitors.

People experience a wide range of mental health problems such as mild to moderate depression, anxiety-related problems, sleep disturbance and addictive problems. Many of these people will only see their GPs for support and medication. Community nurses may have more time to spend with the individual; more time to engage in 'talking therapies' (Stacey et al 2012).

Activity

Prior to undertaking a placement with a mental health practitioner or nurse in the community, it would be helpful to understand more about basic counselling. The following websites are a good starting point to develop your understanding of counselling approaches:

■ http://www.howto.co.uk/wellbeing/counselling-skills

■ http://www.basic-counseling-skills.com.

It is important to note that these are only information sites and the content must be discussed with your mentor and/or personal tutors to ensure safe practice, as a student, is undertaken.

Reading the information on these sites will help give you an insight into this field and support your achievement of both generic and field-specific competencies (if undertaking a mental health nursing pathway) in the NMC Domain 2: Communication and Interpersonal Skills.

During placements with the community nursing team, it may be possible for you to spend some time with the specialist mental health nurses or attend a day care centre where you may be able to observe basic counselling skills in action.

Role of the community psychiatric nurse (CPN)/ community mental health nurse (CMHN)

The following definition illustrates the key aspects of this role:

The CPN is a qualified mental health nurse who works as part of a team of professionals to provide mental health services in the community. The role of the CPN is to work with the people referred, to define what they see as the problem and to agree whether or not further action or further contact with the CPN is needed. At the end of this assessment the CPN and the client may agree an action plan to address any needs identified and the CPN will continue to work with the client until the plan is finished. CPNs have a broad knowledge of mental health problems and

a wide range of skills that they can use to enable clients to work through any programmes agreed. As well as working directly with people experiencing mental health problems, the CPN will try to ensure that the needs of carers are considered. This may mean working directly with a carer or may be related to making sure that the carer is able to access the support needed from other sources.

NHS Tayside Nursing Services
(http://www.nhstayside.scot.nhs.uk/
services/nursing/index.shtml)

 Activity

■ In discussion with your mentor, and through independent research, identify those mental health problems, and their key features, that community mental health nurses would predominantly play a major role in supporting.

■ Make sure you explore the specific reasons why certain clients will be cared for and supported by a CPN/ CMHN.

Continued

- Write up your research and notes on mental health problems in your on-going learning diary or portfolio.

This activity will help you to work towards achieving competencies in the NMC Domain 3: Nursing Practice and Decision Making and NMC Domain 4: Leadership, Management and Team Working.

Having observed the management and delivery of care to people with mental health problems in the community, we now explore in more detail some of the main mental health problems that people can experience. It may be worth starting with mental health as opposed to mental illness. The Mental Health Foundation describes mental health as:

- *Mental Health affects us all. How we think and feel about ourselves and our lives impacts on our behaviour and how we cope in tough times.*
- *It affects our ability to make the most of the opportunities that come our way and play a full part amongst our family, workplace, community and friends. It's also closely linked with our physical health.*
- *Whether we call it well-being, emotional welfare or mental health, it's key to living a fulfilling life.*

The Mental Health Foundation
(http://www.mentalhealth.org.uk)

It can be seen from the above that mental health is about coping with life on a day-to-day basis, it is about having satisfying relationships and it is about having a realistic understanding of your own self-worth; being able to cope with uncertainty, the ability to manage both positive and negative emotions and deal with disappointment. It is clear that mental health is more than the absence of mental illness. Mental illness arises when

stress, whether that be physical, social or psychological overwhelms an individual and interferes with those very aspects of living that are identified above and seen as aspects of good mental health. Therefore, when an individual is mentally ill, they may not be able to manage their emotions and their relationships can become strained or broken. A person can become unable to work or manage their affairs; their concentration can be poor and their thinking distorted or delusional.

Different types of mental illness

Psychiatric diagnoses are categorised by the *Diagnostic and Statistical Manual of Mental Disorders*, 4th edn., otherwise known as the DSM-IV (American Psychiatric Association 1994). The manual is published by the American Psychiatric Association and covers all mental health disorders for both children and adults. It also lists known causes of these disorders, statistics in terms of gender, age at onset and prognosis, as well as some research concerning the optimal treatment approaches. The World Health Organization has its own classification; ICD-10 (WHO 1993), which fulfils a similar purpose; both of these were revised in the early 1990s and are currently being reviewed. Classification manuals/schedules such as these are used by mental health professionals for epidemiological and research purposes to enhance their understanding of mental illness. Nonetheless, it is helpful outwith that context in providing a structure which helps patients, and professionals alike, to understand and describe mental illness.

All the following descriptions and explanations of a range of mental illnesses are followed by specific activities which will support your achievement of a number of competencies across all four NMC domains of: Professional Values; Communication and Interpersonal Skills; Nursing Practice and Decision Making and Leadership, Management and Team Working.

Students in all four fields of practice should use this chapter to learn about mental health problems and how they can gain exposure to the knowledge and skills to be able to manage care situations where patients/clients may present with the behaviours associated with each illness.

It is important to note that, although 'labelling' a person who has a mental illness with an attached 'condition' is considered inappropriate in practice, in the context of this section of the chapter, it is more related to the actual underpinning health problem that the terminology is used. This is to enable the student to understand possible symptoms and behaviour that a person may experience with these diagnosed mental health problems.

Disorders of mood such as depression and bipolar disorder

These conditions are categorised as disorders where the primary symptom is disturbance of mood, whether that be an inappropriate, limited or exaggerated expression of feelings. Elevation or depression of mood and feeling is an experience common to most people. However, to receive a diagnosis of mood disorder, one's feelings must be extreme in terms of both level and duration. This can manifest itself by frequent and prolonged periods of crying, feelings of depression, anxiety, guilt and suicidal ideation. The corollary to this, mania or hypomania, is characterised by the opposite extreme, where someone has excessive energy and hyperactivity with severely disturbed sleep

and grossly disrupted decision-making, often driven by a sense of grandiosity.

A major category within DSM-IV is bipolar disorder (manic-depression). Research has shown a strong biological component for this disorder, with environmental factors playing a role in the exacerbation of symptoms. The implication being that some people are genetically predisposed to bipolar disorder but environmental factors such as stress can play a major role in its manifestation (Elder & Mosack 2011).

Activity

In a person with a genetic or familial predisposition to bipolar disorder, illness can often be triggered by a precipitating factor, often stress, and these factors are referred to as 'stressors'.

Consider the role of individual stress as a precipitant to a depressive episode and from your placement experience and discussion with your mentor, identify the range of potential stressors that can lead to an individual experiencing a depressive episode.

Think of factors that may be physical, psychological or social in nature.

While on placement in the community, consider the role of the environment and how it may play a part in contributing to individual stress.

This activity can help you to achieve knowledge in relation to competencies in NMC Domain 3: Nursing Practice and Decision Making, in particular Competence 3.2 and 3.7.

DSM-IV separates bipolar disorder into two types: Bipolar I and II. To receive a diagnosis of Bipolar I disorder, a person must have at least one occurrence of mania. Mania, the opposite extreme to depression, is characterised by episodes of extreme euphoria; this feeling of high is often accompanied by irresponsible behaviour such as sexual disinhibition and lavish spending, which can be quite destructive to personal relationships, business and finances. They may have elevated self-esteem, flight of ideas, insomnia and be easily distracted. The high, although it may sound appealing, is often fragile and associated with agitation and restlessness, which can result in interpersonal conflict; particularly when challenged by others. The disinhibited behaviour can at times be dangerous and can lead to harm from inappropriate use of drugs and or alcohol. The fluctuations in mood experienced by someone with Bipolar I disorder can lead to sudden swings of mood from elations to depression and vice-versa.

Bipolar II disorder is similar to Bipolar I, in that there are periods of highs that are often followed by periods of depression. The difference with Bipolar II disorder however, is that the periods of mania are less intense and are described as hypomania. People with this condition have similar symptoms but they are not as severe and may not require hospitalisation (Videbeck 2009). People with hypomania can often remain at work, maintain social relationships and therefore do not necessarily require inpatient care. In many cases, they will be seen by their GP, CPN/CMHN or other community-based nurses.

In severe cases of either mania or depression, the symptoms can be such that they will be described as psychotic (see below).

Treatment and care

Medication, commonly known as mood stabilisers, such as lithium carbonate or carbamazepine, can be typically prescribed for this disorder and is the mainstay of pharmacological treatment. Medication reduces the severity and duration of periods of low and high mood. This in turn enables

some people to engage in therapy, which can be useful in helping a sufferer understand the illness and its consequences and thus be better able to know when a manic or depressive episode is imminent and to prepare for this. As with many mental health problems, poor coping skills and lack of social support will make the condition more difficult to cope with.

▮ Student reflection

Consider what resources you had access to on placement that you could have used to learn more about medication, its specific uses, side effects and contraindications.

What strategies could you use in the future to ensure you keep up-to-date with developments in medication? Learning about medication and medication management are core skills for student nurses and they can then engage in delivery of these to patients in their care.

(See NMC (2010) Essential Skills Clusters (ESCs) 33–38, on medicine management for additional learning outcomes to be achieved.)

Prognosis for the individual

The prognosis for people with more severe cases is poor in terms of a 'cure' and many people need to remain on medication for the rest of their lives, with failure to adhere to prescribed medication often resulting in relapse and hospital admission. Medication does assist many people to cope with the condition for long periods without relapse. There is also some evidence to suggest manic episodes slow down because of the natural ageing process (Coryell et al 2009).

Bipolar disorder presents in varying degrees and therefore misdiagnosis and confusion with other mental health problems, particularly mood disorders, can occur. In many circumstances, counselling and family support can be of significant value to people, therefore reducing the reliance on medication.

Major depressive disorder (unipolar depression)

Research by Elder and Mosack (2011) has shown that depression is influenced by both biological and environmental factors. First-degree relatives, regardless of whether they were raised by their relative, have a higher incidence of depression supporting the influence of biological factors. Environmental factors can exacerbate a depressive disorder in significant ways. Factors include stress, lack of a support system and physical illness in self or loved one; viruses can be a significant trigger for depressions in susceptible individuals. Social factors such as legal difficulties, financial struggles and job problems can also play a major role.

Symptoms of the illness

Symptoms of depression include the following:

- Depressed mood such as feelings of sadness, unhappiness or emptiness, often described as a dark cloud that descends over the patient
- Reduced interest in activities they used to find enjoyable
- Disturbances, either not being able to sleep well or sleeping too much, with a loss of energy or feelings of a major drop in energy levels
- Problems with volition, concentration and engaging in conversation as well as reduced levels of attention
- In extreme cases, and not common, patients can experience suicidal ideation and attempt self-harm.

Treatment and care

Treatment can either combine both pharmacotherapy and psychotherapy, and most likely, cognitive behavioural therapy (CBT) or utilise one or other individually. Many people with depressive symptoms who see their GP, will be prescribed antidepressant medication in the first instance. Access to psychological therapies can take several months to acquire due to limitations in service availability. A significant number of people achieve relief by medication alone and expect to see improvement in their mood over the first month of treatment. They may have to continue with the medication for 6 months or more. Medications used to treat this disorder include selective serotonin reuptake inhibitors (SSRI) such as paroxetine. Patients often attribute experiences of physical, emotional and/or sexual abuse as factors that contribute to their depression. Underdeveloped coping skills and other factors such as poverty, social circumstances, housing and unemployment, are also factors that play an important part in the development of a depressive illness. Psychotherapy can help the patient understand the factors that contribute to their depressive illness, whether that is in terms of CBT can help patients deal with the 'here and now' and prepare people to deal more directly with the challenges they experience in their lives (Gallagher-Thompson et al 2008).

Prognosis for the individual

The prognosis for a major depressive disorder tends to be better than other mood disorders in that medication and therapy are very successful in alleviating symptoms. However, for many people, the disorder can become episodic, often caused by stressors that bring back symptoms. This is why it is important that community health professionals, such as the community nurse, CPN and the GP, work closely in partnership to ensure they detect any recurrence of symptoms and ensure that the right interventions are activated as soon as possible. A key issue is that the health professional that detects the relapse may not be the CPN, thus highlighting the importance of knowledge of mental health issues being spread across the primary care team.

Remember when you come across patients in community practice learning, their health problems do not fall neatly into boxes, which often appears to be the case within the confines of a textbook. People present with mixed physical, psychological and social problems that are quite often complicated by family dynamics (Kilbourne et al 2004). The community nurse cannot readily untangle this presentation and has to deal with all aspects of the person's health. Equally, it is wrong to see the patient through a singular lens and in particular, view someone with a mental health problem in a judgemental or stigmatising way.

 Activity

In discussion with your mentor and university tutor, explore the challenges associated with caring for people who have multiple health problems that span both physical and psychological domains. Ensure that you learn the basic principles underpinning both the physical and psychological aspects of the patient's illness in order to be able to deliver holistic care.

■ Reflection

Stigma is an experience that is devaluing and unnecessary

Consider this statement and the potential impact of judgemental attitudes you might have observed on placement and experienced by people with mental health problems in their engagement with health services. What could nurses do to reduce the levels of stigma experienced by people with mental health problems?

The NMC Domain of Professional Values includes two competencies focusing on respecting others and their beliefs and practices: Competence 1.2 and 1.4:

1.2 *All nurses must practise in a holistic, non-judgmental, caring and sensitive manner that avoids assumptions, supports social inclusion; recognises and respects individual choice; and acknowledges diversity. Where necessary, they must challenge inequality, discrimination and exclusion from access to care.*

1.4 *All nurses must work in partnership with service users, carers, families, groups, communities and organisations. They must manage risk, and promote health and wellbeing while aiming to empower choices that promote self-care and safety.*

Consider how learning to reduce the potential for stigma of mental illness will enable you to meet these competencies in practice.

Psychotic disorders (including schizophrenia)

Common characteristics

Psychotic disorders are characterised by symptoms that relate to cognition and perception; thought disorders such as delusions and perceptual disorders such as hallucinations are key features of psychotic disorders.

Delusions are false beliefs that would not normally be held by people of a particular culture; they are not open to reasonable argument and significantly influence a person's ability to function on a day-to-day basis. For example, believing that people are plotting against you when there is no evidence of this, or believing that you have special powers; such as an ability to read other peoples thoughts or that you are some famous person either living or dead, such as the US President or Napoleon.

Hallucinations are false perceptions, sensations that exist in the absence of external stimuli. They can be auditory (hearing), such as voices telling someone what to do; visual (seeing things that are not there); tactile (feeling sensations on your skin that are not there), such as the feeling of bugs crawling on you; olfactory (smelling) or taste.

Psychotic disorders are characterised by a loss of contact with reality and people with schizophrenia and bipolar disorder can be so severely affected by their symptoms that they are unable to separate reality from fantasy. This can be to such an extent that they are a danger to themselves or others. In people with severe depression, psychosis can be manifested by suicidal intent. In people with schizophrenia, it can lead to acts of self-harm or behaviour that shows no regard for personal safety. In people with mania, it can lead to sexual disinhibition and or major personal embarrassment. It is circumstances like this that people may become detainable within hospital, under the relevant mental health legislation.

Schizophrenia

Over the years, a number of theories have emerged in the attempt to explain this disorder. In the 1960s and 1970s, much was written about family dynamics as a cause (Dell 1980). More recently, research evidence points towards biological factors being the most likely factor, with life stressors playing a significant role in whether an individual who is susceptible to the illness actually succumbs (Cannon 2009).

Symptoms

The onset of symptoms of schizophrenia usually follows a period of stress such as beginning university or college or starting a job for the first time. The transition from adolescence to adulthood appears to be a critical period for onset, particularly in males. Typically, the onset occurs slightly later in life for females. Onset that occurs later in life can often be of a paranoid nature, where sufferers are severely incapacitated due to delusions of persecution.

Initial symptoms may include delusions; experiences of thought control or thought insertion and hallucinations; hearing voices either instructional or persecutory, both of which can lead to disorganised, and often bizarre, behaviour and/or speech. Symptoms such as flattening or inappropriate affect (where emotional responses are either lacking or not congruent with the situation) may develop as the condition progresses. Motivational levels can drop, with attention to self-care impeded. Symptoms of schizophrenia tend to be divided into two categories: positive, e.g. hallucinations and delusions; and negative, e.g. the loss of volition, motivation and drive.

Treatment and care

In the acute phase of the illness, medication is the most important part of the treatment, as it can in many cases reduce and sometimes eliminate the psychotic symptoms.

In a number of cases, ongoing medication is required to prevent relapse. Ongoing health and social care input is often needed to assist with daily living skills, financial matters and housing, with CBT helping some sufferers learn better coping skills and improve social and occupational skills.

 Activity

Non-adherence to medication is cited as one of the most common reasons for relapse in people with schizophrenia:

- Discuss with your mentor/tutor and or fellow students the signs that might indicate that a person was failing to take their medication and possibly approaching relapse.
- Why do you think people taking antipsychotic medication stop their medication?

People with a psychotic illness such as schizophrenia can become reluctant to take their medication when they are feeling well. Those who are unfortunate to experience problematic side-effects, e.g. weight gain, a drop in libido, dry mouth, blurred vision and gastrointestinal upset, can feel that they are now well and that they no longer need the medication that causes all the negative effects they experience. It is vital that nurses in the community take every opportunity to educate the patient, and their relatives, about the importance of adherence to medication when well and to notice the signs of deterioration and relapse.

Prognosis for the individual

When compared with many physical conditions, schizophrenia does not have a cure as such, therefore the prognosis is poor for many with this condition. However, medication can be extremely effective against many of the symptoms but

particularly the 'positive' symptoms as mentioned above. The commonly used antipsychotic medications such as flupentixol or haloperidol have been shown to be effective against psychotic symptoms and CBT can help the individual cope with the illness better and improve social functioning. Absence of 'negative' symptoms (flattened affect, loss of volition and poor social interaction) improves the prognosis significantly. Negative symptoms are marginally affected by the antipsychotic medication that is available.

 Activity

People who experience long-term mental health problems such as schizophrenia often have associated health behaviour issues to deal with, such as lack of activity, excessive smoking and poor diet:

- Explore behaviour change models that a nurse may use to help her to work in partnership with such patients to improve their health status.
- Access websites such as: http://www.publichealth.hscni.net/news/spring-positive-mental-health (Public Health Agency) and http://www.nice.org.uk/guidance/index.jsp?action=download&o=44524 to consider the evidence available on behaviour change rationale.

Nurses working in the community are in an excellent position to promote healthy lifestyles across the population and this can be extremely important when caring for people with mental health problems. Whether it is about healthy eating, exercise, reducing smoking, healthy sleeping; all of these and other areas can be problematic for people with mental health problems. This can be due to medication side effects or the symptoms of the illness itself, which can result in reduced motivation and energy levels. In a recent meta-analysis, Robertson et al (2012) were able to identify that walking has a significant effect on depressive symptoms in some patient populations and recommended that further research be carried out specifically within primary care to see how effective exercise might be.

Case study

During your community placement, your mentor organises a short taster experience for you in a mental health resource centre. While on placement there, you are introduced to Frank, who is a 60-year-old man who spent a lot of his younger years in hospital. At a young age, he was diagnosed with schizophrenia and spent many years receiving antipsychotic medication. Frank lives alone in sheltered housing and attends the day centre 3 days per week.

You are asked by your mentor to try to get to know Frank and find out from him how he is coping with meeting his daily needs:

1. From your classroom sessions on communication skills how would you go about building a conversation with Frank?
2. From your knowledge of schizophrenia what sort of challenges would you expect Frank to encounter as he lives alone at home?
3. How could you as a nurse in the community assist Frank to live an independent life?

Make notes of all the answers alongside the questions in your notebook and discuss any areas where you are unclear about the care of Frank, with your mentor and/or personal tutor.

Guidance for answers to the questions on Frank's case study

1. You need to be aware of verbal and non-verbal communication skills
   - Sit in an open position
   - You need to ask open questions
   - Lean slightly forward
   - Maintain appropriate eye contact
   - Try to stay relaxed.
2. Stigma
   - Self-conscious of medication side-effects, such as tremor
   - Reduced motivation towards self-care
   - Poor diet and excess smoking
   - Personal hygiene.
3. Guidance around self-care
   - Medication education
   - Social skills training.

Anxiety disorders

Common characteristics of anxiety disorders

Anxiety disorders encompass a large number of disorders where the primary feature is abnormal or inappropriate anxiety. Anxiety is a normal experience that everyone has from time to time and is key to the 'flight or flight' phenomenon that is seen as a survival mechanism that enables humans in periods of stress, to mobilise energy to deal with threatening situations. When you experience a fright, such as a near miss when driving, you will have felt increased heart rate, tensed muscles and perhaps an acute sense of focus, as you dealt with the immediate threat to your wellbeing. These are all symptoms of anxiety.

These symptoms, particularly the racing heartbeat, tense muscles and rapid breathing, when they occur in the absence of a discernible threat, can be problematic. The absence of both an overt stimuli and a medical cause, meaning that the response is inappropriate, can result in significantly disabling experiences for an individual.

Disorders in this category

- Obsessive-compulsive disorder (OCD)
- Generalised anxiety disorder (GAD)
- Phobias (including social phobia)
- Post-traumatic stress disorder (PTSD).

Obsessive-compulsive disorder (OCD)

The cause of OCD is uncertain and probably relates to the underlying factors that have led to the individual experiencing anxiety. Some of this may relate to either childhood experiences or more recent life experiences. Biological factors may make some people more susceptible to experiencing anxiety but the relationship between biological and psychological factors is not clear.

Symptoms

This condition is characterised by two key features: obsessions (persistent, often irrational and seemingly uncontrollable thoughts) and compulsions (actions that are used to neutralise the obsessions). Critical to understanding this condition is the realisation that the actions are performed as a coping mechanism to deal with the obsessions; the intrusive ideas that intrude into consciousness. A good example of this would be an individual who has thoughts that he is dirty and unclean, which are persistent and uncontrollable. In order to reduce the anxiety caused, he washes his hands numerous times throughout the day, often after touching objects he deems to be contaminated, gaining temporary relief from the thoughts each time. For these behaviours to constitute OCD, it must be disruptive to everyday functioning such as causing skin irritation in someone washing their hands excessively or the inability to leave the house in someone who constantly checks the gas, security, taps, etc., because of a fear that something catastrophic will happen if they leave the house and they have forgotten to do something.

Treatment and care

The mainstay of treatment for OCD is CBT, often combined with medication in the form of SSRI antidepressants such as paroxetine. CBT can be useful in helping sufferers to learn new ways to feel more in control and cope better with stressors. CBT will focus on assisting the patient to realise that the anticipated catastrophes that are associated with the obsessive ideas are not a reality and for them to gradually face up to the challenges and cope independently. Psychotherapy can assist people to explore the underlying issues associated with the obsessive thoughts.

Prognosis for the individual

This condition can become deep rooted in individuals who may have experienced significant disturbances to their lives over a number of years before seeking help, if they indeed seek help. In some cases, it is relatives that put pressure on sufferers to seek help. The condition can have far-reaching impacts on family life, particularly that of children who may not be able to experience normal family life if one of their parents is affected. Medication can help along with CBT but access to the latter can prove problematic if waiting lists are long. One programme that has helped a number of patients and is available through a GP is 'Beating the Blues', see: http://www. beatingtheblues.co.uk/.

General anxiety disorder (GAD)

GAD is a condition where an individual experiences a wide range of anxiety symptoms usually triggered by the stressors of everyday life. GAD seems to be caused by a combination of biological and psychological, otherwise known as predisposing factors, and psychological precipitating factors (triggers). Some individuals do appear more biologically susceptible to anxiety and some have personality traits that make them more prone to having a negative response to stress.

Symptoms

The symptoms of GAD can be wide ranging. GAD can manifest itself as an acute phenomenon, whereby panic is the key feature or a more chronic form, where the sufferer experiences a wide range of physiological experiences such as increased heart rate, blurred vision, excess sweating, gastrointestinal disturbance, sleep disturbance, tremor, shortness of breath and muscle pains. Panic is characterised by hyperventilation, feelings of impending doom, racing heartbeat to the extent they think they are going to have a heart attack and die. Panic attacks will often result in the sufferer collapsing or fleeing the locality.

Treatment and care

The mainstay of treatment for GAD and panic attacks is behavioural with some assistance from anxiolytic medication. CBT teaches individuals to cope with the symptoms of anxiety by helping them to challenge the disordered thinking that leads to negative reactions to stress. Therapy also focuses on helping people cope more effectively with the interpersonal aspects of their lives and can involve activities such as assertiveness training.

Prognosis for the individual

With CBT treatment, sufferers can substantially improve the quality of their life. Accepting the major role played by personality traits in the development of GAD, the focus on treatment is the development of new coping skills. Where this works well, within the context of a supportive personal and social network, most people will do well but there may be a propensity for the condition to return if the stressors in an individual's life recur. Ongoing therapy may be required to support people in such circumstances.

 Activity

Relaxation therapy is often identified as a self-help strategy for people who suffer from anxiety-related health problems.

Review your knowledge of the autonomic nervous system and explain how the symptoms of anxiety occur and why relaxation therapy can help an individual to counteract these symptoms.

Make notes about the relationship between the physical and psychological changes that take place in anxiety problems.

Phobias and simple phobias (including social phobia)

Phobic illness can often be triggered, in susceptible individuals, by a traumatic event, whether at a conscious or subconscious level. It is an inappropriate or exaggerated reaction to an object or situation, which then leads to avoidance. Social phobia is a condition where people who engage in social activity as part of their everyday life become unable to do so because of the fear of an expected catastrophe, the avoidance becoming the key problem.

Symptoms

Symptoms include an acute anxiety reaction and or avoidance triggered by an identified stimulus, e.g. open spaces, insects, enclosed spaces and crowded spaces. To receive a diagnosis of phobic disorder, the symptoms must be disruptive to everyday functioning such as giving up a job because you have to cross a bridge to get to work. The critical factor is the resultant avoidance; the consequence of the anxiety that ultimately becomes life disrupting.

Treatment and care

Treatment is based on behavioural principles, where the individual is exposed to the fear by the therapist in a number of ways, some of which are graded in nature, other more direct. The therapist guides the client through activities where anxiety management techniques are learned to enable the sufferers to cope and confront the anticipated fear stimulus. As with OCD, SSRI antidepressant medication can be used to augment behavioural therapy.

Prognosis for the individual

As with OCD, phobias can go on for years without effective treatment and so cause long-term damage to family dynamics and functioning. Where treatment is introduced, the prognosis is good with relapses often managed effectively by short periods of 'top-up' support from a therapist.

 Activity

Cognitive behavioural therapy is the most widely used intervention to support patients experiencing both phobias and OCD:

- Consider and discuss with your mentor/tutor and fellow students how phobias and or OCD can impact on a family's functioning and outline how the nurse can work with family members as partners and co-therapists in care.

- If possible, discuss with a service user who experiences OCD behaviour, what it is like to live with this problem and how it affects their lives and those of others.

Post-traumatic stress disorder (PTSD)

As the diagnosis suggests, PTSD is triggered by a traumatic event that causes intense fear and/or helplessness in an individual. The symptoms usually develop soon after the event, but may appear many years later. Circumstances that can lead to PTSD might be: involvement in an accident; exposure to warfare; exposure to acts of terrorism; any situation where an individual's life has been threatened. The triggers are often of a magnitude usually only experienced by a small number of people in society but it is not uncommon to see it in situations such as natural disasters and warfare. To receive a diagnosis of PTSD, the symptoms should be present for at least 1 month.

Symptoms

Symptoms include; flashbacks where the sufferer feels as if they are actually in the traumatic situation again; sleep disturbance with re-experiencing the trauma through nightmares; ruminative thoughts. Avoidance is a key feature where an individual avoids situations and people who remind him or her about the traumatic event, e.g. a person experiencing PTSD after a serious car accident might avoid driving. Finally, there is increased anxiety and irritability in general, possibly with a heightened startle response. Sufferers can become aggressive, demonstrating low tolerance to stress.

Treatment and care

The main approach to treatment is based on CBT, with anxiety management and cognitive therapy being central to the approach. CBT is designed to help people understand their reaction to stress and to contextualise their anxiety reaction and to learn coping skills to deal with the triggers and avoidance. As with all anxiety-related conditions, medications such as anxiolytics (diazepam and chlordiazepoxide) can help alleviate some symptoms during the treatment process, but care should be taken due to the addictive potential of these drugs.

Prognosis for the individual

Prognosis can vary depending on the nature of the trauma – for acute trauma of a one-off nature, such as a car accident, patients often respond well to treatment. Where trauma is of a more chronic nature, such as sexual abuse, exposure to war or where the magnitude of the trauma was extensive, such as being kidnapped or raped, the prognosis can sometimes be less positive.

 Activity

Consider how PTSD may impact on the function of a family unit.

You may want to think particularly about issues such as the long-term nature of the effects and sometimes delayed onset.

From your knowledge of 'talking therapies', consider which interventions may be particularly relevant in such cases. Discuss with your mentor during placement and access the Mental Health Foundation Website to learn more about this approach to care: http://www.mentalhealth.org.uk/help-information/mental-health-a-z/T/talking-therapies (accessed July 2012).

Addictive disorders

There are two elements to addictive disorders: that of addiction and that of abuse. Nurses encounter many people who have substance misuse problems due to either of these two categories. Addiction is characterised by a physical dependence on a substance, whereas abuse may not constitute addiction. Physical dependence is when the body reacts, sometimes quite dramatically, to the removal of the drug. Both abuse and addiction can, for example, lead to an individual presenting with ulcerated wounds from infected injection sites. As a nurse, you may be caring for the consequences of abuse/addiction but not necessarily the substance problem itself. A substance can be anything ingested in order to produce a high, alter one's senses or otherwise affect functioning. Alcohol is probably the most common substance of abuse/addiction but other drugs such as

heroin, cannabis and cocaine are also major drugs of concern. DSM-IV also recognises nicotine and caffeine as drugs of addiction.

Disorders in this category

The most commonly held theories on addiction relate to individuals' use of substances as a means to cover up or gain relief from problems such as relationship difficulties, stress, financial problems or coping with the experience of other mental health conditions, such as depression or schizophrenia. There is also evidence to indicate a genetic predisposition to addictive behaviour as a way of coping with stress.

Symptoms
According to DSM-IV, a pattern of substance use leading to significant impairment in social and or physical functioning, one of the following must be present within a 12-month period:
- Recurrent use resulting in a failure to fulfill major obligations at work, school or home
- Recurrent use in situations which are physically hazardous, e.g. driving while intoxicated
- Legal problems resulting from recurrent use
- Continued use, despite significant social or interpersonal problems caused by the substance use.

The symptoms do not meet the criteria for substance dependence as abuse is a part of this disorder.

Treatment and care
Whether the approach adopted is one of controlled use (such as controlled drinking or methadone replacement in heroin addiction) or abstinence, research suggests that no treatment method is superior, but that social support is very important. An openness to accept the abuse as a problem and a willingness to engage in treatment is also paramount in successfully treating the illness. The results of organisations such as Alcoholic Anonymous, Alateen and

Narcotics Anonymous, have proven better than average at reducing relapse.

Prognosis for the individual

The prognosis for people who abuse alcohol or drugs is extremely variable. Social support often plays a critical role in enabling individuals to remain abstinent. People often have cycles of abstinence and misuse that punctuate their lives, often associated with stressors in their lives, whether they are the cause of the relapse or a result of their relapse.

 Activity

In reviewing the role alcohol plays in the admission of people to hospital with physical health problems, discuss with your mentor and fellow students the role of the community nurse in both detecting alcohol/drug-related problems and reducing admissions to hospital.

The following NICE resource will give you an excellent starting point for your research in alcohol use disorders and physical complications: http://guidance.nice.org.uk/CG100/QuickRefGuide/pdf/English

Remember to think about what the community nurse can do to prevent health problems becoming worse for the person.

Sleep disorders

Common characteristics

There are two main categories of sleep disorder: dyssomnias and parasomnias, and they make up the **primary** disorders of sleep. This term is used to differentiate these particular sleep disorders from those that are associated with other factors such mental health or physical problems. **Dyssomnias** are those disorders relating to the amount, quality and timing of sleep.

Parasomnias relate to abnormal behaviour or physiological events that occur during the process of sleep or sleep–wake transitions, such as sleep walking and hypnagogic hallucinations.

Primary insomnia

The cause of primary insomnia can vary from individual to individual but often people possess a preoccupation with the inability to sleep or excessive worry about sleep, which in turn becomes a vicious circle where an individual believes they cannot get off to sleep, so they don't. Up to 10% of adults and up to 25% of elderly adults experience primary insomnia and it appears slightly more common among women.

Symptoms

To meet the criteria for a diagnosis of primary insomnia, at least one of the following should apply:
- Difficulty in falling asleep
- Difficulty remaining asleep
- Receiving restorative sleep for a period no less than 1 month.

The disturbance in sleep must affect social, occupational or other important functions in a significant manner and not appear as a consequence of another mental or medical disorder or during the use of alcohol, medication or other substances.

Treatment and care

The main focus of treatment is the restoration of a normal sleep cycle. It involves learning relaxation techniques and the establishment of a regular behaviour pattern associated with preparing for sleep. The individual should establish a routine based on a set bedtime and wakening time and must adhere to this at all times, and there should be no sleeping outwith this routine. For example, bedtime can be set at 11 pm each night and getting out of bed set at 6 am every morning, regardless of the amount of sleep that occurs. The individual should engage in activity, healthy eating and then use relaxation techniques prior to the scheduled sleep time and avoid napping.

Prognosis for the individual
With the goal of treatment being the establishment of a normal sleep pattern, the refreshment that acts as positive feedback gives encouragement to adopt the new pattern of sleeping. When combined with addressing stressors and improved activity and diet, the prognosis for most is very good.

Activity

'Sleep hygiene' is a term referred to in the literature (Chen et al 2010) and on some online support sites, e.g. http://www.patient.co.uk/health/Insomnia-Poor-Sleep.htm

Explore this issue further and discuss your findings with your mentor/tutor.

Guidance for your answers to the questions on Janice's case study
1. Conclusions
   - Janice is finding having two toddlers in the house and living on her own very challenging
   - This is affecting her self-esteem
   - She is coping with the children but is not taking care of herself
   - She is possibly depressed
   - Low mood, lack of self-care, poor motivation
   - She is smoking excessively and the children may be affected by passive smoking.
2. Advice
   - Try to establish a routine in the house
   - Try to take some exercise
   - Take the children to the park; go to a children's adventure area
   - Try to get some 'Janice' time, for exercise and meeting friends
   - Find out about nursery provision or mother and toddler groups.
   - Sleep hygiene: avoid coffee and other stimulants and alcohol, particularly late at night; avoid late meals; avoid excessively long periods of sleep during the day; exercise during the day; choose a regular bedtime; take a warm milky drink prior to bedtime; get some fresh air during the day; reduce smoking; keep a well ventilated and not too hot bedroom.

Case study

While on placement with a public health nurse, you visit a household where there is a single mother, Janice, who has two toddler children, Darren, aged 15 months and Stephen, aged 3. You are there to check up on the children's developmental milestones, as Janice has not been to the clinic for at least 9 months. The children are lively when you arrive in the house and are both very keen for you to play with them. On further observation, you note that Janice looks tired and hasn't been taking care of herself; her hair is untidy, her clothes dirty and there is evidence that she has been smoking excessively in the house. Janice does not have any major financial problems.

1. What conclusion might you draw from your observations?

   On talking with Janice you discover that she has not been sleeping well and finds looking after the children increasingly difficult. You also find out that she has found it challenging to get out of the house and take the children for a walk.

2. What advice can you give to Janice that would help her address some of the challenges in her life?

- Advise regarding passive smoking. Provide guidance on smoking cessation programmes.

Nursing interventions in the community

Clinical interventions for people with mental health problems should be based upon the best available evidence. Both the NHS in Scotland and the rest of the UK use clinical guidelines: SIGN (Scottish Intercollegiate Guideline Network) and NICE (National Institute for Health and Clinical Excellence); both sets of guidelines are used across the UK where one country does not have specific guidelines for a condition or illness.

Of particular interest is the SIGN guideline for the non-pharmaceutical treatment of depression, which will give you an excellent and evidence-based insight to those treatments that are appropriate for someone with depression (SIGN 2010). Recommendations are graded A, B, C, D, to indicate the strength of the supporting evidence, with A being the strongest.

 Activity

Consider the interventions proposed by SIGN 114 shown in Table 8.2 with key in Table 8.3. Carry out some independent study in addition to reading both SIGN and NICE guidelines in detail.

Address the following key questions:

- Which therapies seem to work the best for people with depression and why?
- What are the potential pitfalls and benefits associated with natural/herbal remedies?
- What are the pitfalls and potential benefits of patients seeking guidance and support on the internet? Consider both self-help sites and social networking sites.

Table 8.2 Non-pharmaceutical treatment of depression

This list of all recommendations from the guideline are summarised below, to assist integration of SIGN recommendations into local audit or pathway documents, with the aim of supporting their implementation. The wording of the recommendations should not be changed.

Behavioural activation

A   Behavioural activation is recommended as a treatment option for patients with depression.

Cognitive behavioural therapy

A   Individual CBT is recommended as a treatment option for patients with depression.

Interpersonal therapy

A   Interpersonal therapy is recommended as a treatment option for patients with depression.

Mindfulness-based cognitive therapy

B   Mindfulness-based cognitive therapy in a group setting may be considered as a treatment option to reduce relapse in patients with depression who have had three or more episodes.

Problem-solving therapy

B   Problem-solving therapy may be considered as a treatment option for patients with depression.

Psychodynamic psychotherapy

B   Short-term psychodynamic psychotherapy may be considered as a treatment option for patients with depression.

Self-help

A   Guided self-help based on CBT or behavioural principles is recommended as a treatment option for patients with depression.

Computerised self-help

A   Within the context of guided self-help, computerised CBT is recommended as a treatment option for patients with depression.

Activity

B   Structured activity may be considered as a treatment option for patients with depression.

Table 8.3 Scottish Intercollegiate Guidelines Network (SIGN) key to evidence statements and grades of recommendations

Levels of evidence

1++	High-quality meta-analyses, systematic reviews of RCTs or RCTs with a very low risk of bias
1+	Well-conducted meta-analyses, systematic reviews or RCTs with a low risk of bias
1−	Meta-analyses, systematic reviews or RCTs with a high risk of bias
2++	High-quality systematic reviews of case–control or cohort studies
	High-quality case–control or cohort studies with a very low risk of confounding or bias and a high probability that the relationship is causal
2+	Well-conducted case–control or cohort studies with a low risk of confounding or bias and a moderate probability that the relationship is causal
2	Case–control or cohort studies with a high risk of confounding or bias and a significant risk that the relationship is not causal
3	Non-analytic studies, e.g. case reports, case series
4	Expert opinion

Grades of recommendation

Note: The grade of recommendation relates to the strength of the evidence on which the recommendation is based. It does not reflect the clinical importance of the recommendation.

A   At least one meta-analysis, systematic review or RCT rated as 1++, and directly applicable to the target population; or

     A body of evidence consisting principally of studies rated as 1+, directly applicable to the target population, and demonstrating overall consistency of results

B   A body of evidence including studies rated as 2++, directly applicable to the target population, and demonstrating overall consistency of results; or

     Extrapolated evidence from studies rated as 1++ or 1+

C   A body of evidence including studies rated as 2+, directly applicable to the target population and demonstrating overall consistency of results; or

     Extrapolated evidence from studies rated as 2++

D   Evidence level 3 or 4; or

     Extrapolated evidence from studies rated as 2+

Good practice points

 Recommended best practice based on the clinical experience of the guideline development group.

Dementia

Many people experience forgetfulness as they grow old. In fact it is more common than not as one progresses through their 50s and into the later years of life. Dementia, in its many forms is a clearly defined set of illnesses with features that are distinct and not part of the normal ageing process. Older people therefore experience the processes of normal ageing which are generally characterised by a physical and mental slowing down. What sets dementia apart from normal ageing is the progressive nature of the symptoms and in some cases, the rapid progression and fluctuating nature. When someone develops dementia, it is often mistaken for normal ageing but it must be recognised that dementia, whatever the cause, is not part of normal ageing. In most cases, the onset of dementia occurs in people aged 70 and above. It is uncommon in people under the age of 60

but where this does occur, it can often be aggressively progressive; in such cases, the term pre-senile dementia is used.

Alzheimer's disease is the most common form of dementia, affecting around half a million people in the UK. People who suffer from this condition experience a general decline in their mental functioning due to the gradual death of brain cells, as well as a reduction in certain neurotransmitter chemicals within the brain. The main features of Alzheimer's disease are:

- Loss of memory
- Mood changes
- Problems with communication and reasoning.

Vascular dementia is a form of dementia that is related to fluctuating levels of blood supply within the brain. This can be due to small strokes caused by either small haemorrhages or microscopic blood clots that result in the death of brain cells and differs in its presentation from Alzheimer's disease mainly by its fluctuating nature. Vascular dementia affects different people in different ways and the speed of the progression varies from person to person. Many symptoms are similar to those of other types of dementia. However, people with vascular dementia may particularly experience:

- problems with concentrating and communicating
- symptoms of stroke, such as physical weakness or paralysis
- memory problems (although this may not be the first symptom)
- a 'stepped' progression, with symptoms remaining at a constant level and then suddenly deteriorating
- periods of acute confusion.

In some circumstances, people can suffer from a combination of both Alzheimer's and vascular dementia and it is not uncommon for depression to feature, particularly in the early stages of the illnesses.

The Alzheimer's Society Website is an excellent resource for information and guidance on all forms of dementia: http://www.alzheimers.org.uk.

DSM-IV describes dementia as the development of multiple cognitive deficits manifested by both memory impairment (impaired ability to learn new information or to recall previously learned information) and one or more of the following cognitive disturbances:

- Aphasia (language disturbance)
- Apraxia (impaired ability to carry out motor activities, despite intact motor function)
- Agnosia (failure to recognise or identify objects, despite intact sensory function)
- Disturbance in executive functioning (i.e. planning, organising, sequencing, abstracting).

The cognitive deficits described above cause significant impairment in social or occupational functioning and represent a significant decline from previous levels of functioning. The course is characterised by

gradual onset and continuing cognitive decline.

The cognitive deficits are not due to any of the following:

- Other central nervous system conditions that cause progressive deficits in memory and cognition (e.g. cerebrovascular disease, Parkinson's disease, Huntington's disease, subdural haematoma, normal-pressure hydrocephalus, brain tumour)
- Systemic conditions that are known to cause dementia (e.g. hypothyroidism, vitamin B or folic acid deficiency, niacin deficiency, hypercalcaemia, neurosyphilis, HIV infection)
- Substance-induced conditions.

The deficits do not occur exclusively during the course of a delirium.

Treatment and care

Many people with dementia are cared for at home by family carers with support provided by a range of health and social care professionals, including specialist community mental health nurse input. Care is often a combination of social support in the home with periods of attendance at a day care facility. The nurse's role in caring for someone with dementia is focused on supporting both the sufferer and their immediate family. Carers can find life extremely tiring and stressful when their loved one has a tendency to wander, turn day into night and often continually seek reassurance. Respite care can be an important part of care packages, enabling family carers to go on caring for as long as they possibly can. Most families want to care for their loved ones at home and avoid nursing/care home or hospital care but inevitably some form of institutional care is required.

The key to supporting families with a dementia sufferer is understanding and respect. The nurse should strive to ensure that individuals retain their dignity in circumstances that are often challenging, confusing, frightening and at times, dehumanising. Short-term memory loss can be a frightening experience, particularly in the early stages of dementia, thus it is important to support individuals to retain their sense of identity and feeling of self-worth.

   Activity

Explore the literature and relevant websites to see what strategies nurses and carers can employ to support individuals with dementia to retain a sense of self-worth and dignity.

Discuss with your mentor and fellow students, strategies, supported by evidence, that promote memory retention and orientation.

You may find it helpful to explore both NICE and SIGN 2006 guidelines to learn more about the recommendations and evidence base to support care of people with dementia:

SIGN: http://www.sign.ac.uk/pdf/sign86.pdf

NICE: http://www.nice.org.uk/CG42

Prognosis for the individual

The prognosis for any form of dementia is poor. It is a progressive and life-shortening condition. People with vascular dementia often have further complications due to vascular disease affecting other organs in the body. As a result, their condition may fluctuate as they experience transient ischaemic attacks, ultimately succumbing to a major stroke or organ failure such as heart or renal failure. Many illnesses that previously caused death in younger people, such as cancers, have become increasingly treatable, with the consequence that people living longer are more likely to suffer from dementia and experience a range of other conditions such as type 2 diabetes, renal failure and arthritis. This multiple pathology results in increasingly more complex healthcare scenarios, which are challenging for both sufferers and carers alike.

Activity

Discuss with your mentor the challenges experienced by health and social care professionals in ensuring people with dementia receive care and support in their homes that maintains their dignity and ensures their safety.

Case study

While on placement with a district nurse, you are visiting a patient's home to assist an elderly gentleman called Peter, who has type 2 diabetes, and the nurse is giving him some advice on his diet and foot care. You have been to the house on two occasions before and Peter recognises you and you seem to be getting on well with him. Peter tells you and the district nurse that his wife has been getting increasingly more forgetful and that she was recently at the hospital where she received a diagnosis of Alzheimer's disease. Peter is finding it increasingly more difficult to cope with Helen on his own, as she tends to forget that she has put food in the oven and sometimes goes out of the house and has to be brought back by one of the neighbours. Peter is quite anxious about all of this and is asking for some advice:

1. Consider what advice and guidance a nurse might be able to give Peter to help him cope with Helen's deteriorating mental state.

Guidance for answers to the question on Peter's case study

- Provide reassurance to Peter but also make sure he understands the progressive nature of the condition
- Try to establish a routine with Helen

- Report back to the family GP and seek additional specialist nurse input and or social care input
- Find out about day centres/drop in centres, so that Peter and Helen can get a break from the house and meet others
- Explain Helen's behaviours to Peter so that he may understand better.

Legal aspects of mental health

Mental health legislation differs across the four countries of the UK and in particular between Scotland and England. In England and Wales, the Mental Health Act 2007 and the Mental Capacity Act 2005 are the main pieces of legislation that govern the detention and treatment of people with mental illness and or mental incapacity.

In Scotland, the main pieces of legislation are the Mental Health (Care and Treatment) (Scotland) Act 2003 and the Adults with Incapacity (Scotland) Act 2000. In Northern Ireland, the main piece of legislation is the Mental Health NI Order (1986). Mental capacity legislation is currently being considered.

Mental health legislation tends to deal predominantly with people who have mental health problems of a psychotic nature. Capacity, sometimes referred to as incapacity, legislation is designed to protect the interests of people with dementia or other illnesses that result in progressive or sudden loss of mental capacity. It is this type of legislation that deals with issues such as power of attorney and guardianship. In addition to covering people with dementia, the legislation is used to support people with a learning disability.

With regard to people with psychotic disorders such as schizophrenia and bipolar disorder, the use of mental health legislation is reserved for circumstances where an individual is a danger to himself or others; circumstances where insight is severely compromised and where hospital care is deemed essential to ensure treatment. This can result in detention in hospital initially for a short period, commonly referred to as emergency detention, and for longer periods where detention against the person's wishes is deemed necessary and may last for a period of weeks or months. The legislation also allows for compulsory treatment in the community, where people are obliged to adhere to an agreed treatment plan.

The whole focus of the legislation is to protect the person from abuse and harm but also to ensure any loss of liberty is for as limited a period of time as possible. People's rights are paramount at all times and health and social care practitioners are constantly mindful of this fact when considering the extensive powers that exist within the legislation.

Activity

1. Access the relevant Department of Health websites and download the relevant guides to the mental health and capacity legislation in the UK.

2. When on placement, discuss with your mentor the relevant mental health legislation that applies to the patients in your care. In particular, explore the following:
   - Adults with incapacity
   - Emergency detention
   - Community treatment.

3. Access the websites related to mental health and capacity in other countries and compare them to those in the UK.

Summary of learning points from this chapter

The student should have gained:
- knowledge of a range of mental health problems which may affect people living in the community
- an understanding of the role of the community mental health nurse and other members of the team caring for the mental health and wellbeing of people in the community
- an understanding of the importance of recognising mental health problems in the community and ensuring effective care is provided
- knowledge of treatment options available in the community for individuals with a mental health problem.

References

American Psychiatric Association, 1994. Diagnostic and statistical manual of mental disorders, fourth ed. APA, Washington DC.

Cannon, T.D., 2009. What is the role of theories in the study of schizophrenia? Schizophr. Bull. 35 (3), 563–567.

Chen, P., Kuo, H., Chueh, K., 2010. Sleep hygiene education: efficacy on sleep quality in working women. J. Nurs. Res. 18 (4), 283–289.

Coryell, W., Roy, J., Carver, L.A., 2009. Age transitions in the course of bipolar I disorder. Psychological Medicine: Journal of Research in Psychiatry and the Allied Sciences 39 (8), 1247–1252.

Dell, P.F., 1980. Researching the family theories of schizophrenia: an exercise in epistemological confusion. Fam. Process 19 (4), 321–335.

Elder, B.L., Mosack, V., 2011. Genetics of depression: an overview of the current science. Issues Ment. Health Nurs. 32 (4), 192–202.

Gallagher-Thompson, D., Steffen, A.M., Thompson, L.W. (Eds.), 2008. Handbook of behavioral and cognitive therapies with older adults. Springer Science and Business Media, New York.

Kilbourne, A.M., Cornelius, J.R., Xiaoyan, H., et al., 2004. Burden of general medical conditions among individuals with bipolar disorder. Bipolar Disord. 6 (5), 368–373.

NHS, 2009. Adult psychiatric morbidity in England, 2007: results of a household survey. NHS Information Centre for Health and Social Care, Leeds.

NHS Tayside Nursing Services, Role of the CPN. Online. Available at: http:// www.nhstayside.scot.nhs.uk/services/ nursing/index.shtml (accessed Jan 2013).

NMC, 2010. Standards for pre-registration nursing education. Online. Available at: http://standards.nmc-uk.org/ PublishedDocuments/Standards%20for %20pre-registration%20nursing% 20education%2016082010.pdf.

Robertson, R., Robertson, A., Jepson, R., et al., 2012. Walking for depression or depressive symptoms: a systematic review and meta-analysis. Mental Health and Physical Activity 5 (1), 66–75.

Scottish Intercollegiate Guideline Network (SIGN), 2006. Management of patients with dementia. Guideline No. 86. SIGN, Edinburgh.

Scottish Intercollegiate Guideline Network (SIGN), 2010. Non-pharmaceutical management of depression. Guideline No. 114. SIGN, Edinburgh.

Stacey, G., Felton, A., Bonham, P., 2012. Placement learning in mental health nursing. Bailliere Tindall, London.

Videbeck, S., 2009. Mental health nursing. Lippincott, Williams and Wilkins, London pp. 297–337.

World Health Organization (WHO), 1993. The ICD-10 classification of mental and behavioural disorders: Diagnostic criteria for research. WHO, Geneva.

Further reading

Griffith, R., Tengnah, C., 2010. Law and professional issues in nursing, second ed. Learning Matters, Exeter.

Hardy, S., Gray, R., 2012. The primary care guide to mental health: a practical and theoretical guide for nurses and AHPs. M&K Update, Keswick.

Thornicroft, G., Szmukler, G., Mueser, K.T. et al. (Eds.), 2011. Oxford textbook of community mental health. Oxford University Press, Oxford.

Wrycraft, N., 2009. An introduction to mental health nursing. Open University Press, Maidenhead.

Websites

Mental Health Foundation, http://www.mentalhealth.org.uk.

National Institute for Health and Clinical Excellence (NICE) Guidelines, http://www.nice.org.uk/guidance/cg/published/index.jsp?d-16544-p=2. Anxiety, depression in adults, bipolar disorder, depression with a chronic physical health problem, obsessive compulsive disorder and body dysmorphic disorder, psychosis with coexisting substance misuse, schizophrenia, drug misuse, alcohol dependence and harmful alcohol use, alcohol use disorders, physical complications.

SIGN (Scottish Intercollegiate Guideline Network), http://www.sign.ac.uk/guidelines/published/index.html.
- Non-pharmaceutical management of depression
- Management of patients with dementia
- Bipolar affective disorder
- The management of harmful drinking and alcohol dependence in primary care
- Postnatal depression and puerperal psychosis
- Psychosocial interventions in the management of schizophrenia.

Section 3. Professional issues

9 Communication in community practice

CHAPTER AIMS

- To revise the student nurse's communication skills in relation to assessment of a client
- To develop knowledge and understanding of the specific communication skills required in giving advice and support by telephone, including nurse triage
- To examine the skills required in teaching clients and carers
- To review the teaching skills in health promotion
- To review the importance of record-keeping and its significance in promoting effective communication in community practice
- To examine the utilisation of telehealth and telecare strategies to support patients

Introduction

Through a variety of activities and case studies, a variety of communication strategies will be examined to equip you with a greater understanding of the range of responsibilities you have as a student nurse, particularly with regard to communication.

The NMC identifies communication and interpersonal skills (NMC Standards: Domain 2) as one of the core competencies for entry to the register, and state that:

All nurses must use excellent communication and interpersonal skills. Their communications must always be safe, effective, compassionate and respectful. They must communicate effectively using a wide range of strategies and interventions including the effective use of communication technologies. Where people have a disability, nurses must be able to work service users to obtain the information needed to make reasonable adjustments that promote optimum health and enable equal access to services.

NMC (2010: 15)

Activity

Access the NMC for Pre-Registration Nursing Education (http://standards. nmc-uk.org) and consider the competencies within Domain 2: Communication and Interpersonal Skills. With your mentor, try to identify examples within your community learning experience which will demonstrate your progress or achievement with each of the competencies. Each of the four fields of practice pathways have both generic and field-specific competencies to achieve at key points at the end of Year 1, Year 2, and Year 3. Please refer to these as well as those that are specific to your own university curriculum expectations.

Communicating with clients and carers

Communication is an interactive process, which consists of the significant exchange, through verbal or non-verbal means, of important information that may include thoughts or emotions; this can include the written word as well as face-to-face interactions. Communication skills are essential to develop rapport with the client and to facilitate comprehensive data collection with the intention of developing an appropriate schedule of care to meet the client's needs (Webb 2011). Developing a therapeutic relationship to achieve this requires a variety of communication skills such as the ability to initiate discussion, listen and respond appropriately, reassure, reduce anxiety, empathise. Effective questioning is also a skill which helps to determine the client's perception of the problem, facilitating questions from the client is also essential to provide an opportunity to explore their concerns. Careful observation of body language such as facial expression and the professional's awareness of body language and the therapeutic use of touch are also essential components of effectively communicating. Remember that communication is two-way, the client is also reading the body language of the practitioner. Good communication skills are also essential in the facilitation of liaison with other professionals and services and in the promotion of continuity of care (Webb 2011).

 Activity

Reference was made in Chapter 6 to the Report of the Health Service Ombudsman on 10 investigations into NHS care of older people. Access this report at: http://www.ombudsman.org. uk/care-and-compassion and review some of the case studies. In what way could any of the incidents be attributed to ineffective communication?

The report refers to a 'theme of poor communication', which appears within most of the case studies; examples of this include lack of communication with relatives of the seriousness of their loved one's condition; failure to inform relevant personnel about discharge arrangements; and failure to establish patients' concerns.

 Activity

Reflect on the different client/ practitioner interactions you have encountered during your community practice experience and consider if there are different stages to the process of interaction. Also re-visit Chapter 5 regarding patient assessment.

Similar to most first nurse–client interactions, one of the aims of the first encounter is to develop a rapport. You may have mentioned friendliness and calmness to portray this. It is important to have time: the first visit, if possible, should be planned taking this into account. You may have referred to the commencement of the interaction as the 'introductory' phase, where the practitioner introduces themselves and in the community context, this will also include how the practitioner is invited into the person's home. An example of this interaction is given in Chapter 3.

Once the introductory aspects of home visiting are addressed, the next stage includes questioning and listening to find out the client's immediate problem, concerns and expectations. It is important to listen to the client's 'narrative' about their experiences. This requires the practitioner's skills to initiate discussion, to listen effectively and then to summarise the key issues (Miller & Webb 2011). The skills of questioning will be required again to gather more data in relation to the client's needs; this will usually include general observations about the client and if required, clinical examination. Once this has been achieved, information can be reviewed and checked with the client and in collaboration with the client, a plan of care with achievable aims and objectives can be devised. The way you conclude your first home visit is important and can determine future visits. This is an opportunity to summarise the plan of action following the visit, to give information regarding the time and purpose of the next visit and to give contact details should the client or carer need to get in touch before the next visit.

Good listening skills are an essential component of the practitioner's communication skills and are particularly significant when attempting to plan appropriate individualised palliative care. Listening to the clients' personal wishes and beliefs to develop understanding of their perspective regarding their situation will greatly assist in the development of appropriate care. Reaching a satisfactory plan of action from the client's perspective will only be achieved by listening, discussing and negotiating.

Hamilton and Martin (2007) have developed a framework for effective communication skills practice, this includes the following:

1. **Interact** with the patient: this stage usually commences the assessment process, the nurse at this stage is using a variety of communication skills, to gather relevant information, help put the patient at ease or reassure patient. Skills such as questioning, reflecting, listening and summarising are required at this stage. Remember that within the community setting, this stage may occur within the client's home; this creates an additional aspect to the consultation, the practitioner is also observing the surroundings and assessing the 'dynamics' of family life.

2. Establish the **Intention** of the interaction: nurses should remember the 'goal' of communication to maximise the interaction; this usually includes gathering data related to physical and psychological need.

3. Decide on the **Intervention** to be used: nurses will use a variety of skills to reassure a client or show concern.

4. Assess the **Impact** of the interventions: nurses should always reflect on interactions to evaluate.

5. Evaluate the **Implications** of the subsequent information obtained and then act accordingly.

Hamilton and Martin (2007) also summarise the communication skills of the nurse using the acronym **EDUCATE**:

E. Engagement: by engaging with clients nurses can reassure

D. Demonstration of skills: the safe and proficient delivery of a variety of clinical skills also demonstrates to the client the professional competence of the practitioner

U. Understanding: practitioners as far as possible should attempt to empathise, i.e. to consider the experience from the client's perspective

C. Clarification, Communication, Collaboration, Confidentiality: nurses should clarify their role with clients and colleagues, collaborate efficiently to enable effective multidisciplinary team working and must adhere to their professional code of conduct regarding the boundaries of confidentiality

A. Assessment and the ability to Adapt: nurses must continually observe and communicate with the client to adapt to changing needs and problems as they arise

T. Teaching: nurses need to educate and inform clients, carers and colleagues

E. Evaluation: nurses must evaluate the results of their interactions by reflecting on the skills they have used and the impact of such interventions.

Information giving

Within the context of managing long-term conditions, community practitioners are often required to communicate multifarious information to patients. Such information may include factors related to treatment regimes, advice regarding diet, rest and exercise or instructions regarding medication – often this information is delivered in a face-to-face meeting. This kind of interaction with the patient provides the practitioner with a valuable opportunity to gain feedback from the patient, to review and check the patient's understanding and to encourage and support them. To ensure effective information giving, it is important to also consider where and when the information is delivered and also what family members, relatives, carers need to be involved.

Reflecting on your communication skills

 Activity

To enable the development of your communication skills, it is essential that you reflect on your interactions with patients. With your mentor, try to regularly reflect on your communication skills by addressing the following questions:

- What skills did I use? (Listening, questioning, summarising)
- What was my rationale for using them? (Checking understanding, enabling the patient to verbalise concerns)
- Did I achieve my intended goals?
- What would I do differently in the future to facilitate effective communication?

To assist you in the development of your communication skills, access the NHS Evidence website: www.evidence.nhs.uk, which provides access to evidence-based health information regarding a range of topics to assist in the delivery of quality care.

Collaborative working

The skills of collaboration, co-ordination and communication are often referred to within the management of long-term conditions. Collaboration is about working together to resolve issues and achieve common aims. The significance of collaborative working is referred to by the Department of Health (DH 2003) and the Nursing and Midwifery Council (NMC 2010). The Healthcare Quality Strategy for

NHS Scotland also emphasises the importance of professionals working collaboratively. The benefits of working collaboratively include the following:

- Involvement of appropriate expertise to address client need appropriately, you are working with people, making joint decisions with the client and colleagues
- Provides motivation for staff
- Collective responsibility for planning and generating ideas to provide innovative high-quality care
- Changing becomes easier as everyone is involved.

Working in a collaborative way necessitates a specific 'way' of working, which includes respecting and trusting the abilities of all of the practitioners/people participating in care and taking a shared responsibility in the delivery of care. Good communication skills play a major contribution in developing collaborative working relationships, which enables appropriate holistic care.

Activity

See the case study regarding Mr Jones in Chapter 10 in order to identify the instances of collaborative working occurring in the delivery of palliative care. Using this case study, discuss with your mentor how collaborative working can be facilitated in the care of a patient to ensure an holistic approach.

Effective record-keeping to promote effective communication

Good record-keeping is an essential professional requirement of all healthcare practitioners and is an essential part of your learning and achieving competence (NMC Standards: Domain 2: Competency 2.7).

Comprehensive records help to facilitate effective communication between agencies to enhance continuity of care and can also assist in the process of clinical supervision and audit. Patient records can provide valuable evidence to defend and support the actions of healthcare staff if legal action is instigated. You may only visit a patient once, yet your record of that visit is significant and is often a valuable aspect of that patient's overall care.

Good record-keeping is identified as Competency 7 within Domain 2 of the NMC Standards for Entry to the Register:

> 7. All nurses must maintain accurate, clear and complete records including the use of electronic formats, using appropriate and plain language.
> NMC (2010: 16)

Most health records are now held electronically; this facilitates the provision of up-to-date, significant health-related information about clients to relevant healthcare professionals and is particularly useful when urgent medical care is required and the GP surgery is closed or if the client is admitted to A&E. Some community nurses will record their visits on their rounds using laptops or even assist patients to use new technology in their home (see the Queen's Nursing Institute Report: Smart New World: Using technology to help patients in the home, at: http://www.qni.org.uk/docs/smart_new_world_final_web.pdf). However, within some practice areas, written records may still be utilised, it is therefore important that you review your responsibilities to ensure comprehensive and thorough records.

Activity

> Access the RCN Guidance (2009) for Nursing Staff on 'Making nursing visible', to review your responsibilities and good practice in relation to the maintenance of electronic record-keeping, at: www.rcn.org.uk
> (See the full report at: http://www.rcn.org.uk/__data/assets/pdf_file/0003/372990/003877.pdf (accessed July 2012).

The importance of accurate written record-keeping: an example

Reference was made earlier in the book to the use of the Liverpool Care Pathway, which can be implemented within the advanced stages of terminal illness to enable the provision of appropriate end-of-life-care. The documentation is completed by healthcare professionals every time they make a visit to the patient's home. This is to enable communication on every aspect of care between all the professionals who are involved with the patient and family. This document also includes contact details of all the services involved with the patient's care, which can be used by the family or by different members of the care team. Contingency medication can also be documented in case there are any changes in the patient's condition.

At weekends, staff who visit may not have previously met the patient and family it is therefore imperative that all documentation is completed comprehensively to communicate care need.

 Activity

> In discussion with your mentor, consider some of the common errors in written record-keeping but also consider the essential elements of good record-keeping.
> What actions can practitioners take to facilitate the keeping of comprehensive patient records?

The following summary of common errors in record-keeping is discussed by Dimond (2005):

- Times omitted
- Illegibility
- Lack of entry regarding abortive visits
- Ambiguous abbreviations
- Lack of detail regarding phone calls (name of social worker)
- No signature
- Absence of information about child
- Inaccuracies, especially dates
- Record completed by person who did not do the visit
- Unprofessional terminology or meaningless statements
- Opinion mixed up with facts
- Reliance on information from neighbours without identifying the source
- Subjective comments.

Activity

> Access the Royal College of Nursing website, at: www.rcn.org.uk to review the guidance for nurses regarding the principles of good record-keeping. One example for student nurses is a presentation by Bird and Robertson 2010, see: http://www.rcn.org.uk/__data/assets/pdf_file/0006/292227/Recordkeeping.pdf (accessed July 2012).

Good records normally include factual, clear, accurate and comprehensive information.

Good record-keeping practice includes the following:

- Writing down all your observations and discussions as they happen
- Carefully recording your judgements and any actions or decisions taken
- Including details and outcomes of healthcare contacts as well as follow-up arrangements
- If appropriate, using a body map to identify specific anatomical marks, injuries, patterns of pain distribution
- Always add the date and time for every entry in your records
- Non-attendance and all significant incidents should always be recorded
- Referrals to other agencies should also be recorded and the outcomes of each referral should also be made.

 Activity

Consider some of the specific record-keeping activities that community practitioners are involved with, e.g. assessment documentation related to the first assessment visit by the community nurse. Negotiate carrying out a patient assessment with your mentor and ask your mentor to review the assessment with you. Do not forget to ensure that the patient/client has been made aware that you are a student nurse and that they have given permission for you to undertake the assessment with the supervision of your mentor.

Writing and preparing for a case conference

Case conferences are often conducted in relation to aspects of care involving children and their health or care of the older adult in residential care. This is an opportunity for all professionals working with a specific client and family to meet to clarify roles and responsibilities. It is also time to review progress with the patient/client and carer or family in order to make an informed choice about future care.

 Activity

With your mentor, it may be possible to attend a case conference to observe the written information required for such an event; or you could also discuss the issues of report writing with, e.g. the public health nurse or school nurse within your placement area who may be involved in writing for case conferences related to child protection. You may like to refer to RCN (2010; www.rcn.org.uk), which provides guidance for nursing staff in 'Safeguarding children and young people – every nurse's responsibility'; this document contains some useful guidelines for report writing within this specific area of care. You can also discuss report writing for case conferences with the GP, community psychiatric nurse or district nurse within your community learning placement.

Additional website resources to help you:

1. Scottish Border Child Protection Procedures: http://www.online-procedures.co.uk/scottishborders2012/contents/what-to-do-if-you-have-concerns-about-a-child/case-conference/preparing-for-case-conference (accessed July 2012)

2. An NHS Trust Guideline: http://www.oxfordshirepct.nhs.uk/about-us/documents/260Non-Clinical GuidelinesforCase Conference ReportsforChildrenandYoung PeopleDecember2010.pdf

3. Angus Adult Protection Multiagency Guidance: http://www.aapc.org.uk/professionalscaseconf.cfm

For a written report for a case conference, consideration should be given to:

- The introduction which should outline the purpose of the report, e.g. to update or monitor concerns or evaluate on-going care
- Information regarding the details of subjects, patient, informal carers, main carer, other healthcare practitioners and other agencies who are involved with care
- Significant other family members; profile of family members
- GP, social worker, chronology of significant events
- Recent history of care and patient's condition, including any significant events or any changes in care
- A professional assessment of the current situation.

Remember that to achieve a well-presented professional document, you should always think about who you are writing for, i.e. your 'target audience'; this may be the patient, carer, colleagues or mentor.

A well-presented document, a clear succinct e-mail, and an informative report, are all part of good professional practice to facilitate inter-professional communication and ultimately to facilitate comprehensive patient care.

Confidentiality and communication

The assurance of confidentiality of verbal and written communication is the responsibility of all practitioners (see NMC 2008: The Code: Standards of conduct, performance and ethics for nurses and midwives.)

 Activity

You must be careful with regard to your response to queries from neighbours and friends of a patient whom you are

Continued

visiting as part of your community placement practice learning. Often when visiting someone at home, those around them are curious and concerned as to their friend or neighbour's state of health and what care they are receiving.

If asked about the condition of a patient being visited either in the home or hospital, construct an appropriate response to:

- A curious neighbour
- A worried family member
- A concerned friend.

Discuss this with your mentor and set a goal for achieving a similar communication activity under the supervision of your mentor.

Remember also your responsibility to the maintenance of confidentiality with electronic health records; always remember to log off; always keep passwords private and where possible take steps to ensure that information regarding a patient on a computer screen cannot be seen easily by passers-by.

Telephone communication within primary care

Community nurses are increasingly involved with telephone work as a means of monitoring clients or as a form of contact for clients and carers seeking advice. Telephone communication within primary care may be used to give general support and advice for specific conditions or during and after treatment, to review repeated medications, to organise investigations, to offer counselling when, e.g. giving encouragement when making lifestyle changes or to triage calls. If you have already had experience of a clinical placement in the acute care sector/hospital environment, you will be familiar with dealing with telephone calls professionally and courteously. Telephone etiquette is therefore one of the transferable skills which you can use while on your community placement.

Nurse-led triage in general practice

As the general practitioner patient numbers and patient expectations increase, many health centre practices are exploring other ways to manage the staff workload. The development of nurse-led telephone triage is one such development that aims to improve patient access to treatment and advice for new and existing conditions. Triage services normally involve the nurse assessing the severity of a patient's symptoms and then deciding on which service and healthcare personnel are most appropriate to meet their needs. NHS Direct is the largest telephone consultation system in the world (see: http://www.nhsdirect.nhs.uk, accessed July 2012).

Nurse-led triage duties can include:

- Face-to-face consultations to treat or triage patients who have initially requested a GP appointment
- Screening requests to prioritise patients who require home visits.

◗ Activity

Access the Nursing and Midwifery Council website to read the paper by Sally-Anne Pygall (2010) regarding the communication skills and systems required in telephone triage work, at: http://www.nmc-uk.org/Nurses-and-midwives/The-code/The-code-in-

Continued

practice/Professional-accountability/ Telephone-triage-QA-with-Sally-Anne-Pygall-Nurse-Training-Consultant-/ Consider some of the Conduct cases involving triage communication that the NMC Conduct panels have listened to and made judgements about.

Great skill is required by the nurse undertaking telephone triage. You will probably find within your community practice placement, that many of the nurses undertaking this activity have completed an extended programme of training, which includes extended nurse prescribing and on-going clinical supervision and mentoring from a GP.

◗ Activity

Consider your concerns as a caller to the triage nurse within each of the following case scenarios and in discussion with the triage nurse within your community practice placement, consider what information the triage nurse should include during each of the calls. Imagine that you are the caller in each situation as well as the triage nurse. Compare the responses of caller and triage nurse in the communication involved:

a. Your 5-year-old son David woke up screaming with pain. He appeared to be alright when he went to bed last night. The pain seems to be in his tummy but he will not let you look at it or touch him. He is curled up crying on his bed. You are extremely anxious and request a visit by the doctor as soon as possible. As the triage nurse begins to take details, you become very angry and frustrated saying that you just want a doctor.

b. It is 4pm and your wife, who is 65 years old, has been complaining most of the

Continued

afternoon, of a slight pain in her chest. You don't want to be a nuisance, as you know how busy doctors are, but you want some advice.

c. You had a sore throat all day yesterday and went to bed with a hot drink but on wakening this morning you notice that the pain has got worse; you can hardly swallow and you feel awful. You have an important day at work today and you want a doctor to give you something to help.

d. You have had a headache for 2 days now, with bouts of nausea, although you haven't been sick yet. Proprietary pain killers have not worked and you are now worried because you feel as if you have difficulty controlling your eyes, i.e. blurry vision. You are very tired.

e. Your husband fractured a rib 1 week ago during a hill climbing accident; he has felt the pain worsening today and has woken up from a sleep complaining of severe pain and difficulty in breathing. You are very anxious and request a visit from the doctor. His breathing is worsening while you are on the phone.

f. Your husband has been complaining of indigestion this morning, which has not been relieved by antacids. The pain feels worse and he can now feel it in his jaw. You phone to request advice.

g. Your daughter had a baby 3 weeks ago. She is staying with you, as she has not been coping very well and you have been doing most the feeding and changing. This morning, she will not get out of bed to see to the baby. You are very worried and don't know what to do. You phone the surgery for advice.

The NHS Direct Website offers some guidance and insight into potential decision-making in these situations: http://www.nhsdirect.nhs.uk/

Telephone consultation requires different skills from face-to-face consultations. Some of the calls may also be made by a third party, a carer or relative, which means that the healthcare practitioner needs to use their communication skills to illicit sufficient information from this third party to accurately assess the problem. The tone of your voice, how you say things, listening actively and good questioning techniques are some of the communication skills which require further development when undertaking this work.

It is the practitioners' responsibility to effectively utilise their communication skills to enable a comprehensive assessment of the patient's problem. To enable this, specific forms of documentation are normally employed and can include a consultation pro-forma or protocol, which will include information such as:

- Name, date of birth and phone number of patient or caller if this is not the patient; time and date of the call; access information from clinical database
- Identification of the problem, taking history, referring to protocols
- Action to be taken
- Advice with guidance to contact again if condition worsens *or*
- GP to advise over phone
- A request that the patient be brought to surgery
- Ask GP to visit
- Detailed records, which should always be made regarding the action that was taken.

The triage nurse will often refer to different assessment questions, which help in providing an organised framework to elicit data from the patient or relative, which will help towards appropriate clinical decision-making, e.g. for the assessment of pain, the practitioner might refer to the PQRST pain assessment:

P. **The position and pattern** of the pain: where it is

Q. **The quality of the pain**: is it dull/sharp, burning?

R. **Does the pain radiate** to other areas?
S. **Severity**: on a scale of 1–10, 10 being excruciating, how severe is the pain?
T. **Timing**: when did the pain start, have you had the pain over a few days or has it just occurred?

Reference has already been made to the importance of good record-keeping: the information in Table 9.1 should be recorded with each nurse triage patient contact.

Table 9.1 Triage patient contact information

Date of contact

Time of contact

Initials of nurse

Patient name

Telephone number patient is calling from

Patient address

Patient's GP or practice

Nature of complaint

Advice given

Outcome

   999 Emergency Ambulance

   Attend accident unit

   GP visit

   Nurse visit

   Same day appointment with GP

   Same day appointment with nurse

   Future appointment with GP

   Future appointment with nurse

   Telephone advice by GP

   Telephone advice by nurse

   Prescription issued

Other comments

Telemedicine within the community

Telemedicine, telecare and e-health systems have the potential to support and enhance the quality of health care and are increasingly utilised as a way of communicating with specialist areas for advice and guidance regarding client care. This mode of communication can provide immediate specialised care to clients in remote or rural settings.

It is also used in the care of critically ill clients in emergency situations where immediate access to specialised hospital care is difficult due to either time or distance to travel. It provides the opportunity for the hospital physician to manage the client's condition pre-admission, which can be vital for the survival of a critically ill patient. Telemedicine includes video-conferencing but also the transmission of vital signs such as ECG, blood pressure and pulse measurements and images from relevant scans. Within the community setting, telemedicine can assist GPs working in very remote areas to gain access to specialist clinicians for their clients, avoiding unnecessary travel to distant specialised clinics. Mobile multimedia transmission systems can send video, scan images and patient's records to facilitate telemedicine consultations.

Activity

- Access the King's Fund website for examples of the use of telemedicine and telecare: http://www.kingsfund. org.uk/topics/technology_and_ telecare/index.html
- Consider the implications for improving the quality of patient care in the community.

Digital dictation, voice recognition and the opportunity to enable clinicians to quickly review scans and documents electronically has already resulted, in some areas, in a significant reduction in document turnaround times. The need for numerous different paper copies of patient documentation is reduced, sometimes enabling reports being sent out in under 12 hours, thus ensuring patients and GPs receive correspondence as efficiently and quickly as possible.

Utilisation of the internet by the patient

The increasing use and management of electronic databases, telemedicine, teleconferencing and electronic patient records in the primary care setting has necessitated the development of information technology skills for community nurses. However, clients have also developed their information technology skills to access the internet in relation to their health. Before their GP consultation, patients can consult the internet to find out more about their symptoms. Although there are a number of benefits for clients utilising the internet for health advice, this activity depends on the client's ability to separate the valid, authoritative sources from sensationalised stories. There is also the danger that patients may misinterpret online advice. The internet cannot replace the clinical judgement and experience of the healthcare practitioner who is dealing with the individual medical history. Patients may also jump to unnecessarily frightening conclusions about their symptoms.

The Scottish Care Information Diabetes Collaboration has become involved with an NHSS website entitled 'My Diabetes, My Way' (www.mydiabetesmyway.scot.nhs. uk). This is a patient information website,

which has so far enabled 100 patients to pilot the programme. Users have access to relevant parts of their electronic diabetes record such as biochemistry tests, BP body mass index, foot risk scores, eye screening results and prescribing. Alongside is patient friendly information, which helps to explain what their data means. This enables greater patient involvement in their care and could significantly empower clients to control their care.

Many e-health initiatives are being developed to inform and support people in their own homes to better manage and control their health condition. Secure websites can be developed to allow patients access and update their own records. Patients can request appointments online, request repeat prescriptions and access test results.

 Activity

> Consider the possible benefits and risks to patients accessing the internet regarding health matters.

The benefits of patients using the internet include the availability of useful advice and information. Official online support groups, such as Young Survival Coalition (www.youngsurvival.org) offers support and advice regarding breast cancer in young women. Use of the internet by cancer patients at several different stages throughout their illness can be made use of, from the time of diagnosis, to developing knowledge regarding the different stages of disease and to seek information regarding the management of the side-effects of treatment. The internet can also be used to share experiences and advice and gain support from support groups and chat rooms. Diabetic Connect (www. diabeticconnect.com) provides a forum for patients to gather and help each other find answers and share information and news. The utilisation of websites like this can be extremely helpful to patients and carers and can offer support 24/7. FDA Drugs (www. accessdata.fda.gov) provides useful information regarding medication. The most authoritative health information is normally offered on .gov or .org sites.

 Activity

Discuss with different members of the primary healthcare team the websites they may recommend to patients and carers to search for information about their illness. Find some of these yourself in order to learn more about certain health problems.

Discuss with your mentor and members of the team how they judge such advice for reliability.

Access these sites for information on website evaluation:

International Journal of Communication article: http://ijoc.org/ojs/index.php/ijoc/article/view/636/

Multiple Sclerosis Trust website: evaluation of health information questions and answers: http://www.mstrust.org.uk/information/opendoor/articles/0511_02.jsp

The use of telehealth and telecare for people with long-term conditions

Reference was made earlier in the book to the care of people with long-term conditions. This increasing aspect of care for community nurses has resulted in many innovative ways to enhance care, such as the use of telecare and telehealth.

Telecare refers to a range of different devices installed in people's homes which, if necessary, raise an alarm back to a monitoring centre. Such devices include bed occupancy monitors, falls sensors and medication reminders.

Telehealth includes equipment installed in the patient's home that enables them to take their own readings, such as blood pressure and blood oxygen levels. This is accompanied by a list of individualised questions specifically related to their condition, which they can answer and will be fed back via the phone line to a computerised system, which is monitored by a key worker. Lyndon and Tyas (2010) refer to the positive aspects of such monitoring systems revealed in a number of patient's experiences in Cornwall:

- Improved management of their condition as they can monitor their readings
- Feeling more independent and empowered
- Feeling that this may have prevented hospital admission.

Such positive telehealth experiences they argue is significant in facilitating community care of this particular client group in the future.

The following are some examples of how telemedicine can facilitate the management of long-term conditions:

Video-conferencing

A recent development within Orkney enables patients who have complex diabetes to have consultations with the consultant based in Aberdeen via video-conferencing. They can discuss their progress, review their home glucose monitoring results and agree actions to improve self-care at home.

Self-monitoring for patients with chronic obstructive pulmonary disease

Self-monitoring in chronic obstructive pulmonary disease can support patients to self-manage and self-care, to enhance quality of life and reduce unplanned hospital admission. This is enabled with the use of telehealth monitoring to keep track of patients. Patients test their oxygen levels daily and have the opportunity to answer questions on sputum levels and medication and update healthcare staff if they commence any anticipatory medication. Telephone information from patients can be directly recorded onto the community nurses computer; the nurse can then at a glance, monitor signs and readings, if necessary ask a patient or carer to do a specific test again and then if necessary, make a home visit.

Activity

Read the case study below and discuss the outcome with your mentor and/or tutor and consider how telehealth and telecare could have enhanced the care of some of the patients you have visited.

Case study

Mary has dementia and lives with her husband. She tends to walk around the house during the night. Recently, she was admitted to hospital after a fall during one of those night-time events. Before going home, a sensor system was placed in the home with a pager system. If Mary tried to leave the house during the night, the exit sensor would raise an alarm on her husband's pager, which also turns on the bedside light. This enables Mary's husband to get down to the front door to try to encourage his wife to go back to bed. He will get a better sleep, knowing he will be alerted if needed.

Educational skills in community nursing: for patients and healthcare professionals

The nurse as teacher

Nurses often fulfil an educational role within their work and, during your community practice placement, you will observe many interactions when, for example, the community nurse is teaching the patient and carer specific aspects of care to maintain and promote health and self-care. The health visitor may inform a parent about the significance of childhood immunisation or the practice nurse may instruct a patient about the schedule of their new medication regime. This educational role also often includes the facilitation of professional development opportunities for colleagues. Meeting the educational needs of patients suffering from a long-term condition is important to enhance their self-care abilities (Linsley et al 2011).

The educational role of a nurse is therefore essential to:

- Assist clients to adopt healthier lifestyle changes
- Enable patients to self-care and enhance patient and carer's ability to manage day-to-day care
- Facilitate a smooth transition from hospital to home
- Enable patients and carers to manage proactively.

Patient education is therefore a vital component in providing high-quality care and the development of a patient teaching plan centred on the client and family should be part of this.

When developing a patient teaching plan, it is advisable to adopt a systematic process approach which will include:

Client assessment: collecting and organising the data about the client; their level of understanding about their disease or condition and working with the client to consider their concerns. The client with a new diagnosis will usually have several questions

Planning: identify the client's goals. Remember that greater client involvement in determining goals normally results in greater client motivation which leads to greater achievement of gaols. Goals must be realistic and achievable. Ensure that you consider how the teaching plan will be integrated, taking into consideration any resources, which may help with the development of the client's new knowledge or skills, e.g. leaflets, information sheets, videos

Implementation: implement the plan and monitor the patient's response, checking the client's understanding and development of new knowledge and skills

Evaluation: evaluation of outcomes, the client's new knowledge, behaviour, attitude and skills.

When making a teaching plan, consideration should also be given to issues which may affect a client or carer's ability to learn. Table 9.2 show the factors which may affect the

patient and or carer's ability, readiness and motivation to learn.

To assist in meeting the patient and carer's educational needs appropriately, it is also advisable to identify and negotiate with the patient and carer realistically attainable objectives which will maintain motivation and build confidence and a sense of achievement. Healthcare practitioners will also look at prioritising learning needs into the following categories:

- *Acute educational needs:* the information needs or skills the patient and carer must have, e.g. to manage their condition
- *Preventative needs:* the information needs or skills necessary to prevent complications or to be able to manage acute exacerbations or complications of illness at an early stage (proactive, anticipatory care)
- *Maintenance educational needs:* the information needs or skills of the patient and or carer necessary for the everyday management of their condition.

🔊 Activity

Identify the learning needs of a newly diagnosed diabetic client or a client with hypertension and consider the specific knowledge and or skills to be addressed in meeting their educational needs.

Table 9.2 Factors to consider to assess the patient or carer's readiness to learn

Age	Sensory difficulties: hearing, sight, dexterity
Cognitive state	Comfort
Educational level	Stress – *remember the stress of the carer*
Language barriers	Time restrictions, many learning needs of patients and carers are quite complex with little time to achieve

You may have considered some of the following issues.

Meeting the educational needs of the client with diabetes

Patient education is a significant part of the health professional's role within the management of diabetes, and is referred to within the National Service Framework for Diabetes (DH 2001). Remember that before embarking on any educational interaction with clients, you should check your own level of knowledge and understanding about the condition. Do you have an appropriate level of knowledge to be able to address the client's concerns?

Meeting the educational needs of the client with diabetes may commence with an explanation regarding the difference between type 1 and type 2 diabetes and then going on to address issues related to:

- Developing an appropriate dietary regime
- Developing skills related to the administration of insulin, measuring glucose levels
- Making contingency plans; how to avoid and treat hypoglycaemic episodes, adjusting insulin requirements during illness
- Adopt a healthier lifestyle; increasing exercise activities
- Recognising and participating in preventative care such as regular podiatry care and ophthalmic screening.

Remember that the above issues are only the 'core' issues to be addressed and that your 'teaching plan' needs to be planned according to the individual needs of the client, e.g. the district nurse may need to initially visit the patient on a daily basis in the morning to supervise insulin administration.

Meeting the educational needs of the client with hypertension

Similar to the teaching plan above, there will be some issues which are relevant to most management plans to reduce hypertension, however, risk factors are different with each client, resulting in the need for individualised client assessment to tailor appropriate teaching plans. One of the main educational needs of the client with hypertension is to recognise lifestyle changes, which may help control blood pressure. Lifestyle changes may include:

- Developing an appropriate dietary regime, to reduce weight and sodium intake

- Adopting a healthier lifestyle, increase exercise activities
- Limiting alcohol intake
- Smoking cessation.

Knowledge and advice may also be given regarding medicinal interventions and personal risk factors. Remember also that clients are not always receptive to making changes.

The educational needs of carers can be quite complex, with the little time and the stress of being a carer. It is therefore important that healthcare practitioners' teaching skills are sufficiently competent to fulfil these educational roles.

Activity

Consider the educational needs of **the carer** within the following case scenario:

Case study

Educational needs of the carer

Mrs Hunter is an 82-year-old widow who lives with her daughter Emma, son-in law Alex and their two teenage children. They occupy a very small semi-detached house in the middle of a large council estate.

Mrs Hunter is thin, frail and underweight. She gave up her council flat after a succession of falls, which eventually resulted in her sustaining a fractured femur. Since her hospitalisation, she has become increasingly dependent, unsteady on her feet and more and more forgetful. Alex, her son-in law, offered accommodation in his house, although this meant his two teenage daughters sharing a bedroom. Mrs Hunter was also to pay for her keep and give some of her personal effects (TV and several items of antique furniture) to her daughter. The extra money coming into

Continued

the house eased some of the family's financial problems. Unfortunately, the family situation has deteriorated as Mrs Hunter's dependency has increased. She has become more and more forgetful and a diagnosis of Alzheimer's disease has recently been confirmed. Her increasing dependency has resulted in her daughter resigning from work to look after her mother full-time.

From the discussions within the above activity and from your observations of practitioner/client–carer interactions during your community practice experience, you may have concluded that the educational needs of the client and or carer may be identified from the general details of the patient's present situation and the questions and comments from the patient and or carer.

The practitioner may also use their professional knowledge about the patient's condition to identify potential problems and needs and to prioritise learning needs. It is also imperative for a successful educational interaction to identify how able and willing the patient/carer is to learn. The identification of learning needs will also be influenced by the patient and carer's present state of knowledge and what they say they need to know.

Using your teaching skills in health promotion

Health promotion (also referred to in Chapter 5) is an activity which usually has a specific goal to achieve and which relates to the prevention of ill-health, improving or enhancing health (Linsley et al 2011).

 Activity

During your community experience, take note of all the health promotion activities that you come across and in discussion with your mentor, consider what the specific aims of these activities are. You might also use one of these health promotion areas in a university assignment which asks you to consider the health of the local community and how the nurse is involved in addressing this generally and more specifically in one health need, such as obesity in young people or sexual health in young adults. (See Linsley et al 2011 for examples on both these topics. Also access the OUP online Resource Centre for a range of resources linked to health promotion, such as the Health Promotion Tools: http://www.oup.com/uk/orc/bin/9780199561087/resources/health/.)

You will probably have included a number of activities, some of which may be identified within the following list:
- Smoking cessation
- Immunisation – information for informed consent
- Well-man/well-woman screening clinics
- Clinics related to specific conditions such as hypertension, diabetes, COPD, asthma
- Weight reduction clinics
- Organisation of 'awareness days', e.g. AIDS awareness, breast cancer awareness
- Baby weight clinics.

Health promotion activities can range from one-to-one discussion with a patient or client, to promoting health for a specific client group or community, such as promoting healthy eating in schools. There are a number of skills required by the practitioner to facilitate health promotion activities. Ewles and Simnett (2003) identified the following core competencies, in health promotion:

- **Managing, planning and evaluating:** managing resources for health promotion activities, planning appropriate health promotion strategies and evaluating outcomes
- **Communicating:** competence is needed to work in groups and in a one-to-one situation
- **Educating:** health educators need to be competent in a range of educational skills such as delivering a talk about a specific health promotion issue, teaching a specific skill and planning ways in which knowledge and information can be delivered effectively and clients motivated to utilise this to enable, if required, behaviour change
- **Marketing and publicising:** skills in using marketing to raise public awareness such as using local radio or getting local press coverage
- **Facilitating and networking:** sharing skills, building confidence and trust, working with other agencies
- **Influencing policy and practice:** health promoters require skills to enable them to influence policies and practices which affect health, including national and local government plans.

Consider these principles in the Betty's case study.

Case study

Health promotion – Falls prevention

Betty, aged 72 years, lives on her own in a small bungalow about 2 miles from the town centre, which she shared with her husband until his sudden death from a heart attack 1 year ago. Since her husband's death, Betty has become quite isolated; she does not have many friends and has few other interests apart from reading and watching the television. Betty has one son, Andrew, who lives 30 miles away and visits whenever he can. Andrew works full-time as a primary school teacher and has three young children. Betty feels her son is too busy to bother but is always happy to see Andrew whenever he visits.

Betty was admitted to A&E after falling and hitting her head on the pavement when trying to catch a bus into town. Although she sustained no bone injuries, a cut on her chin required three sutures. Apart from a persistent slightly raised blood pressure, all other neurological observations were satisfactory. A physical examination detected no other obvious problems. However, there was a slight trace of glucose in her urine, which was not there at subsequent testing. She is quite a large lady and appears to have slight difficulty in mobilising; this may be due to her obesity. While in the A&E department, she was very quiet and rather withdrawn, needing a great deal of encouragement to answer any questions from the nurse practitioner. On discharge, the A&E staff have requested a visit by the community nurse to review her blood pressure and check her blood glucose levels; she has also been referred to the local 'Falls Prevention Service', as this is her third recent fall.

Nurse's health promotion and nursing activities for Betty and her family

An assessment of Betty's normal dietary intake and general lifestyle should be initiated. Betty's knowledge regarding a balanced diet should be assessed in order to give relevant advice regarding this. Assessment of dietary intake should also assess alcohol intake; this can increase calorie intake and add to depression. Advice should also be given regarding salt restriction in view of hypertension. Other factors which can impact on dietary intake, should be reviewed such as availability of shops and problems with shopping, such as transport.

The community nurse could offer dietary advice depending on assessment information regarding a healthy diet, which could be supported with a range of relevant leaflets. Consideration should also be given to strategies which may increase Betty's general activity levels, some local leisure centres offer specialist fitness sessions relevant to Betty's requirements. This would also provide an opportunity for more social contact.

Summary of learning points from this chapter

If you have read this chapter and undertaken the numerous learning activities included, you should have been able to achieve the following actions, which will support your achievement of many learning competencies and knowledge to meet NMC Standards (NMC 2010):

- Communication skills in relation to assessment of the client and family in the community
- Knowledge and understanding of the specific communication skills required in giving advice and support by telephone
- The importance of record-keeping and its significance in promoting effective communication across multidisciplinary and multi-agency teams
- The use telecare and telehealth to enhance quality of care
- The skills required in teaching clients and carers in their own homes
- The importance of health promotion activities essential to the role of the nurse in the community setting.

References

Department of Health (DH), 2001. National Service Framework for Diabetes. DH, London. Online. Available at: www.dh.gov.uk.

Department of Health (DH), 2003. Learning for Collaborative practice with other professions. DH, London. Online. Available at: www.dh.gov.uk.

Dimond, B., 2005. Legal aspects of nursing, fourth ed. Pearson Education, Harlow.

Ewles, L., Simnett, I. (Eds.), 2003. Promoting health: a practical guide. Bailliere Tindall, London.

Hamilton, S.J., Martin, D.J., 2007. Clinical development: a framework for effective communication skills. Nurs. Times 103 (48), 30–31.

Linsley, P., Kane, R., Owe, S., 2011. Nursing for public health. Oxford University Press, Oxford.

Lyndon, H., Tyas, D., 2010. Telehealth enhances self care and independence in people with long term conditions. Nurs. Times 106 (26), 12–13.

Miller, E., Webb, L., 2011. Active listening & attending: communication and the healthcare environment. In: Webb, L. (Ed.), Nursing: communication skills for practice. Oxford University Press, Oxford.

Nursing and Midwifery Council (NMC), 2008. The Code: standards of conduct, performance and ethics for nurses and midwives. Online. Available at: www.nmc-uk.org/Documents/Standards/nmcTheCodeStandardsofConduct PerformanceAndEthicsForNurses AndMidwives_LargePrintVersion.PDF.

Nursing and Midwifery Council (NMC), 2010. Standards for pre-registration nursing education. Online. Available at: standards.nmc-uk.org.

Royal College of Nursing (RCN), 2009. Record keeping. Guidance for nurses and

midwives. RCN, London. Online.
Available at: www.rcn.org.uk.

Royal College of Nursing (RCN), 2010.
Safeguarding children and young people –
every nurse's responsibility. RCN, London.
Online. Available at: www.rcn.org.uk.

Webb, L., 2011. Communication skills in
practice. Oxford University Press, Oxford.

Further reading

Bach, S., Grant, A., 2011. Communication
and interpersonal skills in nursing
(transforming nursing practice), second
ed. Learning Matters, Exeter.

Department of Health (DH), NHS
Modernisation Agency, London, 2003.
Essence of care. Benchmarks for
communication between patients, carers
and health care. DH, London.

Goodwin, N., 2010. The state of telehealth
and telecare in the UK: prospects for
integrated care. Journal of Integrated Care
18, 3–10.

Lewis, K.E., Annandale, J.A., Warm, D.L.,
et al., 2010b. Home telemonitoring
and quality of life in stable, optimised
chronic obstructive pulmonary disease.
J. Telemed. Telecare 16 (5), 253–259.

Polisena, J., Tran, K., Cimon, K., et al., 2010.
Home telehealth for chronic obstructive
pulmonary disease: a systematic review
and meta-analysis. J. Telemed. Telecare
16 (3), 120–127.

Royal College of Nursing (RCN), 2012.
Using telehealth to monitor patients
remotely. Online. Available at: www.rcn.
org.uk.

Sorknaes, A.D., Madsen, H., Hallas, J., et al.,
2010. Nurse tele-consultation with
discharged COPD patients reduce early
readmissions-an interventional study.
Clinical Respiratory Journal 5 (1), 26–34.

Websites

Communication skills and language used in
communicating. http://www.youtube.com/
watch?v=YIns3DStfIE.

Diabetic Connect, www.diabeticconnect.com.

NHS Evidence Website, www.evidence.nhs.uk
provides access to evidence-based
health information regarding a range
of topics to assist in the delivery of
quality care.

Royal College of Nursing, 2009. Record
keeping. Guidance for nurses and midwives.
www.rcn.org.uk.

Royal College of Nursing, Safeguarding
children and Young People – every nurse's
responsibility. www.rcn.org.uk.

Talking with acutely psychotic people. http://
www.iop.kcl.ac.uk/iopweb/blob/
downloads/locator/l_436_Talking.pdf.

Telecare, www.telecareaware.com presents an
overview of the news and updates about
e-care telecare and telehealth products,
services and technologies.

Young Survival Coalition, www.youngsurvival.
org offers support and advice regarding breast
cancer in younger women and Diabetic
Connect: www.diabeticconnect.com
provides a forum for patients to gather and
help each other find answers and share
information and news. The utilisation
of websites like this can be extremely helpful
to patients and carers and can offer
support 24/7.

10

Leadership, management and team working in community practice

CHAPTER AIMS

- To explore the concept of leadership as a process
- To examine the skills of effective leadership
- To consider the leadership role in relation to teamwork and delegation
- To consider the leadership skills in the management of change
- To explore how the student nurse can gain leadership, management and team working skills within the community placement

As a student nurse, you will be expected to develop the skills of leadership and management, as well as those required to work in a team. At the end of every year (Progression Points) and at other key points in your programme of study, you will be assessed in various aspects of these three areas of practice and will have to achieve all the competencies related to the main NMC Domains by the end of the programme, in order to qualify as a nurse.

Those of you studying in other countries will have similar competencies to achieve, but wherever you are undertaking your programme of study, these three areas are essential to being able to undertake the role of the qualified nurse in today's healthcare systems internationally.

Introduction

Within earlier sections of this book, reference has been made to the significant role of the community nurse in the co-ordination of care. This often includes undertaking a leadership role. One of the core conditions for developing community nursing, identified by the RCN (2010), in their policy position paper on the development of community nursing (Pillars of the Community), refers to leadership capacity.

 Activity

In Chapter 9, reference was made to the Nursing and Midwifery Council (NMC) Standards for Pre-registration Nursing Education. Access this framework again on: http://standards.nmc-uk.org and consider the competencies within Domain 4: Leadership, Management and Team Working. This will guide you in terms of highlighting the leadership responsibilities you are expected to

Continued

achieve for entry to the professional register. With your mentor, identify examples within your community learning experience which might demonstrate your progress or achievement with each of the competencies. In accordance with your specific university requirements for clinical practice, agree specific learning outcomes to achieve the competencies in the community placement.

Leadership, accountability and managing change

As healthcare delivery in the UK moves increasingly to the community setting, development of leadership skills becomes essential, given the complexity of services, multiprofessional working and the co-ordination of packages of care for individuals. The RCN position statement, Pillars of the Community (Royal College of Nursing, 2010: 7) for example, emphasises this need and states that:

> strong, visible and influential community nurse leadership is needed to plan and manage change and to ensure the safe and effective practice of frontline nurses and healthcare assistants.

Activity

Obtain a copy of this paper and consider how community services and nursing care is changing in your own locality in one of the four UK countries. If you are a student in another country, find out how policy in relation to

Continued

community or rural healthcare services is changing the way care is being delivered. The following links will give you access to a number of publications to guide your searching:

1. http://www.rcn.org.uk/_data/assets/pdf_file/0007/335473/003843.pdf (RCN paper)
2. http://www.aihw.gov.au/rural-health-publications (Australian Rural health papers)
3. http://www.scotland.gov.uk/Resource/Doc/222087/0059735.pdf (Report on remote and rural health care in Scotland UK)
4. http://www.who.int/healthsystems/topics/delivery/en/index.html (WHO papers on health service delivery in different countries).

Your community practice experience can provide you with many opportunities to observe community nurses undertaking a lead role in care. For example:

- *The District Nurse* can lead the multidisciplinary team for a client with complex needs and in the day-to-day organisation and delegation of home visits
- *The Public Health Nurse* may take the lead in the organisation of the multidisciplinary team for a family with special needs
- *The Practice Nurse* may take the lead in the development of a nurse-led clinic for a specific long-term condition such as diabetes
- *The District Nurse* may also play a significant leadership role in co-ordinating care with other services such as hospices, in the delivery of palliative care.

Activity

Within your community practice placement, find out the various activities your mentor undertakes on a daily basis which require leadership skills. You may have set a learning goal with your personal tutor to achieve in your placement, which focuses on an aspect of leadership.

To be able to set a goal which focuses on leadership, it is important to have a shared understanding of what leadership is.

Defining leadership

Cooke (2001) defines a clinical nurse leader as a practitioner who is involved in direct patient care and who continuously improves care by influencing others. Leadership therefore includes not only specific skills but is also an 'attitude that informs behaviour' (Cooke 2001) Leaders act as 'visionaries' motivating, encouraging and supporting other practitioners to evaluate practice and plan for appropriate changes (Jooste 2004).

Northouse (2007) considers the following components to be essential within leadership:
- Leadership is a process
- Leadership involves influence
- Leadership occurs in a group context.

Pointer's (2006) definition leadership as:

a process through which an individual attempts to intentionally influence human systems in order to accomplish a goal

He concludes from this that 'leadership resides with a person rather than a position' (Burton 2011: 205). This is an important observation because a student nurse can and must demonstrate skills in leadership to be able to qualify as a nurse (NMC Standards 2010). Although you may hear qualified nurses say that 'she/he is a natural leader' of a student nurse, when asked to explain why, they find it difficult to define. Being a 'natural leader' when it involves taking charge or responsibility for a group of patients in their care, may be one way of demonstrating this trait for some students, while for another student, it may clearly be evident in the way they take the lead in a 'crisis' situation involving one patient. Both situations require leadership skills but will require different leadership style to ensure a successful patient outcome.

You will see many different types of leadership skills and styles throughout your clinical placements, some of which you find unhelpful and others more supportive.

Styles of leadership

There are several different types of leadership identified within the literature:
- **Autocratic leaders**, who set the agenda and goals without the involvement of others. They make the decisions and tell others what they are and what they have to do
- **Transactional leaders** *is almost an authoritarian style whereby the leader establishes the outcomes required in the task and communicates this to the followers or subordinates and then monitors the performance during the delivery of these.* (Burton 2011: 214)
- **Transformational leaders** are charismatic, visionary and inspire others, through shared values and most importantly trust
- **Bureaucratic leaders** rigidly adhere to rules, policies and regulations
- **Laissez faire leaders** leave people to identify and manage their own strategies to meet goals but without a clear direction of what is needed to be achieved

- **Situational leaders** adopt different styles of leadership to suit different situations.

A more detailed review of these various leadership styles can be found in the Further reading list at the end of this chapter.

⬥ Activity

Access the following website and take the Leadership Style Test! There are a number of other resources on this Foundation of Nursing Leadership website, including leadership literature. Discuss your leadership style profile with your personal tutor and set out a learning plan for how you can reflect on your practice learning and identify situations where you have used that style of leadership.

Foundation of Nursing Leadership website: http://www.nursingleadership.org.uk/resources_free.php (accessed August 2012).

Leadership skills

Leadership skills are often discussed in terms of their relevance to quite senior roles, however such skills are relevant to all practitioners especially to those working directly with clients and carers in their everyday practice. Adams (2010) outlines the leadership responsibilities that are required by community practitioners:

All levels of practitioner must be able to lead and deliver services appropriate to client need, working with a variety of practitioners and services to develop a package of care, collecting data and demonstrating outcomes from their practice. Clinicians also need to lead their skill mix team, ensure quality of care being delivered, and deliver in accordance with local organisational needs.

Clinical specialists should have the skills to provide practitioners with support, mentorship and clinical supervision and be able to provide the necessary education and training to ensure that best evidence is implemented into practice. This also requires the dissemination of best evidence and practice.

The leadership skills of nurses on the boards of new commissioning processes are essential to ensure that services are planned to meet the holistic needs of clients. Nurse directors have a significant role in leading service developments, facilitating regular communication with practitioners to understand the realities of everyday practice to inspire changes in practice.

Adams (2010) emphasises the facilitative nature of leadership required by today's NHS services, such 'facilitative' leadership includes the ability and skills to motivate staff, make appropriate decisions and encouraging staff to share and implement new ideas and practices. The leadership attributes of the senior charge nurse for example have been outlined by the National Health Service Education for Scotland (2011):

- **Integrity, honesty and authenticity:** Within your work you are continually observed by a number of people, clients, professional colleagues and managers and a lack of integrity, honesty and authenticity can be instantly identified
- **Courage:** Courage is required to make decisions, to play the role of advocate for your clients and to support your staff and colleagues
- **Inquisitiveness:** You recognise that you have a professional commitment to lifelong learning and support other colleagues with this
- **Inspiration:** Your passion and interest in your work motivates other colleagues
- **Decisiveness:** You prepare to make decisions and when necessary access advice before doing this

- **Meticulousness:** You are conscientious and address detail to achieve good standards and expect this of your colleagues
- **Emotional attentiveness:** You demonstrate sensitivity and understanding to others.

Activity

Refer to the above list of attributes and consider your own potential leadership qualities. The identification of your specific attributes should provide you with an opportunity to review and continue your personnel and professional development with regard to your leadership skills. For those particular characteristics that perhaps you may feel are lacking, this is an opportunity to discuss and identify with your mentor learning opportunities to progress with this in your personnel development plan.

It could be argued that the skills of effective listening, understanding, accountability, empowerment, observation, networking and relationship building, which are built during initial professional training, are also essential within leadership. Adams (2010) argues that community practitioners who are clinical leaders also need to develop skills in:

- Planning
- Business case development
- Systems management
- Resource management
- Prioritising time-keeping
- Data analysis
- Audit and evaluation.

Contino (2004) groups leadership skills into the following four specific categories:

1. **Organisational management:** which includes effective management of time, information, human resources and change.
2. **Communication:** leaders need to have good communication skills to disseminate and interpret information quickly and accurately; an ability to 'inspire' vision. Leaders need to be able to translate policies into practice; they can see the relevance of a policy in relation to practice and patient care and can communicate this to staff to demonstrate the relevance of strategic changes to improving patient care.
3. **Analysis/strategy:** leaders should be able to plan work to meet organisational objectives and to analyse data to make enable effective decision-making.
4. **Creation and vision:** leaders should be creative in finding solutions to problems; this includes utilising the skills and expertise of staff.

Activity

To assist you to examine the leadership skills required by the practitioner, access the Department of Health's online learning project: www.e-lfh.org.uk which is a learning resource to support practitioners to develop the skills required for their leadership role in relation to different aspects of care such as child protection, safeguarding children and end-of-life care. It also hosts many other resources of value for learning in a community placement.

Above, reference was made to Contino's (2004) categorisation of leadership skills, which included organisational management, the effective management of time, information, human resources and change.

Managing the community nursing caseload

Organisational management skills are essential for the community/district nurse when planning the daily schedule of home visits, which may cover a wide geographical area and can range from dispensing medication to wound dressings to palliative care. While planning the schedule of visits, the practitioner has to prioritise the visits, delegate appropriately to the rest of the community nursing team and also consider the distances to be travelled. Time management skills are also required, especially when the unexpected has happened and the nurse is delayed in visiting other patients and has the daily responsibility of completing all relevant patient documentation.

 Activity

All nurses must be able to identify priorities and manage time and resources effectively to ensure quality of care is maintained or enhanced. NMC (2010) Competency 3, Domain 4: Leadership, Management and Team Working.

In discussion with your mentor, find out the methods through which they prioritise and manage tasks, such as the allocation and timing of home visits amongst community nursing staff.

Managing change

To improve an aspect of care normally requires making a change, therefore most nursing staff will take part in managing change or as senior members of staff will be involved with leading and managing change.

 Activity

With your mentor identify a specific aspect of service delivery that has changed recently and discuss the steps that were taken to facilitate that change. Find out what the underpinning evidence was to support the change. This activity could be used as part of your achievement of the NMC Standard related to evidence based practice within Domain 4: Leadership, Management and Team Working.

Exploring the evidence to support change is normally the first step within the change process; this might also include the identification of local or national initiatives to learn how other service areas are managing the particular aspect of care that you wish to change. This would normally be followed by careful consideration and detailed planning of what specifically had to change while also considering the resources this would require; the acceptability to service users; and the skills required by practitioners to implement this change. Opportunities should also be sought to share experiences from other areas; this can also provide a forum to give support and advice. Evaluation and audit are also an essential aspect of the change process and are required to continually monitor the effects of change and for the early identification of any problems.

 Activity

Refer to the Knowledge Network 'Evidence into Practice' Website at: www.evidenceintopractice.scot.nhs. uk which identifies and discusses different aspects of managing change and improvement methodologies.

Resistance to change

Changes in practice can often be considered quite stressful by staff. It is therefore essential that practitioners who are instigating change understand how people react with the intention of looking at how we can minimise resistance. If staff concerns are not considered, this can result in resistance to change, which can manifest in staff paying 'lip service' to the change, being aggressive or even destructive to the new way of working. Staff may be feeling stressed regarding the new skills; new accountability or responsibility concerns; how advantageous the change will be to them; and how much they like the 'old ways'. It is essential therefore that staff acting as change managers, take time to motivate staff and demonstrate the necessity for change but also take time to address their concerns and questions. Good feedback mechanisms to facilitate this include:

- Listening to service users
- Getting feedback from staff
- Reviewing comments, concerns and complaints
- Team meetings
- Monitoring audit findings.

Involving everyone from the beginning

From the commencement of the change process, it is essential that everyone involved feels convinced about the necessity for change. Service users, carers and team members can all be involved in looking at the problem and working together on solutions. Changes are much more likely to succeed if all parties feel involved. Kerridge (2012) states that individuals will also adapt to changes at different times and refers to people in these different stages as innovators, early adopters, early majority, late majority and laggards.

 Activity

Supporting colleagues through the process of change is a significant component in managing change. To help you understand the skills required in this process, refer to the earlier discussion within this chapter regarding styles of leadership and consider which style of leadership might be the most effective in managing change. The following website will also assist you in the consideration of the approaches most likely to succeed in making staff and service users feel involved with change. www.improvingnhsscotland.scot.nhs.uk

Refer also to: www.evidenceintopractice.scot.nhs.uk to examine different ways of managing change.

As a practitioner, you will often be involved in the process of change. The above activity can assist in the identification of skills which will be invaluable to you to facilitate this process.

When developing services, it is important to be receptive to ideas for change from service users, carers and colleagues and feedback mechanisms. This might include:

- Listening to service user's stories
- Getting feedback from students
- Studying complaints, suggestions and audit data
- Team meetings.

 Activity

Access and read the following article to enable you to consider the managing change process:

Bowers B (2011) Managing change by empowering staff. Nursing Times 107:32–33.

Continued

> Summarise the facilitating skills used by the senior nurse to manage change and enable staff to successfully participate within the process.

Within the above activity, you may have identified the importance of:

- Sharing the reason for change with staff to enable commitment
- Scheduling time to give staff the opportunity to discuss some of the weaknesses within the current service/system
- The opportunity to consult each member of the team individually to gain their views on the present service/system
- Joint decision-making after consultation to identify ways to improve
- Continued staff support to sustain change and support with new ways of working.

The above activity should have made you aware of the importance of planning and involving staff with the process of change and this should help in enabling change to be accepted and supported. Supporting individuals before, during and after change, is an essential aspect of managing change and within your role as a practitioner, the persistent need to provide high quality safe care for patients requires continual evaluation, which often requires a change in practice.

Teamwork

During your career as a student nurse, you will be required to work in a number of teams, whether this is with student colleagues while in university or within the nursing team or multidisciplinary team when you are completing your practice placements. Within the community setting, the delivery of client care is often the result of good teamwork, combining the expertise and skills of different practitioners and agencies to provide appropriate care. To work in an effective way within a team requires an understanding of how teams operate, and the skills to engage staff to promote effective team working (see, e.g. Goodall et al 2006).

Within the scenario below, Sarah, a senior district nurse/team leader, reflects on the skills she uses to facilitate team working among the nursing staff:

> *It has been very important for me to regularly communicate with staff and to consult all staff about any changes. Motivating staff is important too, acknowledging all their hard work, just saying thank you regularly is so important. Initial team meetings are vital to develop trust within the team, this enables openness among team members, nobody is scared of bringing something to the group when things have not gone well, we can then learn from mistakes quickly but we always also celebrate when things go well.*
>
> Sarah (A senior district nurse/team leader)

 Activity

Think about the different groups of people you have worked with and consider what made the experience positive and encouraging. In discussion with your mentor and reflecting on Sarah's experience, consider the ways in which teamwork can be facilitated.

Working in teams

Healthcare practitioners often work in multidisciplinary teams. Effective co-ordinated teamwork necessitates that each practitioner has a good understanding of each individual role and a shared understanding of the 'collective' goal of the work of the team. The effective utilisation of expertise within teamwork aims to enhance the delivery of care. For example the client suffering from diabetes may require care from quite an extensive team of specialists:

- Consultant physician
- General practitioner
- Practice nurse
- Dietician
- Ophthalmologist
- Chiropodist
- Psychologist
- Pharmacists.

Competency 6 within the NMC Standards: Domain 4: Leadership, Management and Team Working (NMC 2010), referred to earlier within this chapter, refers to the necessity of nurses being able to work in teams, to work co-operatively within teams and to respect the skills, expertise and contributions of colleagues. If you refer to the Code of Conduct for some of the different professions you have worked with, such as the General Medical Council, you will find similar statements regarding teamwork. Reference is also made to team working within the NMC Guidance on Professional Conduct for Nursing and Midwifery Students (2011).

 Activity

Consider the different professions and services which may be included within the care team for the client and family within the following case scenario:

Case study

Palliative care of Dr Jones

Dr Jones is a 48-year-old man with a malignant brain tumour. He was diagnosed 3 years ago and received surgery and chemotherapy at that time. He has recently suffered from a stroke as a result of radiotherapy treatment for a previous brain tumour several years ago. The stroke has resulted in severe left-sided weakness in his left hand and arm and leg, however, with intensive physiotherapy, he has learned to walk again and has been fairly independent with most activities of living. However, his condition has worsened and the tumour has shown no response to treatment; he is becoming increasingly tired and weak and frequently wakens very early in the morning with excruciating headaches, nausea and vomiting. His mobility has worsened considerably and, recently, he has had a few episodes of incontinence due to his inability to make the toilet in time. His wife who is a lecturer in nursing is his main carer; they also have four young children. Dr Jones is completely aware of the severity of his condition. He wishes to die at home. The district nursing service and local hospice have been contacted to organise assistance for Dr Jones and his family.

Discuss the case scenario with your community mentor to identify within your current practice placement the practitioners who may be involved with this patient's care. How would your mentor facilitate team working with all the possible professionals involved in caring for this family?

You will probably have identified a number of different professionals and services to support this client and his family; your list may have identified the following professionals:

- The pharmacist, GP, consultant oncologist, hospice consultant and specialist nurse, to review medication to alleviate headaches, nausea and vomiting
- Social services for the delivery of practical equipment which may assist Mrs Jones in caring for her husband, such as commode, wheelchair, incontinence supplies, pressure mattress
- The district nursing team, to enable the regular accurate and continued assessment of the client's physical and psychological symptoms, to provide general support and advice and also provide the opportunity for early identification of new problems. Continued visiting also provides the opportunity for staff, client and family to build relationships and to voice any concerns and anxieties
- The Marie Curie nursing service or a night sitting service could give Mrs Jones some much needed rest
- Some emergencies can be anticipated and appropriate arrangements made. There is a chance that this patient's risk of convulsions will increase as intracranial pressure increases. Information should be given to Mrs Jones about whom to contact in an emergency. It may also be appropriate to have a stock of emergency medication within the home for pain relief or to control possible seizures due to raised intracranial pressure
- Dr Jones and his wife may welcome specialist advice from the MacMillan Nurse, hospice staff or health visitor, regarding the support of their young children during this distressing time.

Care teams often include a number of people from different professions and services such as mental health services, community pharmacy services, local authority teams, the independent sector. Increasingly, patients and carers are included in team meetings and case conferences. The roles of a wide range of practitioners are described in Chapter 2.

Multidisciplinary team working: child protection as an example

Within the area of child protection, practitioners are required to work across different agencies such as police, education, social work and health care. The House of Commons Education and Skills Committee report 'Every Child Matters' outlines a set of reforms supported by the Children Act 2004. The development was made mainly as a result of the review of the failings of the Child Protection System which had led to the tragic death of a child called Victoria Climbie in February 2000. One of the challenges identified within the review was around working together with different partner agencies such as health, education and the police. It is essential that agencies work together to improve children's wellbeing. The aim of 'Every Child Matters' is that every child, whatever their background or circumstances has the support they need to:

- be healthy
- stay safe
- enjoy and achieve
- make a positive contribution
- achieve economic wellbeing.

 Activity

Effective partnership working across different agencies such as health services and social care is often emphasised to enhance support for the care of children and young people. Refer to the 'Every Child Matters' website, at: http://every-child-matters.co.uk to examine a number of resources which

Continued

can facilitate multidisciplinary working. If you are a children's nursing student in a children's community placement, organise with your mentor to undertake some specific 'spoke' visits to various services, including a day with a social worker responsible for child protection in the community.

To enable team working to provide co-ordinated client care, it is essential that plenty of opportunities are made to facilitate communication between practitioners.

Activity

- Observe the different ways practitioners communicate as a team within your practice placement, e.g. is there a regular practice team meeting or community nursing team meeting?
- Consider the skills and knowledge needed by the practitioners for effective collaborative working.
- Identify one of the Communication and Interpersonal Domain competencies which you can achieve in your placement, which focuses on communication between you and patients and their families/carers.

The community nurse will often be the 'key worker'; the facilitator, drawing health and social care together, enabling the care team to work together; co-ordinating care and leading the different members of the multidisciplinary team. The National Health Service Education for Scotland (2011) has identified a number of key issues for the nurse who is leading the team:

- Be honest about your own views but also respect and listen to the views of the team

- Discuss and agree on aims and objectives
- Encourage team members to participate and contribute
- Celebrate success with the team.

Many researchers emphasise that to enable good teamwork, a 'team policy' should be agreed upon which should be reviewed regularly, particularly when a new member of staff joins the team. This policy defines the details of the purpose of the team and how it works. Regular meetings and opportunities for on-going communication are also considered essential to facilitate teamwork. Meetings are also helpful if different members of the care team find that their professional role appears to infringe on another role. A meeting can provide the opportunity to develop understanding of the unique contribution of each team member and the team's overall purpose.

Team reflection

Reflection is also considered good practice to facilitate teamwork and includes team members regularly meeting to reflect and critically examine their performance. This however, necessitates a conducive environment, in which team members feel they can safely share their concerns and issues. Zwarenstein and Reeves (2002) have identified the following activities to facilitate teamwork:

- Ensure team members agree on a shared definition of patient care which has included the different perspectives of team members
- Ensure clarity about the roles of each team member
- Understand different challenges each profession may face in delivering care and where possible implement strategies to assist and support
- Acknowledge that delivering care is challenging.

Activity

Within your community practice placement, discuss with your mentor the activities which have been undertaken to facilitate team working within, e.g. the district nursing team or the multiprofessional team.

Delegation

The delegation of work to different team members is often part of the community nurses role, making sure that different levels of nursing staff are utilised effectively and efficiently.

 Activity

With your mentor, discuss the rationale for the decisions she makes regarding the daily delegation of work within the nursing team.

The National Health Service Education for Scotland (2011) has developed a checklist of activities before delegating to different team members. This includes making sure that:

- the task is within the job description of the practitioner's role
- the practitioner has received appropriate training and has the necessary knowledge, skills and competence to carry out the task safely and efficiently
- the practitioner fully understands what they have been asked to do and is happy to do it
- the practitioner's work will be appropriately supervised and the outcomes will be reported.

Remember that within the home setting, care is often delivered by informal carers, relatives and friends; although this carer is not an employee, as a nurse you still have responsibilities with regard to deciding what care activities can be delegated to them and to ensure that they receive the appropriate training. The teaching of carers is discussed earlier in this book. Most community organisations will have a policy regarding the delegation of care to carers.

 Activity

In discussion with your mentor, identify a patient that you have visited who has complex needs and consider the range of services, agencies and people which the community nurse has to communicate and work with to implement appropriate care. Discuss with your mentor how care is delegated to appropriately utilise the skills of the staff. How are staff supported with their professional development to meet changing healthcare needs?

Team working in community settings

Borrill (2002) states that teams that appear to work best have higher levels of involvement, are more successful in delivering high-quality health care, have better team morale and have lower stress levels. Effective teamwork necessitates the skills of good facilitative leadership, which motivates and inspires colleagues but also regularly monitors team arrangements and practices to ensure that members are working collaboratively and therefore effectively as a team. Cornwell (2010) discusses the effectiveness of leadership in enabling good teamwork and declares that team working is beneficial for the mental health of staff and patients. Reference is also made to the importance of staff engagement to facilitate good team working.

The development and delivery of care necessitates that nurses at every level in the community have leadership skills to devise innovative ways to deliver cost-effective quality care.

Adams (2010) provides a summary of the possible results of effective leadership:

- Client focused, quality services
- Sign up to organisational values and vision
- Partnership working with patients or clients
- A motivated, confident workforce
- A workforce fit for purpose
- Evidence-based services
- Outcome driven services
- Financial propriety
- Risk management
- Effective working across organisational boundaries
- Good recruitment and retention in the workforce
- A reduction in health inequalities.

Adams (2010: 106)

 Activity

Earlier in this chapter, we referred to Sarah, a senior community nurse, and her ability to facilitate team working. Reflect back to this scenario to help you summarise some of the skills of Sarah's leadership and management role. To help you with this, also reflect on comments made by the nursing staff within the team:

Sarah always seems to know what's happening in community nursing, what's happening in the big picture of things, she is always telling us about recent policies and changes, she is always enthusiastic and sees a way of developing practice. She always listens to us and takes on board our worries and concerns. We kind of look up to Sarah because we respect her knowledge although she will always discuss new ideas with us and will involve the skills and expertise of other.

Summary of learning points from this chapter

The provision of patient-centred care often demands good multiprofessional team working, and the evaluation of services to improve care often necessitates supporting practitioners through the process of change and being able to lead and manage change. This chapter and the learning activities included, should have helped you to achieve the following actions, which will support your achievement of many of the NMC Standards learning competencies within Domain 4: Leadership, Management and Team Working (NMC 2010):

- Skills in relation to leadership, accountability and managing change
- Knowledge and understanding of the different style of leadership
- Knowledge and understanding of specific leadership skills
- The skills required in managing change and supporting practitioners throughout his process
- The importance of the skills required to facilitate team working.

References

Adams, C., 2010. What leadership skills will community nurses need to improve outcomes in the new NHS? Nurs. Times 106, 47.

Borrill, C., 2002. Team working and effectiveness in health care: findings from the healthcare team effectiveness project. Aston Centre for Health Service Organisation Research, Birmingham.

Contino, D.S., 2004. Leadership competencies: knowledge, skills and aptitudes nurses need to lead organisations effectively. Crit. Care Nurse 24 (3), 52–64.

Cooke, M., 2001. The renaissance of clinical leadership. Int. Nurs. Rev. 48, 38–46.

Cornwell, J., 2010. Caring for patients means caring for nurses. Nurs. Times 16 March, 1–6.

Goodall, E., Lowry, L., Jones, C., 2006. Facilitating collaboration using a clinical teams programme. Nurs. Times 102 (5), 32–34.

Jooste, K., 2004. Leadership: A new perspective. J. Nurs. Manag. 12, 217–223.

Kerridge, J., 2012. Leading change. Nurs. Times. Online. Available at: www. nursingtimes.net.

NHS Education for Scotland, 2011. Leading accountable and professional care: a companion for senior charge nurses and midwives in Scotland. NES Delegation, Scotland.

Northouse, P.G., 2007. Leadership: theory and practice, fourth ed Sage, Thousand Oaks.

Nursing and Midwifery Council (NMC), 2010. Standards for pre-registration nursing education. Online. Available at: http://standards.nmc-uk.org.

Nursing and Midwifery Council (NMC), 2011. Guidance on Professional Conduct for Nursing and Midwifery Students.

Pointer, D.D., 2006. Leadership a framework for thinking and acting. In: Shortell, S.M., Kaluzny, A.D. (Eds.), Health care management: organization design and behaviour, fifth ed. Thomson Delmar Learning, New York.

Royal College of Nursing, 2010. Pillars of the community. RCN, London.

Zwarenstein, M., Reeves, S., 2002. Working together but apart: barriers and routes to nurse-physician collaboration. Jt. Comm. J. Qual. Improv. 28, 242–247.

Further reading

Binney, G., Wilkie, G., Williams, C., 2009. Living leadership – a practical guide for ordinary heroes. Prentice Hall, Harlow.

Bolton, S., 2003. Multiple roles? Nurses as managers in the NHS. International Journal of Public Sector Management 16 (2), 122–130.

Department of Health, 2008. High quality care for all. DH, Norwich.

Department of Health, 2009. Inspiring leaders: leadership for quality. DH, London.

Department of Health, 2010. Equity and excellence: liberating the NHS. DH, London.

Huber, D., 2010. Leadership and nursing care management. Elsevier, Edinburgh.

Huston, C., 2008. Preparing nurse leaders for 2020. J. Nurs. Manag. 16, 905–911.

Masterton, A., Gough, P., 2010. Adaptable leaders are crucial to the new NHS. Nurs. Times 106 (34), 23.

McKenna, H., Keeney, S., Bradley, M., 2004. Nurse leadership within primary care: the perceptions of community nurses, GPs, policy makers and members of the public. J. Nurs. Manag. 12 (1), 69–76.

McMurray, R., Cheater, F., 2004. Vision, permission and action: a bottom up perspective on the management of public health nursing. J. Nurs. Manag. 12 (1), 43–50.

Poulton, B., 2000. Barriers and facilitators to the achievement of community focused public health nursing practice: a UK perspective. J. Nurs. Manag. 17, 74–83.

Royal College of Nursing, 2008. Carers of children. RCN, London.

Scottish Executive, 2006. Modernising nursing careers – setting the direction. Scottish Executive, Edinburgh.

Williamson, C., 2009. Using life coaching techniques to enhance leadership skills in nursing. Nurs. Times 105, 20–23.

Yoder-Wise, P., 2011. Leading and managing nursing. Elsevier, Edinburgh.

Websites

The Foundation of Nursing Leadership, http://www.nursingleadership.org.uk/resources_free.php.

The Healthcare Foundation, www.health.org.uk is an independent charity working to continuously improve the quality of health care in the UK.

www.improvingnhsscotland.scot.nhs.uk – considers the approaches most likely to succeed in making staff and service users feel involved with change.

Knowledge Network 'Evidence into practice', www.evidenceintopractice.scot.nhs.uk provides a range of evidenced based information in relation to improving quality in health care and facilitating patient safety

Modernising Nursing in the Community, at: www.mnic.scot.nhs.uk is an informative website offering a range of information and support on a variety of different aspects of care for community practitioners

Nursing and Midwifery Council Code, 2011, at: www.nmc-uk.org provides information on a range of different aspects of care as well as the code of conduct for nursing and standards for nursing education

11 Promoting clinical effectiveness and maintaining quality of care

CHAPTER AIMS

- To examine the concepts of clinical effectiveness and clinical governance
- To examine a variety of different factors which can contribute to maintaining quality of care
- To develop the student's knowledge and understanding of the audit process
- To explore how an understanding of clinical effectiveness can support the student's achievement of specific Nursing and Midwifery Council Standards and Competencies

Introduction

All healthcare practitioners are involved with continually examining ways in which care can be improved to enable the continuous delivery of high-quality care. This chapter examines a range of issues which are related to improving quality in care such as clinical effectiveness, audit, clinical governance, evidence-based care and quality indicators and outcomes. The student nurse needs to ensure that the knowledge and skills to deliver quality care need to be attained as an ongoing part of their learning and continued throughout their future practice as a qualified nurse in order to ensure competence in delivering and promoting quality in healthcare.

Figure 11.1 demonstrates the wide range of issues that can contribute to achieving quality in health care. This chapter refers to each of these issues with specific reference to the community nursing role.

 Activity

In Chapters 9 and 10, reference was made to the Nursing and Midwifery Council Standards for Pre-registration Nursing Education (NMC 2010). Access this framework again at: http://standards.nmc-uk.org and consider Competencies 2 and 3 within Domain 4: Leadership, Management and Team Working. These directly relate to improving quality of care and are an essential part of its promotion by the student nurse. With your mentor, try to identify examples within your community learning experience which demonstrate your progress towards achievement of learning outcomes that relate to the quality improvement process.

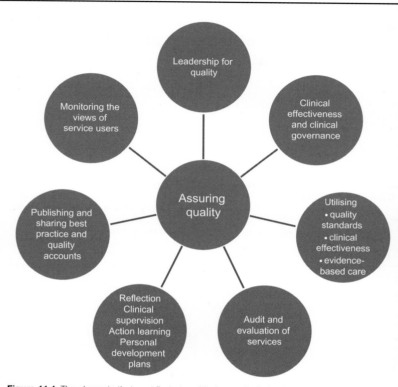

Figure 11.1 The elements that contribute to achieving quality in healthcare services.

Policy drivers

The Department of Health's publication, 'High Quality Care for All' (DH 2008a) emphasised the significance of quality in health care for all practitioners and stated that service provision should centre on three essentials of quality:

- Clinical effectiveness
- Safety
- Patient experience.

In addition, the Healthcare Quality Strategy for NHS Scotland (Scottish Government 2010) focuses on similar ambitions for the quality of healthcare, namely, safe, effective and person-centred care. These strategic documents set the direction for achieving excellence in healthcare quality and drive forward initiatives at all levels of health and social care organisations.

 Activity

Access the government website in the country you are undertaking your course of study (the UK government

Continued

websites are listed at the end of Chapter 1) and pick out the key policy documents that relate to quality in health care. Read the overall aims and ambitions of the strategy and reflect on their relevance to community nursing practice. You may like to discuss this with your mentor or university tutor to identify the implementation of such policy documents to everyday practice.

Clinical effectiveness

You will have come across a number of key phrases that are involved in the promotion and sustainability of quality in care, including reference to clinical effectiveness. Clinical interventions are deemed clinically effective when they do what they are intended and achieve the best possible outcomes for people within the resources that are available. Bowers and Cook (2012) refer to the importance of district nurses being able to demonstrate their effectiveness and role within the multidisciplinary team in supporting health outcomes for patients. Clinical effectiveness requires an analytical and questioning approach at all levels of the organisation and a willingness to make changes according to the evidence of what works best. Methods to promote clinical effectiveness include clinical audit and different strategies to develop and utilise skills, knowledge and experience of staff. The continual evaluation of practice is also an essential part of clinical effectiveness and includes gaining feedback from service users, carers and members of the clinical team.

NHS Quality Improvement Scotland (NHS 2005; www.clinicalgovernance.scot. nhs.uk) describes clinical effectiveness as the right person (you) doing:

- *The right thing (evidence-based practice)*
- *In the right way (skills and competence)*

- *At the right time (providing treatment/ services when the patient needs them)*
- *In the right place (location of treatment/ services)*
- *With the right result (clinical effectiveness/ maximising health gain).*

 Activity

To develop your knowledge and understanding of the clinical effectiveness process in practice, in discussion with your mentor:

- Identify an aspect of care which requires changing in order to improve; your mentor will be able to help you with the identification of an aspect of care
- Consider the evidence that supports the change, e.g. evidence-based guidelines, clinical audit, feedback from service users, local or national initiatives
- Find out if specific resources are required, e.g. the development of skills among practitioners
- Identify how this change has or will promote better care and how it can be evaluated.

From the above activity, you will see that clinical effectiveness consists of a series of actions and changes which necessitates the management of change, the implementation of evidence-based care and the continuous monitoring and supervision of practice.

Assuring quality

The provision and promotion of quality services are an essential part of the healthcare practitioner's role. As professionals, nurses are personally accountable for their actions and omissions and must adhere to the Nursing and Midwifery Council Code (NMC 2008b).

 Activity

Access The Code: Standards of Conduct, Performance and Ethics for Nurses and Midwives, at: www.nmc-uk. org and consider aspects of the code which relate directly to quality of care.

Some characteristics of professional behaviour are essential to ensure quality, safety and effectiveness of care. These include a commitment to learning and updating of knowledge and skills; willingness to accept responsibility and to stand accountable for one's own practice; respect; compassion and empathy for clients and colleagues; and being able to act in the best interest of service users and carers. As a student, you are personally accountable for the care you provide and this includes saying 'No' to something for which you feel unprepared or inexperienced. Access the Guidance on Professional Conduct for Nursing and Midwifery Students, at: www. nmc.org which outlines your professional responsibilities as a student nurse.

 Activity

- Can you recall a situation in clinical practice where you were asked to do something which made you feel uncomfortable? Did you say 'No'? Did you undertake the task?
- Try a short reflective exercise using this experience or try testing out how it would feel to say 'No'. You might find it helpful to discuss the issues this raises with other students when you all meet for a reflection on practice session that many of you will experience on return from placement to the university.

The significance of regularly reflecting on practice in promoting quality of care is discussed later in this chapter.

Quality in health care

Quality can mean something different to different people, whether healthcare users or healthcare providers. The Institute of Medicine (2001) identified six dimensions of quality and these have been used widely in the UK to clarify the meaning and establish a shared understanding of quality in healthcare and are relevant to all practitioners. The Healthcare Quality Strategy for NHS Scotland (Scottish Government 2010) refers to the six dimensions, which are shown in Table 11.1.

Table 11.1 The dimensions of quality in health care

1. Person-centeredness: care which addresses the individual needs and values of the client

2. Safety: care which is safe and avoids injury to the patient

3. Effectiveness: care which is based on scientific evidence

4. Efficiency: care which avoids waste and utilises resources appropriately

5. Equitable: all care is available to all clients and patients whoever and wherever they are

6. Timely: care is delivered when it is required whenever that may be without undue delay.

Institute of Medicine (2001).

Person-centred care, involving patients and the views of service users

Person-centred care was referred to in Chapter 5 and was defined as the provision of care that is responsive to individual needs and values. There are a number of programmes which place people at the centre of care and support the development of relationships between them, their carers and healthcare providers. This results in shared decision-making, better experiences of care and greater job satisfaction for staff. The Department of Health (DH 2010a) referred to the importance of patient involvement in decisions about their health care; emphasis has also been placed on the facilitation of this with the provision of information to help patients make informed choices.

An important aspect of quality healthcare provision is the attainment of feedback from people who use the health service. In England, patient reported outcome measures (PROMs) are used to measure a person's health status or health-related quality of life and provide a way of assessing the effectiveness of care from the patient's perspective. In Scotland, the Better Together programme is using the public's experiences of NHS Scotland to improve health services.

Activity

Refer to the PROMs, which are now published on a monthly basis, and can be accessed at: www.ic.nhs.uk/proms or the Better Together Website, at: www.bettertogetherscotland.com. This feedback provides insight to you as a practitioner about the quality of the care that we deliver from the perspective of people who experience it as patients. Read some of the patients perceptions of care and discuss with your mentor if some of these stories change your perception of the quality of care that is delivered. Also, consider how patients' feedback is obtained within your community learning placement.

Continued

The Care Quality Commission (CQC; www.cqc.org.uk) is a new independent regulator of all health and adult social care in England, which emphasises the importance of the patient's perspective by listing a range of essential standards that clients should expect from health and adult social care services in England. This includes client expectation to:

- be respected, involved in your care and support and told what's happening at every stage
- receive care, treatment and support that meets their needs
- be safe
- be cared for by staff with the right skills to do their job properly
- know that the services you receive are continually monitored and checked for quality.

Registration with the CQC provides assurance that essential levels of safety and quality are being met. An increasing number of healthcare providers are now registered with CQC in reference to healthcare associated infection. This requires that providers ensure clients and workers are protected against identifiable risks of acquiring a healthcare-associated infection. Service users can be reassured that quick action will be taken against those providers that fail to meet the requirements. (In Chapter 1, you will find reference to the organisations that perform this function in the other UK countries.)

During your placement you will be expected to contribute to the development of quality of care delivered to the patients and their families/carers – this will be relevant to all students regardless of which pathway they are pursuing towards registration as a nurse.

The role of the community nurse in promoting quality

The Department of Health publication, 'The Nursing Roadmap for Quality: a signposting map for nursing' (DH 2010b) has demonstrated the nurse's essential role and contribution to promoting and achieving quality. Seven elements to maintaining quality are identified within this publication:

- *Bringing clarity to quality*
- *Measuring quality*
- *Publishing quality performance*
- *Recognising and rewarding quality*
- *Leadership for quality*
- *Safeguarding quality*
- *Staying ahead.*

DH (2010b: 4)

Quality standards

The first stage of the quality process 'bringing clarity to quality' is to ensure that practitioners and service users are clear about the standard of care to be achieved. This is facilitated by the utilisation of quality standards. Quality standards have been mentioned within earlier sections in relation to their role in practice placement educational experiences. The National Institute for Health and Clinical Excellence (NICE) has devised quality standards in relation to a range of different aspects of care. Those that are particularly relevant to community nurses include diabetes in adults, end-of-life care in adults, stroke and dementia. Healthcare practitioners can use quality standards to consider the quality of care to be achieved and clients can use the standards to consider the care they should expect.

 Activity

Access some of the following websites to review some of the practice standards for care. You may focus on a specific aspect of care that you have been involved with during your community practice placement or a learning outcome that you are working towards achieving for your ongoing portfolio requirements:

1. NHS Evidence: www.evidence.nhs.uk
2. The National Institute for Health and Clinical Excellence (NICE) Clinical Guidelines: www.nice.org.uk/guidance
3. Scottish Intercollegiate Guidelines Network (SIGN): www.sign.ac.uk
4. The Nursing and Midwifery Council: www.nmc-uk.org

Evidence-based care

Evidence-based care is an essential aspect of quality care; to deliver care which is based on recent evidence and not on out-dated thinking and which is safe and appropriate for the patient. It is the responsibility of all healthcare practitioners to provide care based on the best available evidence. The practice of evidence-based care requires specific skills which include the ability to:

- Appraise practice
- Identify questions/criteria
- Search for evidence
- Assess quality of evidence
- Assess local applicability.

 Activity

Review your learning outcomes for this placement and note where you are expected to demonstrate provision of

Continued

evidenced-based care. Discuss with your mentor and other members of the team the types of evidence, and their sources, that are used to inform and deliver evidence-based care in the community. Identify one specific area of care that you have encountered and write a goal for finding out the evidence base to the nursing practice related to the care. An example could be the use of honey in wound care.

Clinical guidelines

From your discussion with your mentor regarding the above activity, your mentor will have referred you to The National Clinical Guidelines Centre (NCGC), which is a multidisciplinary health services research team funded by NICE to produce evidence-based clinical practice guidelines which aim to improve the quality of patient care within the NHS in England and Wales. Scottish Intercollegiate Guidelines Network (SIGN) develops evidence-based clinical practice guidelines for the National Health Service (NHS) in Scotland. The clinical guidelines refer to many different aspects of clinical care, including: management of deficit disorder in children and young people; non-pharmaceutical management of depression; falls; pressure ulcers and venous leg ulcers, and are used by the NHS and health and care organisations across the UK. Other organisations also develop evidence-based guidelines for specific clinical conditions often in partnership with others, e.g. the British Thoracic Society (BTS) and SIGN.

 Activity

The British Thoracic Society (BTS) and SIGN have recently published their revised British guidelines on the

management of asthma (BTS/SIGN 2012) for implementation in England, Wales, Scotland and Northern Ireland. (See: www.brit-thoracic.org.uk/guidelines/asthma-guidelines.aspx and www.sign.ac.uk/guidelines.)

Discuss opportunities with your mentor to spend time with a general practice nurse or community respiratory nurse to observe how this guideline is used in practice.

Clinical Quality Indicators (CQIs) are evidence-based process indicators that support practitioners to focus on quality, safety and reliability of care (NHS 2008b). The transforming community services (TCS) programme identified 43 indicators for quality improvement of community services in England (DH 2009). The programme supports: the development of services by setting out clear ambitions and the actions to achieve these; the development of people to design, deliver and lead change; the reform of systems to put in place the strong organisations and incentives that are needed to respond to the needs of people in their communities. The indicators cover many aspects of community services that interface with GPs, secondary care and social services and are very relevant to community nurses as part of the community multidisciplinary team. Their use is voluntary and, consequently, they are not used in all localities. (A link to the indicators for quality improvement is provided at the end of the chapter.)

 Activity

If you are a nursing student in community practice in England, ask your mentor about the impact of the TCS community indicators for quality improvement locally. If you are based in another part of the UK, ask your mentor

Continued

Continued

about the clinical quality indicators that may be in place in that country. This should give you an insight into the practical implementation of quality indicators in practice to enhance specific aspects of care.

The improvement of work processes to enhance care

The productive series: releasing time to care (RTC)

The productive series is a module improvement programme based on lean methodology, which assists teams to look at ways of improving work processes and the working environment to release more time to spend on direct patient care. To begin with, this initiative focused on ward processes (NHS 2009c) but it is equally applicable to the community setting, where it is now becoming established (NHS 2009b). In community nursing, looking at issues such as the organisation of the working environment, caseload management, the patient perspective and working effectively with key partners, has the potential to release capacity and capability within the service (NHS 2009a). A close and questioning look by the team at working practices can lead to simple but effective ways of utilising time and resources to better effect and increasing the focus on the client. For example, district nurses working in geographical clusters may reduce time and effort spent on travel and free up time to spend with service users and families. RTC has also provided the opportunity to examine traditional practices such as completing all home visits in the morning and utilising time more effectively. Even simple changes to the work environment can save time. Reference was made earlier in the book to the promotion

of self-care; time invested in developing a care plan with the patient to identify mutually agreed goals can make a significant contribution to a patient's quality of life. RTC can be utilised as an effective tool to facilitate safe, effective, evidence-based and person-centred care, supporting practitioners to develop quality community services.

 Activity

To develop your understanding of how RTC can enhance practice, access the Modernising Nursing in the Community website, at: www.mnic.nes. scot.nhs.uk to read examples of good clinical practice.

The NHS Institute for Innovation and Improvement identifies five key aims of 'productive community services':

- *To increase patient contact time*
- *To reduce inefficient work practices*
- *To improve quality and safety of care*
- *To motivate the workforce*
- *To enable staff to re-design their services.*

NHS (2009b)

 Activity

You may like to access some of the NHS Institute for Innovation and Improvement's Productive Series, at: www.institute.nhs.uk to see the range of areas covered and to examine how quality in care within these different areas can be developed.

Also, refer to: www.institute.nhs.uk or the Leading Better Care/Releasing Time to Care Website, at: www. evidenceintopractice.scot.nhs.uk to review some of the innovative initiatives to facilitate safe and effective care.

Continued

> You may also like to consider discussing with the community team how they see the effectiveness of their work practices and discuss how they would change anything and what resources they would need to do this.

The Department of Health's 'Transforming Community Services Transformational Guides' are a series of best practice guidelines developed with clinicians, which relate to the following six key specific areas of practice:

- Rehabilitation services
- End-of-life care
- Long-term conditions
- Acute care closer to home
- Services for health, wellbeing and reducing inequalities
- Services for children, young people and their families.

All of the guidelines include reference to three important components to promote the development of quality care and include: the improvement of services; developing the skills and knowledge of the people who deliver the service and aligning systems to underpin the change required to improve services. (See: http://www.dh.gov.uk/en/Publicationsandstatistics/Publications/PublicationsPolicyAndGuidance/DH_124178.)

Enhancing quality of care at home: the experience of palliative care

The example of palliative care is taken as a major component of community care and of the district nurses' workload, and demonstrates implementation of the three components identified above in the development of quality care.

Utilisation of guidelines to improve care

Earlier in the book, reference was made to The Liverpool Care Pathway (www.liv.ac.uk/mcpcil/liverpoop-care-pathway) and the Gold Standards Framework (www.goldstandardsframework.org.uk/TheGSFTollkit); both are evidence-based guidelines to ensure dignity and comfort and quality of care for patients suffering from terminal illness. Reynolds and Croft (2010) stress that the Gold Standards Framework can enhance staff confidence and facilitate teamwork to plan and implement good individualised home-based care which enhances quality of life and death. The Liverpool Care Pathway is normally implemented within the last few days of life and focuses on the physical, psychological and spiritual comfort of the patient and family. A vital element of the care pathway is also the care after death in relation to verification and certification. The pathway provides guidance on different aspects of care such as pain relief, nausea and vomiting, respiratory secretions and agitation. The Liverpool Care Pathway also assists in providing carers with information about bereavement services (see: http://www.liv.ac.uk/mcpcil/liverpool-care-pathway/).

Improving the skills of the practitioner to improve palliative care

With reference to the Department of Health's components to promote the development of quality care, a range of strategies need to be considered to enable practitioners to improve their skills in palliative care. Reynolds and Croft (2010) outline a number of initiatives which may enable staff development with this specific aspect of care such as:

- Shadowing a specialist practitioner or a practitioner with extensive experience in relation to palliative care

- Spending time at hospice/specialist palliative care units
- Utilising a significant event analysis approach to enable staff to reflect and discuss with colleagues their current palliative care experiences and responsibilities.

Services also have to be aligned to support carers in the community. Rapid response services such as 'Hospice at Home' may enable carers to continue with care and avoid admission to acute care.

 Activity

> Three initiatives suggested by Reynolds and Croft (2010) for developing practitioners' skills in palliative care are equally relevant for nursing students. Discuss with your mentor the opportunities for shadowing specialist palliative care nurses, including Macmillan nurses, spending a day at a local hospice and being involved in any local palliative care learning sessions. A reflective account of your learning experience could be used as evidence in your portfolio.

Within Figure 11.1, reference is made to clinical audit as part of enhancing quality of care. Please refer back to this before reading the next section.

Clinical audit

Clinical audit is the process that seeks to improve client care through the comprehensive review of care against specific criteria. It is a rigorous check to ensure that what should be done is being done.

The National Institute for Health and Clinical Excellence (NICE), within their paper 'Principles for Best Practice in Clinical Audit', defined clinical audit as:

> *a quality improvement process that seeks to improve patient care and outcomes*

> *through systematic review of care against explicit criteria and the implementation of change. Aspects of the structure, processes and outcomes of care are selected and systematically evaluated against explicit criteria. Where indicated, changes are implemented at an individual, team or social level and further monitoring is used to confirm improvement in healthcare delivery*

NICE (2002: IX)

There are several different types of audit:
- *Standards-based audit*: defining standards, collecting data to measure current practice against the standards
- *Adverse occurrence screening and critical incident monitoring*: peer review of specific incidents in practice which have caused concern; within primary care this is referred to 'significant event audit'
- *Peer review*: this is similar to the 'significant event audit' but also includes interesting and unusual events
- *Patient surveys and focus groups*: obtaining service users views of quality of care they have received.

 Activity

> In discussion with your mentor, identify and discuss some of the types of audit that have carried out within your community learning practice placement and discuss how this has contributed to enhancing care.

Significant event audit in primary care

Within primary care, many teams of practitioners find 'significant event auditing' provides a useful and practical way to examine issues within practice and from this, identify practice learning needs. Regular protected time can be arranged for 1–2 hours on a monthly or bi-monthly basis. Topics to be discussed within significant event auditing can include almost anything which the team feels closer examination to improve practice. Topics could include:

- A template for review on the computer
- Computer audit for asthma
- Telephone message book for the district nurse
- Staff resourcing for flu immunisation clinics
- Developing the learning environment for students.

 Activity

> In discussion with your mentor, find out if significant event audit is carried out; how is this implemented? Reflect on the specific aspects of care which have been developed and improved as a result of this process. To help you to understand this process, it may be beneficial to consider your personal reflections of significant events which have resulted in you reviewing your own personal and professional development. Undertake this in relation to your own field of practice but also consider the way in which there may be differences in other fields of practice with regards to the type of significant events that can occur and which are then audited.

Significant event audit normally commences with the selection of a topic or issue to be audited and normally includes measuring adherence to healthcare processes that have been shown to produce best outcomes for clients. The second stage normally includes the formulisation of the aims and objectives of the audit, resulting in a series of statements about what is being measured with specific reference to aspects of care which can be objectively measured. The third stage is the data collection phase which may consist of the collection of the views of service users. The fourth stage includes the comparison of data collected with criteria and standards which results in the fifth stage, the dissemination of audit findings and an action plan compiled to if necessary make changes to service delivery to enhance care.

Reflection on significant events is also an aspect of the process of clinical supervision which is discussed later in this chapter.

Clinical governance

In the pursuit of developing quality care, practitioners must take a continuous improvement approach developing a working culture which encourages and supports the on-going examination of service improvement, continuously attempting to find better ways of doing things. Clinical governance is the system by which NHS services are accountable for continuously improving the quality of services and which emphasises the practitioner's responsibility with regard to accountability for their practice. Clinical governance supports and encourages clinical effectiveness, research and evidence-based care, clinical supervision, personal and professional development and clinical audit. Improving the quality of care and outcomes

 Activity

> Discuss with your mentor the research findings and clinical guidelines that are utilised within a specific aspect of care and consider the audit practices that are carried out to evaluate that care. Also try to find out what opportunities are organised to facilitate the sharing of good practice with colleagues within your community placement area.
>
> Refer to the Scottish Government 'Supporting Improvement' website, at: www.improvingnhsscotland.scot.

Continued

nhs.uk to access a continuous improvement 'toolkit'. The website: www.knowledge.scot.nhs.uk/making-a-difference is also a resource for NHS staff to support the enhancement of service user experience.

for people who use nursing services also depends on the quality of the workforce (DH 2008b). A number of initiatives are in place to support this and the following are examples that relate specifically to community nursing.

Career and development frameworks

These guide practitioners in the development of their roles and careers. As part of the Modernising Nursing in the Community programme in Scotland, career and development frameworks have been developed for the following:
I. District nursing
II. Public health nursing: health visiting and school nursing
III. Community mental health nursing
IV. General practice nursing
V. Community children's nursing
VI. Community learning disabilities nursing
VII. Nursing in occupational health
These are available on the 'Modernising Nursing in the Community' website, at: www.mnic.nes.scot.nhs.uk/. They map progress through the Career Framework for Health and include examples of the roles associated with certain levels of the framework and the sphere of responsibility, key knowledge and skills and educational development required.

 Activity

Access the 'Modernising Nursing in the Community' website, at: www.mnic.nes.scot.nhs.uk/ and type career and

Continued

development frameworks into the search box. Alternatively, choose one of the platforms: children, young people and families; adults and older people; work and wellbeing. Then go to the resources section where you will find the career and development frameworks. You can find information about the role, aspects of practice and the key knowledge, skills and behaviours that are expected of the registered nurse working in each of the community nursing teams. If you aim to work in the community, this will apply to you!

The image of nursing

Specific reference was made to modernising the image of community nursing in 'Modernising Nursing Careers' (DH 2006) and the 'Front Line Care' report on the future of nursing and midwifery in England (DH 2010c). The King's Fund – a charity which seeks to understand how the health system in England can be improved – also refers to modernising nursing careers and makes reference to the increase of autonomy within the nursing role and to a provision of care, less centred around hospital provision.

NHS Education for Scotland has created 'Extraordinary Everyday', in partnership with practitioners from across Scotland. Photographs, video stories and text leaflets/templates show the real faces and stories of nursing and midwifery careers in hospitals, in communities, in prisons and in people's homes. The resources will be available for Higher Education Institutions, NHS Boards and all stakeholders to use to support greater understanding of nursing and midwifery career opportunities.

Pre-registration nursing

The NMC standards for pre-registration nurse education (NMC 2010) require all nursing programmes to be at a minimum of degree level and also to include a greater emphasis on public health and health improvement but also nursing in the community.

Preceptorship

The development of new nurse registrants as confident, autonomous practitioners with life-long learning skills for continuous professional development has been supported UK-wide. The governments in England and Scotland have invested in a universal development programme, 'Flying Start NHS' in Scotland and 'Flying Start England', which provide a 1-year programme of preceptorship and online support. This has helped promote the appointment of newly qualified nurses in community setting and given them opportunities to contribute to quality improvement in community nursing.

Leadership

The role of leadership in community nursing has been recognised in a number of leadership development programmes as instrumental in achieving high-quality, person-centred, safe and effective care. Leadership is discussed in more detail in Chapter 10.

Skill-mix

As skill-mix has developed within community nursing teams, when community nurses are delegating care within the nursing team, they must be assured that the team member is competent to deliver the type and standard of care required. For example NHS Education for Scotland (2009) published a set of nationally agreed educational requirements and core skills for clinical healthcare support workers. This has helped to strengthen and standardise

the role of the healthcare support worker in Scotland and promote the quality of care in the community.

 Activity

If you have not already done so, discuss with your mentor organising time with a healthcare support worker (HSW) within the practice area and find out what specific roles and responsibilities they have and how they have been prepared for these. Consider how they both differ and complement your own role as a student nurse and that of your mentor who is a registered nurse. Discuss with the HSW how they view their role in the team.

Learning from experience

Part of being professional is also being able to learn from experience and from making mistakes. Reflection has been discussed in Chapter 4, as a significant skill to develop to help you think objectively about an experience and to utilise experience as an opportunity for personnel and professional development. Engaging in dialogue with a supervisor, mentor or peer can facilitate reflective discussion and help you develop an understanding of different situations and plan how you might manage these situations in the future. This can assist in promoting quality care. Clinical supervision is a formalised way to encourage reflection on a regular basis.

Clinical supervision

Clinical supervision is a means of formal professional support and learning, which enables individual practitioners to reflect on their everyday practice to develop their knowledge, skills and competence to ultimately maintain quality of care for clients. This support mechanism is an opportunity to enable practitioners to discuss key issues in relation to their work and to then consider a plan for future action.

Neil Gopee (2011) refers to the health care practitioner's peer support role within clinical supervision, utilising expertise and experience to support and enable peers with their own continuing professional development.

The Nursing and Midwifery Council (NMC 2008a) identify the following aims of clinical supervision to:

- *Identify solutions to problems*
- *Increase understanding of professional issues*
- *Improve standards of patient care*
- *Further develop their skills and knowledge*
- *Enhance their understanding of their own practice.*

This supportive and educative process is important to practitioners in an increasingly busy NHS, in which practitioners face a number of challenges including the managerial challenge, ensuring practitioners are able to work to appropriate standards.

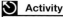 **Activity**

In discussion with your community practice mentor, find out how clinical supervision is achieved within your community practice placement. Try to find out if the implementation of clinical supervision differs within different fields of nursing practice. For example, is this support strategy different in mental health nursing, public health or in adult nursing?

Table 11.2 identifies the responsibilities of the clinical supervisor and some of the ways in which clinical supervision can be achieved.

 Activity

Discuss with your mentor, what might be the advantages and disadvantages of participating in clinical supervision in their workplace.

Your list of advantages may have included some of the following:

- Develops clinical competence and knowledge base and reflective skills
- Facilitates improvements in patient/client care

Table 11.2 Clinical supervision

Responsibilities of the clinical supervisor	How clinical supervision can be achieved
Establish a safe environment to share information, experience and skills. Help explore and clarify thinking processes. Provide constructive and clear feedback. Challenge ideas and practice issues. Establish and adhere to ground rules in relation to the supervision meeting.	Regular one-to-one sessions with a supervisor from the same profession. Regular one-to-one sessions with a supervisor from a different discipline. One-to-one peer supervision; working with people of a similar grade and expertise. Group supervision; a group of practitioners with similar expertise and interests who do not necessarily work together, meet on a daily or regular basis.

- Makes staff feel supported/'a place of safety'
- Staff feel less stressed
- Helps reduce number of NHS complaints
- Makes you feel more confident
- Is a good support to newly qualified staff
- Reduces guilt, loneliness and fear
- Motivates, increases morale
- Enables collective solution finding.

Clinical supervision can be an invaluable opportunity for community practitioners who may feel relatively isolated, such as practice nurses in small practices or district nurses who work in quiet rural areas or for staff who face the daily challenges of working in very deprived areas. Reference has been made to the significant role of the community nurse in palliative care. Clinical supervision can provide an important restorative function for staff in this emotionally challenging area of work.

Regular meetings among community practitioners in a clinical supervision forum encourage reflection and learning from experience, and provides an opportunity to consider appropriate improvements in care; the overall result being improved quality in care.

Continuing personal and professional development

Ensuring you are up-to-date and competent is a significant component in facilitating the delivery of high-quality care.

 Activity

In discussion with your mentor, try to identify the different ways that both of you can develop your practice and keep yourselves up-to-date. You will already be maintaining a Personal Development Plan (PDP) and portfolio, which will be an added advantage when having to continue this practice once qualified during your preceptorship period.

There is a variety of different ways of keeping up-to-date and developing your practice, such as reading widely in your area of work; being an active member of a professional society; attending conferences; shadowing colleagues; discussing issues with peers; participating in action learning sets; taking part in courses within higher education.

Your mentor has probably also referred to personal development planning (PDP), which provides an opportunity for practitioners to review their professional learning needs. The PDP process also provides an opportunity to identify small steps which have enabled your development and which can contribute to future learning. PDP also provides an opportunity to review the development of specific clinical skills and subsequent training needs and development and can be extremely useful in helping you as a student with your on-going record of achievement, as well providing an opportunity to facilitate career progression once you are qualified.

Action learning sets

Action learning has been referred to earlier in this section and can be a valuable tool for personal, professional and organisational development. It is an active process which provides group support, the action learning set, which provides practitioners with the opportunity to reflect and review. Action learning works with the realities of practice, focusing on the identification and development of solutions to real work-related issues. A further strength of action learning is also the opportunity to learn in a positive way from work that has met with success. This is often the mode of learning within clinical supervision and significant event analysis (Figure 11.2).

⊘ Activity

You will find out more about action learning by accessing the International Foundation for Action Learning Website, at: www.ifal.org.uk. You may have already used action learning sets within your classroom sessions, reflecting on, e.g. a specific significant incident from your practice experience and sharing this with your colleagues to help you identify what you have learned from this experience; what future learning needs you have identified; and how you will manage this aspect of care in the future.

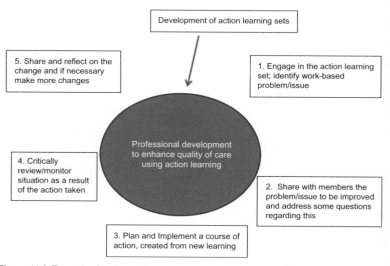

Figure 11.2 The action learning cycle.

Creating a positive learning environment for students and colleagues

NHS Education for Scotland (NHS 2008a) states: *'that good clinical environments are good learning environments and vice versa'*. Creating a positive learning environment for all staff and students therefore enables practitioners to be clinically effective and to deliver high quality care. National Standards to ensure quality practice learning are set out in the NMC Standards for Education for Pre-registration Students (2010), at: http://standards.nmc-uk.org/PreRegNursing/statutory/Standards/Pages/Standards.aspx and those related to the role of mentor in supporting the development of a positive learning environment for you as a student nurse can be found at: http://www.nmc-uk.org/Documents/Standards/nmcStandardsToSupportLearningAndAssessmentInPractice.pdf.

Activity

If you are a student nurse in the third year and approaching your final assessment of practice, this latter document can be used to look at essential skills that you can gain to prepare for mentorship and teaching role once qualified. Set a goal for yourself with regards to teaching another student who may be in the same community placement with you. Discuss with them what they have to achieve and support them through offering to teach them a skill that is within your ability and under supervision can do, or help them to learn about an issue such as evidence-based practice. Have your mentor assess you doing this and in doing so, it will enable you and the other student to both achieve the relevant goals and NMC competencies relating to that goal.

However, a conscious effort is needed to change a working environment into a learning environment in which learners feel 'safe' in revealing their thoughts and feelings, and in which they feel that their knowledge and experiences are respected and valued. The clinical mentor can have considerable influence over the arranging of opportunities for learning in the practice setting.

 Activity

Reflect on your clinical learning experiences including your current experience in the community and consider what you have felt as useful in supporting and guiding your learning.

You may have identified some of the following points which have helped in creating a positive learning environment:
• A comprehensive orientation
• Demonstration of interest in your personnel and professional learning needs
• Identifying clinical opportunities to assist enable your professional development
• Giving regular constructive feedback
• Having a person centered approach, showing interest, concern and understanding.

 Activity

Access the following article, which outlines student nurses perceptions of a good learning environment: Tremayne P (2007) Improving clinical placements through evaluation and feedback to staff. Nursing Times 103 (25):32–33.

Chapter 3 referred to the Quality Standards for Practice Placements (NHS 2008a). Refer to this again here and look at the standards in relation to creating a good learning environment. Use these as a guide for evaluating the quality of your current learning environment.

The NMC gives very specific guidelines regarding your support during your practice placement experiences, and includes reference to areas such as the role of your mentor in supporting your learning in practice and identifying and organising valuable clinical learning opportunities which will assist you as a student to achieve your learning practice objectives.

This chapter has focused on a variety of different aspects of developing quality in care. However, earlier chapters have made reference to aspects of care such as holistic assessment; patient-centeredness; evidence-based practice; the enhancement of patient

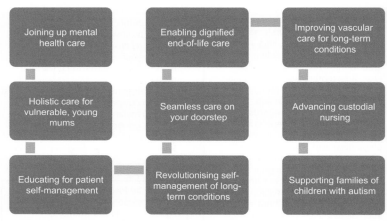

Figure 11.3 Examples of community nursing developments which enhance the quality of care.

empowerment; the utilisation of specific guidelines, e.g. in palliative care; preventing and controlling infection; preventing falls; medicines management and case management, all of which are concerned with improving quality in care.

Figure 11.3 outlines some of the recent developments in community nursing, which are presented by the Royal College of Nursing (RCN 2010) as evidence of outstanding community nursing developments that have substantially contributed to the quality of care in the community.

Summary of learning points from this chapter

After reading this chapter and completing the learning activities you should have been able to achieve the following, which will support your achievement of the NMC Standards (NMC 2010):

• Knowledge and understanding regarding the principles of clinical effectiveness and clinical governance in the provision of quality care

• Knowledge of professional behaviour which ensures quality, safety and effectiveness of care

• Development of your knowledge regarding person-centred care and the role of the Care Quality Commission

• An understanding of the skills required to deliver evidence-based care including the utilisation of clinical quality indicators and guidelines

• Knowledge and understanding of different types of clinical audit

• Knowledge and understanding of the principles of significant event audit and its relevance to primary care

• The principles of reflective practice and clinical supervision

• The importance of a quality learning environment.

References

Bowers, B., Cook, R., 2012. Using referral guidelines to support best care outcomes for patients. Br. J. Community Nurs. 17 (3), 134–138.

British Thoracic Society/Scottish Intercollegiate Guidelines Network (BTS/SIGN), 2012. British Guideline on the management of asthma: a national clinical guideline. Online. Available at: www.brit-thoracic.org.uk/guidelines/asthma-guidelines.aspx.

Department of Health, 2006. Modernising nursing careers: Setting the direction. DH, London.

Department of Health, 2008a. High quality care for all. Online. Available at: http://www.dh.gov.uk/en/Publicationsandstatistics/Publications/PublicationsPolicyAndGuidance/DH_085825.

Department of Health, 2008b. NHS next stage review: a high quality workforce. DH, London.

Department of Health, 2009. Transforming community services: ambition, action, achievement. DH, London.

Department of Health, 2010a. Equity and excellence: liberating the NHS. Online. Available at: www.dh.gov.uk.

Department of Health, 2010b. The nursing roadmap for quality: A signposting map for nursing. DH, London.

Department of Health, 2010c. Front line care: the future of nursing and midwifery in England. DH, London.

Gopee, N., 2011. Mentoring and supervision in healthcare. Sage, London.

Institute of Medicine, 2001. Healthcare quality strategy. Online. Available at: http://www.evidenceintopractice.scot.nhs.uk/healthcare-quality-strategy.aspx.

NHS, Education for Scotland, 2008a. Quality standards for practice placements. Online. Available at: www.nes.scot.nhs.uk/media/323817/qspp_leaflet_2008.pdf.

NHS, Institute for Innovation and Improvement, 2009a. High impact actions: the essential collection. Online. Available at: http://www.institute.nhs.uk/building_capability/general/aims/.

NHS, Institute for Innovation and Improvement, 2009b. Productive community services: releasing time to care. Online. Available at: http://www.institute.nhs.uk/quality_and_value/productivity_series/the_productive_series.html.

NHS, Institute for Innovation and Improvement, 2009c. The productive ward: releasing time to care. Online. Available at http://www.institute.nhs.uk/quality_and_value/productivity_series/productive_ward.html.

NHS, Quality Improvement Scotland (NHS), 2005. Online. Available at: www.clinicalgovernance.scot.nhs.uk.

NICE, 2002. Principles of best practice in clinical audit. Online. Available at: www.nice.org.uk.

Nursing and Midwifery Council, 2008a. Clinical supervision for registered nurses. Online. Available at: www.nmc-uk.org.

Nursing and Midwifery Council, 2008b. The Code: Standards of Conduct, Performance and Ethics for Nurses and Midwives. Online. Available at: http://www.nmc-uk.org/Publications/Standards/The-code/Introduction/.

Nursing and Midwifery Council, 2010. Standards for pre-registration nursing education. Online. Available at: http://standards.nmc-uk.org.

Reynolds, J., Croft, S., 2010. How to implement the Gold Standards Framework to ensure continuity of care. Nurs. Times 106 (32), 10–13.

Royal College of Nursing, 2010. Community nursing: transforming health care. RCN, London.

Scottish Government, 2010. The Healthcare Quality Strategy for NHS Scotland. Online. Available at: http://www.scotland.gov.uk/Publications/2010/05/10102307/0.

Further reading

Burton, R., Ormrod, G., 2011. Nursing: transition to professional practice. Oxford University Press, Oxford.

Care Quality Commission, Patient information surveys. Online. Available at: http://www.cqc.org.uk.

Department of Health, 2003. Essence of care. Benchmarks for communication between patients, carers and health care. Department of Health, NHS Modernisation Agency, London.

Department of Health, 2008. End of life care strategy: promoting high quality care for all adults at the end of life. DH, London.

Department of Health, 2010. Energise for excellence in care. Online. Available at: www.dh.gov.uk.

Driscoll, J., 2006. Practicing clinical supervision, second ed. Elsevier, Edinburgh.

Flying Start Scotland. Online. Available at: http://www.flyingstart.scot.nhs.uk.

Hoffman, T., Bennett, S., Del Marc, C., 2010. Evidence based practice across the health professions. Churchill Livingstone, Edinburgh.

Kenworthy, N., Nicklin, N., 2000. Teaching and assessing in nursing practice: an experiential approach. Balliere Tindall and Royal College of Nursing, Edinburgh.

NHS, The Information Centre for Health and Social Care, Patient reported outcomes measures (PROMs). Online. Available at: www.ic.nhs.uk/proms.

NHS, The Information Centre for health and social care, 2008b. Clinical quality indicators. Online. Available at: http://www.ic.nhs.uk/services/in-development/clinical-quality-indicators.

Websites

Healthcare Improvement Scotland, Making Scotland's Healthcare Better Together: a person-centred improvement programme, at: www.bettertogetherscotland.com, will provide you as a practitioner with an insight of the patient experience.

Flying Start England. Online. Available at: http://www.flyingstartengland.nhs.uk.

National Clinical Guideline Centre (NCGC), Developing clinical guidelines on behalf of the National Institute for Health and Clinical Excellence (NICE). Online. Available at: www.dh.gov.uk.

The Institute for Healthcare Improvement is an International Forum on Quality and Safety in healthcare, www.ihi.org.

The International Foundation for Action Learning, www.ifal.org.uk.

The National Association for Healthcare Quality, www.nahq.org, provides education and support for professionals at all levels of management on continuous improvement methods to enhance quality of care.

NHS Scotland, www.evidenceintopractice.scot.nhs.uk.

NHS Scotland, www.knowledge.scot.nhs.uk/making-a-difference.

NHS Scotland, Modernising nursing in the community. www.mnic.nes.scot.nhs.uk.

NHS/NICE, To review different standards for care, see: www.evidence.nhs.uk and www.nice.org.uk.

NHS Scotland, To access a continuous improvement 'toolkit', see: www.improvingnhsscotland.scot.nhs.uk.

NHS Scotland, Educational Resources, Clinical Governance, http://www.clinicalgovernance.scot.nhs.uk/.

NHS UK, A quick and easy access to quality health and social care information. www.evidence.nhs.uk.

Prevention of healthcare-associated infections in primary and community care. http://tinyurl.com/com/yfagns8.

12 Medicines management in the community

CHAPTER AIMS

- To give an overview of the activities involved in medicines management and the role of patients and practitioners
- To explain the importance of medicines management in the community and primary care
- To illustrate the impact of good medicines management on the quality of care using case studies
- To identify the student's role in medicines management in the community and identify opportunities for learning

Introduction

Medicines make a huge impact on the health and wellbeing of individuals and populations. They enable people to: live longer; help prevent the onset and adverse effects of acute illness; effectively manage long-term conditions; prevent and treat infection and promote health. Not surprisingly, medicines are the most common clinical intervention used in the NHS today (National Prescribing Centre 2008). However, there are also significant costs associated with medicines. There are human costs, resulting from unwanted side-effects or the inappropriate use of medicines, which can lead to serious illness or death. There are also huge financial costs for the health service in paying the medicines bill, which includes medicines that are dispensed and never used. As life expectancy increases and new treatments enter the market, the medicines bill will continue to rise.

Medicines management can be described as:

> *the process of managing the way in which medicines are chosen, bought, delivered, prescribed, administered and reviewed, including appropriate safe, agreed withdrawal, in order to make the most of the contribution medicines can make to improving care and treatment.*
> DH (2008: 1)

Medicines management aims to enable people to get the maximum benefit from the medicines they take, not only by ensuring that they are appropriate and clinically effective but also by balancing safety, cost, tolerability and choice. The term covers a wide range of activities involving doctors, pharmacists, nurses, other members of the health and care team and most importantly, the person and their family. However, the nursing team plays such a pivotal role, that medicine management has been included in the NMC Standards for Pre-registration Nursing Education as one of the five Essential Skills Clusters (ESC) (NMC 2010), Consequently, medicines management underpins a number of your nursing programme learning outcomes.

Medicines management in the community

The safe and effective use of medicines is essential in all healthcare settings. However, there are additional challenges in the community that make it even more important to get medicines management right. For example, people have a great deal

---

 Activity

The Essential Skills Cluster: Medicines management (NMC 2010), states that people can trust the newly registered graduate nurse to:

- *safely and correctly undertake medicines calculations*
- *work within legal and ethical frameworks that underpin safe and effective medicines management*
- *work as part of a team to offer holistic care and a range of treatment options of which medicines may form a part*
- *ensure safe and effective practice in medicines management through comprehensive knowledge of medicines, their actions, risks and benefits*
- *safely order receive and store and dispose of medicines (including controlled drugs) in any setting*
- *administer medicines safely and in a timely manner, including controlled drugs*
- *keep and maintain accurate records using information technology where appropriate within a multidisciplinary framework as a leader and as part of a team and in a variety of care settings including the home*
- *work in partnership with people receiving medical treatments and their carers*
- *use and evaluate up-to-date information on medicines management and work within national and local policy guidelines*
- *demonstrate understanding and knowledge to supply and administer via a patient group direction*

NMC (2010: 134–152)

Not all of the skills and behaviours that comprise the medicines management ESC as listed here will apply to you now, as it depends on your year of study and any specific learning outcomes that have been identified for this placement.

Review the learning outcomes that you are expected to achieve during your community placement and discuss with your mentor the learning opportunities that are available, e.g. the opportunities to learn about the medicines management process from different members of the health and care team in the community and opportunities to use transferable skills and knowledge you may have already acquired in other settings.

more responsibility for managing their own medicines in the community than they would in an inpatient setting. They not only have access to a wide range of medicines on sale in shops, pharmacies and on the internet, but also any medicines that are prescribed. In most cases, the responsibility for the administration of medicines and the day-to-day monitoring of their effect rests with the individual and carer.

When the health and care team is involved in home care, the emphasis is on educating, supporting and empowering people to manage their medicines safely and effectively. The primary care team manages increasingly complex medication regimens for people who would once have been treated in hospital. Older people with multiple health problems, those with long-term conditions and children with very complex healthcare needs are now cared for at home for as long as possible. To be effective therefore, medicines management must involve a wide range of people in a wide range of activities namely:

- Prescribing
- Dispensing
- Administration
- Repeat prescribing
- Promoting partnerships with patients and carers to improve medicines adherence
- Educating health and care practitioners
- Monitoring and evaluating the desired and undesired effects of medication through medication review
- Reporting suspected adverse drug reactions
- Safe storage and disposal of medicines.

 Activity

The NMC (2007) have published Standards for Medicines Management that all registered nurses must comply with. Observing how nurses work

Continued

within the standards in the community is an essential part of your learning and preparation for registration.

Access this booklet and become familiar with the content. Two of the standards relate specifically to student nurses. Pick these out and think about how they might apply to you during learning in practice in the community. Reference will be made to these Standards later in the chapter.

Why is medicines management so important?

Safety, effectiveness and cost underpin medicines management. Medicines aim to control symptoms, help improve a person's health and wellbeing and prevent ill-health of individuals and populations, for example through immunisation programmes. However, we know that people do not always use medicines in the way that was intended by the prescriber. NICE (2009) have estimated that up to 50% of patients do not take their medicines as prescribed. Sometimes, people choose not to take their medicines at all. They may be unclear about their purpose or they may have a physical or psychological problem which prevents them from following the directions they have been given. As a result, far from getting benefit from the medicine, people continue to experience poor health or may be affected by the harmful effects of taking medicines incorrectly. This has a huge personal cost to the individual and family. There is also a cost to the health service, as money wasted in one part of the health service means denying services in other areas.

The overriding reason for effective medicines management is safety. The safety of medicines relates to two different effects: an adverse drug incident and an adverse drug reaction.

An **adverse drug incident** refers to an unsuitable or incorrect procedure. The National Patient Safety Agency (2009) identified three incident types accounting for 71% of the serious harm or fatal outcome of medication incidents. These were:

1. Unclear/wrong dose or frequency
2. Wrong medicine
3. Omitted or delayed medicines.

Four groups of drugs account for more than 50% of the drug groups associated with preventable drug-related hospital admissions: antithrombotics (e.g. aspirin); anticoagulants (e.g. warfarin); non-steroidal anti-inflammatory drugs (e.g. ibuprofen); and diuretics (e.g. hydrochlorothiazide) (Howard et al 2007).

Garfield et al (2009) reviewed the UK literature and found a prescribing error rate of around 7.5% and showed that approximately one in 15 hospital admissions were related to medication, with two-thirds of these being preventable. Barber et al (2009) reviewed the medication of older people living in 55 care homes in England and found that 70% of the residents they studied had one or more medication error.

Adverse events are reported through local and national risk management systems. The National Patient Safety Agency (NPSA) National Reporting and Learning System (NRLS), collects information on reported patient safety incidents from local risk management systems in England and Wales. Scotland has the National Patient Safety Programme coordinated by Healthcare Improvement Scotland, an organisation that directly promotes patient safety within NHS Scotland.

An **adverse drug reaction** (ADR) is defined on the MHRA website as:

an unwanted or harmful reaction following the administration of a drug or combination of drugs under normal conditions of use, which is suspected to be related to the drug. The reaction may be a known side effect of the drug or it may be new and previously unrecognised.

(http://www.mhra.gov.uk/ Aboutus/index.htm accessed December 2011)

Pirmohamed et al (2004) studied hospital admissions in the UK and found that:

- 6.5% of hospital admissions were related to adverse drug reactions
- More than 2% of patients admitted with an ADR died
- Almost three-quarters of ADRs could probably have been avoided.

Reporting adverse drug reactions

The Medicines and Healthcare Products Regulatory Agency (MHRA) is a UK government agency whose role is to ensure that medicines and medicinal devices are effective and acceptably safe. The MHRA is responsible for licensing new medicines and monitoring the use of existing medicines in the UK. Yellow card reporting is the main reporting scheme for suspected adverse drug reactions. Without this scheme, it would be very difficult to monitor the safety of new medicines and also established medicines when they are used in new ways. It relies on the voluntary reporting of suspected adverse drug reactions by healthcare professionals and the public from all over the UK by completing a yellow card.

Yellow card reports enable the MHRA to identify risk factors for certain medicines and evaluate these together with other sources of evidence. As a result, actions can be taken to improve the safety of the medicine, such as making additional information available to prescribers and the public or in cases where the evidence suggests the drug is unsafe. The MHRA has

Activity

Yellow card reporting

It is very important that everyone who suspects an adverse reaction knows what to do and how to make a report. It is just as important to report suspected adverse effects of medicines and herbal remedies that are bought as over-the-counter medicines, as well as medicines that have been prescribed. Reports can be made online, on a free Yellow Card, telephone hotline and on a Yellow Card form, which is available at pharmacies, GP surgeries and at the back of the British National Formulary (BNF). All health professionals and members of the public are encouraged to report a suspected adverse drug reaction in this way.

Go to the MHRA Website and try accessing the frequently asked questions and the link to a yellow card report, at: http://yellowcard.mhra.gov.uk/faqs/

Find out about yellow card reporting from someone who has made a report. Ask your mentor if they have reported an ADR using a yellow card. Ask one of the GPs about their experience of yellow card reporting.

the authority not to license the drug following the trial period or to suspend or withdraw a licensed medicine from the market.

How people get their medicines in the community

The ways in which people access medicines relate to the three main groups of medicines defined by the Medicines Act 1968. This is shown in Table 12.1.

Prescription-only medicines (POMs)

The vast majority of POMs are prescribed by the GP. However, there are other methods of obtaining POMs in the community which enable people to get easier and quicker access to the treatments they need, without having to rely on a doctor being present.

Non-medical prescribing

Since nurse prescribing was first introduced in 1994, people can now obtain prescriptions from a much wider range of

Table 12.1 Three main groups of medicines defined by the Medicines Act 1968

Prescription only medicines (POM)	Medicines that can only be obtained with a prescription
Pharmacy (P)	Medicines that can be bought in a pharmacy but their sale must be supervised by a pharmacist
General sale list (GSL)	Medicines that can be bought over-the-counter without pharmacist supervision in a wide range of retail outlets such as supermarkets, garages and health food stores

healthcare professionals. Unfortunately, the term 'non-medical prescribing' is not straightforward, as different non-medical prescribers can prescribe different medicines in different ways. This is explained in more detail later in the chapter.

Exemptions

These are known as exemptions from the general rules and apply to midwives, podiatrists and optometrists under the Medicines Act 1968. Exemptions permit them to supply and/or administer or sell POMs under specific conditions.

Patient group directions (PGDs)

PGDs are used in hospital and community settings within a legislative framework and make provision for identified groups of patients, rather than individual named patients to obtain prescription only medicines.

 Activity

Who can prescribe?

Doctors and dentists are no longer the only healthcare professionals who can prescribe medicines. Working out which healthcare professional can prescribe which medicine is confusing for patients and they may ask you about this. Make a note of the practitioners that you think are eligible to prescribe. You will be able to determine if your answers are correct by reading the rest of this chapter.

Prescribing and prescribers

Changes in prescribing legislation have given an increasing number of healthcare professionals eligibility to prescribe prescription-only medicines (POMs) under certain conditions. Legislation and professional regulation strictly control prescribing rights and determine who can prescribe and what they can prescribe. This can be confusing for everyone and particularly patients. Essentially there are:

- Two types of prescriber: medical prescriber and non-medical prescriber
- Two types of prescribing: independent prescribing and supplementary prescribing
- Three types of independent prescriber apart from doctors and dentists: Nurse/midwife independent prescriber, pharmacist independent prescriber and community practitioner nurse prescriber.

Medical prescribers are doctors (and dentists) who are licensed to prescribe when they complete their training. Non-medical prescribers must successfully complete a specific course of preparation which meets the standards of their professional regulatory organisation, for the type of prescribing they are eligible to undertake. Table 12.2 lists the practitioners who are currently eligible to become non-medical prescribers. However, further changes in legislation will extend prescribing roles further, particularly in relation to allied health professionals.

Independent prescribers are responsible for assessing the person's healthcare needs, making a diagnosis and using prescribing as one potential component of the treatment plan. They make prescribing decisions independently within their area of competence and are not required to refer to another practitioner.

Supplementary prescribers do not make the initial assessment of the patient. The doctor assesses the patient, makes the diagnosis and then draws up with the patient and supplementary prescriber a clinical management plan for their care. Supplementary prescribers are responsible for continuing care, which includes ongoing evaluation and by prescribing as directed by the clinical management plan. Supplementary prescribing is a

Table 12.2 Practitioners who are eligible to undertake training to be non-medical prescribers

Nurses and midwives	Nurse/midwife independent and supplementary prescribing
	Community practitioner nurse prescribing
Pharmacists	Independent prescribing
	Supplementary prescribing
Optometrists	Independent prescribing
	Supplementary prescribing
Physiotherapists	Supplementary prescribing only*
Radiographers	Supplementary prescribing only
Chiropodists and podiatrists	Supplementary prescribing only*

*Independent prescribing by appropriately qualified practitioners will be introduced in 2014.

voluntary partnership between the independent and the supplementary prescriber and agreed by the patient. *Case study 1* illustrates the role of the supplementary prescriber.

Legal restrictions apply to each professional group regarding the items they can prescribe, either as an

Case study 1

Supplementary prescribing

Sam Barnett is an experienced podiatrist and last year, qualified as a supplementary prescriber. He runs a podiatry clinic at the health centre and also provides a home visiting service. One of his regular patient's, Mr Cook has type 2 diabetes. Mr Cook has limited mobility due to obesity and cardiovascular problems. He lives alone and rarely goes out. He has developed a small ulcer on the underside of one of his toes and the toe is red and swollen, preventing him from wearing his shoes. The GP visited and was concerned about the potentially serious or even life-threatening consequences of a diabetic foot ulcer. The GP discussed the treatment with Mr Cook and when she returned to the surgery, drew up a clinical management plan with Sam. The management plan included directions for Sam as the supplementary prescriber to prescribe, with Mr Cook's agreement, flucloxacillin, the first-line antibiotic for diabetic foot ulcer – and a range of suitable dressings. Sam was then able to write a prescription which was then dispensed by the practice pharmacist and visit Mr Cook that afternoon with the items he required to treat his ulcer. He was able to advise Mr Cook about his medicines; give him information about his lifestyle to promote healing of his ulcer; remove a callus using scalpel techniques and dress the ulcer. Within the management plan, Sam would be able to prescribe an alternative antibiotic depending on the response to flucloxacillin and also analgesia, as required. The tissue viability nurse was also involved in Mr Cook's care and on the days that she dressed his ulcer, contacted Sam if she felt that any changes were required according to the management plan.

Activity

Case study 1 demonstrates how supplementary prescribing can help to ensure safe and effective medicines management for Mr Cook.
Supplementary prescribing requires teamwork with different members of the multiprofessional team being clear about their roles and responsibilities. Ask your mentor about supplementary prescribers in your practice area and arrange to discuss their role or accompany them on home visits to observe their prescribing practice.

independent or supplementary prescriber. For example, community practitioner nurse prescribers are only permitted to prescribe from the Nurse Prescribers Formulary for Community Practitioners. This contains dressings and appliances and a limited number of medicines, including some POMs, which have been selected to support community nursing interventions. Nurse independent prescribers can select items from the British National Formulary (BNF). Table 12.3 summarises the scope of prescribing for each type of prescriber.

Table 12.3 Summary of prescribing

Practitioner	What they can prescribe
Doctors	Any medicine listed in the British National Formulary (apart from Schedule 1 controlled drugs)
Dentists	From a formulary listed in the British National Formulary
Nurse independent prescribers	Any medicine listed in the British National Formulary for any medical condition within the prescriber's competence including Schedule 2–5 controlled drugs
Pharmacist independent prescribers	Any medicine listed in the British National Formulary for any medical condition within the prescriber's competence including Schedule 2–5 controlled drugs
Optometrist independent prescribers	Any licensed medicine for conditions that affect the eye and surrounding tissue, except controlled drugs
Community practitioner nurse prescriber	Only items listed within the Nurse Prescribers Formulary – for Community Practitioners (current edition 2011–2013). This is published as a separate booklet but also listed as an appendix in the BNF
All supplementary prescribers: nurses, midwives, pharmacists, optometrists, radiographers, physiotherapists, chiropodists/podiatrists	Any medicine identified in the clinical management plan, including controlled drugs, for any condition within the prescriber's competence

From nurse prescribing to non-medical prescribing

Community nurse prescribing has led the way for a much wider group of health professionals, namely, midwives, pharmacists, radiographers, podiatrists, physiotherapists and optometrists, collectively known as non-medical prescribers, to gain prescribing rights. As long ago as 1989, the Report of the Advisory Group on Nurse Prescribing (the Crown Report) advised Ministers how patient care in the community could be improved by introducing nurse prescribing. The report identified a number of clear benefits that could arise from nurse prescribing including:

• Improvements in patient care
• Better use of the patients', nurses' and GPs' time
• Clarification of professional responsibilities.

In 1994, teams of qualified health visitors and district nurses in England successfully piloted nurse prescribing using a nurse prescriber's formulary, which is similar to the Nurse Prescribers Formulary for Community Practitioners used today. A nationwide programme to implement nurse prescribing commenced in 1997, and all practicing health visitors and district nurses attended their local universities to complete a 2–3-day training programme. In 1999, nurse prescribing training became part of all health visiting and district nursing programmes. This means that district nursing and health visiting were the first, and remain the only, professional groups for which non-medical prescribing is integral to their role.

In 2001, extended nurse prescribing was introduced and included other categories of nurses and midwives. A new course was developed in accordance with NMC standards, which was more lengthy and in-depth and prepared practitioners for independent and supplementary prescribing. Although the range of prescribable items was much broader than in the formulary for community nurses, prescribing was restricted to specific items for specific conditions and consequently, not applicable to all areas of clinical practice. Not until 2006 did new legislation allow Nurse Independent Prescribers to prescribe from the entire BNF and include allied health professional groups in non-medical prescribing. Although there were limitations regarding controlled drugs at this time, in April 2012, legislation was enacted to allow Nurse Independent Prescribers to prescribe schedule 2–5 controlled drugs for any medical condition within their competence. Nurses continue to be the largest professional group who are qualified to prescribe. In England, 2–3% of the registered nurse and pharmacist workforce are independent prescribers (Latter et al 2011).

Government policy in all four UK countries continues to promote non-medical prescribing as an important method of improving the quality of patient care, giving people easier access to treatments and services they require and making best use of the knowledge and skills of the professionals involved. An evaluation of nurse and pharmacist independent prescribing in England, commissioned by the Department of Health, reported prescribing to be safe and clinically effective, increased the quality of services and was very acceptable to patients (Latter et al 2011).

Community practitioner nurse prescribers

Community nurses who hold the specialist practice qualification for district nursing or health visiting are also qualified community practitioner nurse prescribers. Most find that the items available within the Nurse Prescribers Formulary for Community Practitioners enable them to fulfil the requirements of their role and scope of practice. There are also district nurse and health visitors who do not use their prescribing role, and the reasons for this vary.

Although prescribing legislation was initially enacted to enable only qualified district nurses and health visitors to prescribe, the NMC have since set standards for educational preparation to enable nurses who do not hold a specialist practice qualification to be able to prescribe from the community practitioner formulary. Consequently, some registered nurses working in the community are also qualified community practitioner nurse prescribers.

Nurse independent prescribers and supplementary prescribers

A wide range of nurses working in the community are qualified nurse independent and supplementary prescribers. The role is particularly useful for general practice nurses, community mental health nurses, specialist nurses and some district nurses and health visitors who have found the community formulary too restrictive for their role and have completed the preparation for nurse independent and supplementary prescribing. In general practice settings, practice nurses and nurse practitioners are often the first point of contact people have with the health service and they can be responsible for delivering complete episodes of care for which nurse independent prescribing is an essential element. They also run clinics and services for people with long-term conditions and may use supplementary prescribing in

partnership with the GP as part of the patient's clinical management plan.

Unlike nurses working in hospitals, community nurses often work in settings where doctors are not always available to prescribe, for example in intermediate care facilities, walk-in centres and community hospitals or clinics. Community nurses can also be the contact point for travelling families or homeless people. The nurse's ability to prescribe in situations such as these not only has the potential to improve existing services but can also fill gaps and provide a service to people whose needs were not being met.

Activity

Find an example in your community practice area where nurses are leading or involved in providing a service to people who would otherwise not readily access health services, e.g. people from minority ethnic backgrounds, homeless people. Discuss with your mentor how you might arrange to visit the service and explore the nurses' role in medicines management, focusing on prescribing.

Patient group directions (PGDs)

A Patient group direction (PGD) is a written instruction for the supply and/or administration of a medicine to a group of patients in a specific clinical situation, without individual prescriptions having to be written for each patient. PGDs are developed by doctors, pharmacists and other health professionals according to specific legal criteria and to meet local requirements in NHS Trusts and Boards. A PGD is not a prescription but an alternative way of obtaining prescription-only medicines. They enable practitioners to give medicines and deliver services in situations where a prescriber is not present, for example a health visitor running an immunisation clinic.

Practitioners who are eligible and identified to use the PGD must adhere strictly to the instructions, which include specific criteria against which the patient can be assessed as suitable to be given the medicine. Practitioners who are legally eligible to supply/administer medicines using PGDs are: nurses; midwives; health visitors; optometrists; chiropodists and podiatrists; radiographers; physiotherapists; pharmacists; dietitians; occupational therapists; prosthetists and orthotists; speech and language therapists; paramedics and orthoptists. PGDs serve a useful purpose and the legislation that directs their use has been put in place to make them as safe as possible. However, the preferred and safest method is for an appropriately qualified healthcare professional to prescribe for an individual patient on a one-to-one basis (National Prescribing Centre 2009).

Case study 2

Patient group direction (PGD) for the administration of human papillomavirus vaccine (HPV) (Cervarix)

A schools-based HPV immunisation programme was introduced across the UK in September 2008, to protect girls between the ages of 12 and 18 against the two types of HPV (types 16 and 18), which can cause 70% of cervical cancer cases. The vaccine, Cervarix (POM) is given by intramuscular injection into the deltoid region or anterolateral aspect of the thigh in three doses divided over 6 months. The aim was to offer the HPV vaccine to all 12–18-year-old girls by 2011 and assuming a high rate of uptake, a very efficient and effective way of delivering the programme to such a large number of girls was required. In the absence of a PGD, a prescriber would have needed to assess each individual and write a prescription for them before the vaccine could be given. Here is how a PGD would work in this situation.

In NHS Northland, school nurses Heather Walsh, Sue Ritchie and Grace Otayo were responsible for delivering the programme in their locality. A PGD for the administration of HPV vaccine was developed by the chief pharmacist, consultant paediatrician and nurse consultant, agreed with a wider reference group of clinical experts and signed off according to legislative requirements. Arrangements were put in place to deliver the programme in local schools. This included giving information to school girls and their parents, gaining consent and preparing the premises and the school nurses for their role. The PGD not only specified the details of the medicine, the inclusion and exclusion criteria for recipients and safety and reporting issues but also the criteria for whom could give the vaccine. The PGD stipulated that the vaccine must only be administered by nurses who:

■ *are currently registered on the NMC register*
■ *work within:*
   ■ *NMC (2008) The Code, Standards of Conduct, Performance and Ethics for Nurses and Midwives*
   ■ *NMC (2007) Standards for Medicines Management*

> ■ *NMC (2009) Record Keeping: Guidance for nurses and midwives*
> ■ *are competent to undertake immunisation*
> ■ *are competent in using PGDs*
> ■ *have resuscitation skills and anaphylaxis training*
> ■ *can evidence updates on resuscitation skills, immunisation and the management of anaphylaxis within the community.*
>
> *The school nurses received training in the use of the PGD, human papillomavirus and the vaccine itself and also attended a management of anaphylaxis update. They worked as team in each school, vaccinated up to 100 girls in a morning session and were able to use time in the afternoons or evenings for education sessions with parents and children.*

Patient safety is the priority and this example illustrates the high level of skill, knowledge and experience required of a nurse in order to administer a vaccination under PGD. This is why the NMC make very clear in Standard 1 of the NMC Standards for Medicines Management that a student cannot undertake this role but would be expected to understand the principles of a PGD and be involved in the process (NMC 2007).

◆ Activity

Learning point

It is not unusual for PGDs to be used in clinic and other settings in the community. Learn more about how PGDs are developed and implemented by reading the local guidelines and make arrangements to discuss the advantages and disadvantages with a practitioner who uses PGDs in their practice.

Over-the-counter medicines

People buy over-the-counter (OTC) medicines for a wide range of health issues: to treat minor illness or injury, to improve

health and prevent health problems developing. Over-the-counter medicines fall into two categories:

- Pharmacy (P) medicines, which are only available in pharmacies
- General sales list (GSL) medicines, which are more widely available in places such as supermarkets, convenience stores and petrol stations. Herbal remedies come under this category and are also available in health food shops.

Pharmacy (P) medicines are probably more accurately described as 'behind-the-counter' medicines as they are not freely available on the shelves and must be sold under the supervision of the community pharmacist. Examples of P medicines are Canesten cream (Clotrimazole 1% w/w), which is used to treat fungal skin infections or irritation of the vulva associated with thrush; and Stugeron 15 (Cinnarizine 15 mg), which is used to control travel sickness.

GSL medicines cover a very wide range of minor illness and injury, including, colds and flu, allergies, gastric problems, pain relief and skin problems. They also include minerals and vitamins. The pharmacist has an important role in advising people about all OTCs and people are encouraged to consult the pharmacist if they are in any doubt.

When medicines are first licensed they are usually classified as POMs. However, over time, they may be reclassified as pharmacy medicines and eventually may be considered suitable for general sales and reclassified again. This process may take many years and is only suitable for medicines where there is evidence of a very good safety record and they are deemed appropriate to be used without supervision by a prescriber. The first switch from POM to P in the UK was made for oral ibuprofen 200 mg (for pain relief) in 1983, now a GSL medicine. Another notable example of reclassification from POM to P was chloramphenicol 0.5% w/v eye-drops solution, in June 2005.

 Activity

Visit the supermarket and observe the range of over-the-counter GSL medicines that are on sale there. Make a note of the brand/trade name but also note the generic name or active ingredient of a selection of medicines. You will note that some products are only labelled with their generic name and you may be interested to note the difference in price between this and the branded product, e.g. generic paracetamol and branded paracetamol. Make sure you are familiar with the profile of the medicines that you have selected. The next activity will help you to do this. It is not unusual to find that people you are visiting at home take GSL medicines alongside prescribed medicines when it is not always necessary or safe to do so.

Dispensing medicines

An important part of the remit of the pharmacy team is dispensing medicines. Dispensing means:

to label from stock and supply a clinically appropriate medicine to a patient/client/ carer, usually against a written prescription, for self administration or administration by another professional and to advise on safe and effective use.
NMC (2007)

Nurses and midwives are also legally able to dispense medicines but this is unusual and must be set within local policy and governance arrangements.

Most people collect their prescriptions or have arrangements for them to be collected on their behalf from the community or practice pharmacist. Pharmacist's contracts with the NHS also include ways to enable people to get their prescriptions more easily, for example by offering a delivery service. Arrangements are made locally for medicines to be dispensed out of normal pharmacy service hours and in an emergency. Contact with the pharmacy team at the point at which medicines are dispensed is an important opportunity for the pharmacist or pharmacy technician to assess the person's need for support regarding their medicines, give advice and guidance and for the person to ask any questions about their medicines. Some people ask a lot of questions about their medicines whereas others have a lot of questions but never like to ask.

 Activity

The cartoon in Figure 12.1 shows the things that people need to know and often ask nurses about their medicines. Reflect on a recent situation where you were involved in administering a medicine or discussing someone's medication with them. Could you answer these questions?

Continued

What are my medicines for? What do they do?

Why do I need to take them?

Should I take them before/after/with my meals?

Can I take all my tablets at the same time?

Will there be any side-effects?

Do they come in containers that are easier to open?

Is there anything I shouldn't eat/ drink while I'm taking them?

How will I remember to take the right ones at the right time?

How do I get more when I run out?

How can I find out more about my medicines?

Are there alternative treatments?

What do I do if they are not working?

Where do I store my medicines?

What do I do if I think they are causing side-effects?

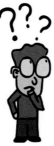

Figure 12.1 Questions people ask about their medicines.

Choose one medicine and find out the answers to the questions using the electronic Medicines Compendium (eMC; www.medicines.org.uk/emc). This contains information about all UK licensed medicines including Patient Information leaflets (PILs) and Summary of Product Characteristics (SPC).
The British National Formulary will also help you with your answers.

The community nurse is often in the best position to advise people and their carers about their medicines during home visits and it is therefore essential that the information they give is accurate and up-to-date. The NMC makes this explicit in Essential Skill 36 of the medicines management Essential Skills Cluster, 'ensure safe and effective practice in medicines management through comprehensive knowledge of medicines, their actions, risks and benefits' (NMC 2010: 137).

According to the Department of Health (DH 2007), approximately 80% of prescriptions in primary care are repeat prescriptions ordered from the GP surgery. This is an indication of the large number of people who are treated for long-term conditions in primary care. People either post or hand in a repeat prescription order slip, or telephone the surgery. Repeat prescribing speeds things up as it is not necessary to make an appointment to see the doctor every time. However, there is risk that people remain on the same treatments when they are no longer effective or appropriate and they order medicines as a matter of routine leading to stockpiling and wastage. This is easily addressed where systems are in place for continuous monitoring and review of the person's condition by the prescriber and vigilance of other members of the team. (This is discussed in more detail later in this chapter.)

Administration of medicines

In the community, people's medicines are their own property and their rights must be respected regarding this. The majority of people take full responsibility for their medicines from getting their prescription from the pharmacy, arranging repeat prescriptions from the doctor, safely storing their medicines, taking them and monitoring their effects. However, some people require assistance with some or all stages of the process, often depending on the route of administration and some rely completely on others.

▮ Student reflection

You will probably have already covered medicines administration theory and either practised the relevant skills in a simulated environment or experienced administering medicines perhaps in a hospital ward. Read over your notes and reflect on any previous experience to identify where you could further develop your knowledge and skills.

Community nurses are frequently involved in medicines administration in the home. As part of a comprehensive assessment process, the patient's medication needs are addressed through the care plan, in partnership with the patient and carer, the GP, the community pharmacist and other health and social care practitioners. The community nurse has the same professional accountability and responsibility as the registered nurse in a hospital ward in relation to administering medicines in the best interests of patients. NMC Medicines Management Standard 8: Standards for

Practice of Administration of Medicines states that all registered nurses must:

- *be certain of the identity of the patient to whom the medicine is to be administered*
- *check that the patient is not allergic to the medicine before administering it*
- *know the therapeutic uses of the medicine to be administered, its normal dosage, side effects, precautions and contra-indications*
- *be aware of the patient's plan of care (care plan or pathway)*
- *check that the prescription or the label on medicine dispensed is clearly written and unambiguous*
- *check the expiry date (where it exists) of the medicine to be administered*
- *have considered the dosage, weight where appropriate, method of administration, route and timing*
- *administer or withhold in the context of the patient's condition (for example, Digoxin not usually to be given if pulse below 60) and co-existing therapies, for example, physiotherapy*
- *contact the prescriber or another authorised prescriber without delay where contra-indications to the prescribed medicine are discovered, where the patient develops a reaction to the medicine, or where assessment of the patient indicates that the medicine is no longer suitable*
- *You must make a clear, accurate and immediate record of all medicine administered, intentionally withheld or refused by the patient, ensuring the signature is clear and legible. It is also your responsibility to ensure that a record is made when delegating the task of administering medicine.*

NMC (2007: 7)

The role of the community nurse in medicines administration varies according to the needs of the patient and family, the route of administration of the medicine and the knowledge, skills and competence of the staff involved. This is set within a governance framework, which includes the NMC Code and Standards for Medicines Management, legislation, local NHS policy and guidelines and national guidelines for practice.

An important part of the medicines management process is the assessment of the patient's capability to take the medicines correctly and as prescribed. In many cases where oral medicines are involved, the patient is completely independent in administering these themselves, perhaps with some assistance from a family carer. Where there is a risk that the correct medicine would not be taken at the right time and in the right dose, compliance aids such as reminder charts and monitored dosage systems supplied by the community pharmacist are often very effective in supporting independence and medicines adherence.

However, if more support is required, and family carers are not able to take on this responsibility, a suitably trained healthcare assistant may provide this assistance rather than a registered nurse. As more skill mix is introduced into community healthcare teams, the role of non-registered staff is developing to include the administration of medicines in the home and treatment room settings. This will be part of the written care plan and will include the consent of the patient and/or carer. In these situations, accountability is retained by the registered nurse and vicarious liability by the Trust or employer. Local medicines administration policy for non-registered staff is usually drawn up jointly by NHS and local authority partnerships. The policy makes explicit the criteria for training, support and supervision of healthcare assistants and the tasks that can be undertaken which commonly include the following:

- Administration of oral, buccal and sublingual medication
- Application of creams, ointments or lotions
- Eye, ear and nasal drops and ointments
- Inhalation devices, nebulisers, oxygen
- Insertion of pessaries, suppositories or micro-enemas.

In all cases, the community nurse or GP will have assessed the patient on an individual basis and determined whether it is appropriate for the task to be undertaken by a member of non-registered staff with the patient's consent. Invasive procedures such as giving injections are not normally delegated to non-registered staff. Pharmacists are responsible for filling compliance aids such as dosage systems and this may never be undertaken by other members of the care team.

Community nurses have an important role in teaching, supervising and monitoring medicines administration, but their direct role in administration tends to focus on invasive procedures such as:

- Insulin injections, given at home for people with diabetes who are unable to get to the surgery and unable to give injections themselves
- Part of a complex care plan, e.g. administering medicines via percutaneous endoscopic gastrostomy (PEG) and jejunostomy sites and continuous intravenous administration of medicines, including controlled drugs using a syringe driver in palliative care
- Immunisation programmes including the childhood immunisation schedule and annual influenza vaccination programme.

 Activity

There are many opportunities for nursing students to gain experience in the administration of medicines in the community. In fact, the scope is probably much wider than it is in the hospital ward because of the variety of clinical situations; from public health interventions such as vaccination to complex medication regimens for end-of-life care in the home.

Discuss with your mentor any specific learning outcomes associated with medicines administration in this placement and the learning opportunities that are available in the community for you to achieve these. For example, there are excellent opportunities for learning about the role that vaccination plays in controlling infectious diseases across the lifespan and for enhancing skills associated with administering medicines by injection. This may involve spending time with health visitors for children's vaccinations, school nurses for HPV vaccination for young people, general practice nurses for travel vaccinations and district nurses for influenza and pneumococcal vaccination. However, NMC guidance must be adhered to at all times (see activity below).

 Activity

Important guidance for students from the NMC Standards for Medicines Management (NMC 2007):

1. Students must be supervised at all times (Standard 18),

   Students must never administer or supply medicinal products without direct supervision. (NMC 2007: 10)

2. Students must not administer medicines that are part of a patient group direction (PGD) and must only administer prescription-only medicines that have been prescribed for the individual concerned (Standard 12)

Continued

3. The student and registered nurse must sign the patient's medication chart or document administration of the medicine in the patient's notes (Standard 18)

4. Administration of medicines is the responsibility of the registered nurse and they will assess the student's readiness and capability to undertake the task before deciding to delegate (Standard 18)

5. Equally, a student may decline to undertake a task if they do not feel confident enough to do so (Standard 18).

Activity

Read the short article which is published by Nursing Standard online, at: http://nursingstandard.rcnpublishing.co.uk/students/clinical-placements/placement-advice/practical-advice/i-felt-pressured-to-countersign-for-controlled-medications.

Here a student is uncertain where they stand in relation to countersigning for controlled drugs. What would you have done in this situation?

Medicines adherence

At all stages of the medicines management process, there are opportunities for the patient, carers and healthcare team member to discuss matters relating to medicines. The aim is to support people to adhere to medicines' regimens, rather than to expect them to comply with instructions. Giving information about medicines and treatment options and trying to understand the reasons why people choose not to take their medicines or cannot take their medicines as prescribed, enables decision-making to be shared between the patient and the practitioners. This approach acknowledges that non-adherence to medicines is not the patient's problem but a breakdown in understanding that can in many cases be rectified.

■ Case study 3

Medicines adherence

George Hay felt fit and well and decided on his 50th birthday that he was going to stop smoking. He made an appointment to discuss this with the practice nurse and on routine examination was surprised to be told that his blood pressure was raised and that he was overweight with a body mass index (BMI) of 28. He was given lifestyle advice and referred to the GP who diagnosed hypertension, prescribed Lisinopril 10 mg daily and asked to see him again in 4 weeks. At the appointment 4 weeks later, George's blood pressure was higher. The conversation between George and the GP went something like this:

Dr Khan *'Mr Hay, as we discussed last time, it's important that we get your blood pressure under control. You have a history of stroke in your family and although you are working on losing weight and stopping smoking, these remain risks to your health. The dose of tablets that I started you on last month has not been as effective as I hoped. I will need to increase the dose and ask you to come back again in 4 weeks time. Is there anything you would like to ask?'*

George *'I don't feel that happy about taking these tablets, Dr Khan. I've never taken anything before apart from the odd course of antibiotics. A chap at work was taking blood pressure tablets and ended up collapsing and falling down a flight of stairs. He's still off work. Could I just go for the lifestyle changes? I've signed up for an exercise course at the gym and I've started a diet with my wife. Cutting out smoking should make a big difference too'.*

Dr Khan *'Were the tablets making you feel unwell Mr Hay?'*

George *'To be honest Dr, I didn't take them. I read the leaflet that came with them and all the side-effects put me off. I'm feeling really good at the moment; probably better than I did when I saw you last month now I'm on the diet. I don't think I need to take them'.*

Dr Khan *'I'm very glad we are having this conversation Mr Hay. I understand where you are coming from. I think if we discuss the risks and benefits and options available we can agree a way forward together'.*

George Hay made a decision not to take the medication that Dr Khan prescribed. His non-adherence was intentional. Non-adherence can also be unintentional when the person wants to follow the treatment but is unable to do so. An example of this is when language is a barrier and information is not translated into a form that the patient can easily understand and use. Another example of unintentional non-adherence is a patient unknowingly using the incorrect inhaler technique to manage their asthma and consequently getting no benefit from the bronchodilator. NICE (2009) have published guidelines to improve medicine adherence. The key principles are shown below and applied to the interaction between Dr Khan and Mr Hay.

Improve communication
When Dr Khan diagnosed hypertension and George was prescribed Lisinopril, George could have been encouraged to ask questions about his treatment and Dr Khan could have used open-ended questions to make it easier to uncover the concerns that George clearly had. Did George give any non-verbal cues that Dr Khan could have picked up, e.g. a concerned or confused facial expression?

Increase patient involvement in making decisions about their medicines
A better understanding of hypertension; the symptoms, risks and different approaches to treatment could have helped to inform George's decision to take his tablets. Dr Khan could have helped George to make decisions based on the likely benefits and risks of the treatment rather than misconceptions.

Increase understanding of the patient's perspective
Could Dr Khan have found out more from George about how he felt about taking tablets on a long-term basis? George clearly was not convinced that he needed or wanted to take tablets and had linked a work colleague's accident to a side-effect of anti-hypertensive therapy. Dr Khan was not aware of George's health beliefs in relation to the positive impact of lifestyle changes on his hypertension.

Provide information

George did not appear to be well informed about his diagnosis or treatment following the first consultation. Perhaps Dr Khan could have given more information at the point of prescribing and checked George's understanding. In reality, appointment times with doctors and other healthcare professionals are short and time to give information during the consultation may be limited. Dr Khan could offer George written information and links to websites such as NHS Choices to back up their discussion and perhaps offer him a follow-up appointment with the practice nurse at the anti-hypertensive clinic.

Assess adherence by asking the right questions

When George returned for his follow-up visit, Dr Khan assumed that he was taking the medication. He could have asked George questions such as, 'Have you taken your tablets every day?' 'Have you missed any tablets?' People are often very reluctant to question the doctor or nurse about their treatment for fear of seeming ungrateful or dissatisfied. Fortunately, George was able to be honest with Dr Khan but many people would find this difficult unless they were asked about it in a way which encouraged them to do so. Without accurate assessment of adherence, there is a risk that the medication will be changed or the dose increased unnecessarily.

 Activity

Choose a medicine, preferably that you are not familiar with, that is prescribed for someone on the caseload. Put yourself in the position of the patient taking the medicine and resource information that is available about the medicine. Try answering the following questions: How easy was this information to find? Was it in a format that would be helpful to this patient? How much of this information would you expect the healthcare practitioner to give to the patient? How important is it that the patient has the information and understands the implications? Discuss your findings with your mentor and think about how you might use the information that you have found to inform the patient.

The patient information leaflet (PIL)

Since 1999, it has been a statutory requirement for pharmaceutical companies to include a patient information leaflet (PIL) with all medicines. The PIL contains essential information for the user about how to take the medicine correctly, its uses,

safe storage and potential side-effects. The PIL is regulated by the Medicines and Healthcare Products Regulatory Agency (MHRA) and only PILs that are judged as providing clear and consistent information are approved. In October 2010, legislation was introduced to ensure that the name of the medicine is displayed in Braille on the labelling and that the PIL is supplied in a format suitable for blind and partially sighted people. Provision for people with a first language other than English or with poor basic skills in language, literacy and numeracy, includes: the use of plain English; avoiding medical terminology or jargon; leaflets in other languages in written or web-based format; telephone helplines; translator services and links and signposts to other sources of information. These methods help to provide a consistently high standard of information which enables people to use medicines safely and derive optimal benefit from them.

Medication review

Medication review can take a number of forms but is essentially a process for scrutinising the patient's medication, evaluating its usage and effectiveness and with the patient and carers agreeing on a plan to maximise the benefits of the medicines in improving or maintaining their health. The process is well suited to people who take medicines on a long-term basis, in the management of long-term conditions. Medication review is seen as the cornerstone of medicines management due to its potential to promote safe, effective and person-centred care. Examples of the benefits of medication review have been identified by Clyne et al (2008):

- Improved health outcomes through optimal medicines use
- Opportunity to develop a shared understanding between the patient and practitioner about medicines and their role in patient treatment
- Reduction in adverse events relating to medicines
- Empower patients and carers to be actively involved in their care and treatment.

Three types of medication review are recommended by the National Prescribing Centre (Clyne et al 2008) and have been linked to pharmacy and GP contracts:

Type 1:*Prescription review* – addresses technical issues relating to the medicines that are prescribed and would probably not involve the patient.

Type 2:*Concordance and compliance review* – addresses issues relating to how the patient takes their medicines and patient would be integral to the discussion.

Type 3:*Clinical medication review* – addresses issues relating to the patient's medication taking behaviour in relation to their medical condition and would involve the patient.

Medication review can result in doses being changed, some medicines being stopped altogether and new medicines being added. Any changes to the regimen would be discussed and agreed with the patient, communicated to other members of the prescribing team and the outcomes of the review clearly documented in the patient's records. Medication review may be undertaken by any practitioner who is competent to do so. Community nurses and particularly non-medical prescribers are well placed to undertake medication review as they are often the practitioner who has most contact with the patient and family, have knowledge of their health condition and medicines and are likely to be aware of the factors that may affect the person's ability to manage their medicines. Any OTC medicines that patients are taking should be included in the review, as they can interact with some prescription only medicines.

This formal process of medication review would normally be set at specific intervals such as once a year, or take place in response to a change in the patient's condition or circumstances, e.g. discharge from hospital, a move to residential care or a concern about their adherence. However, all health and social care practitioners have a responsibility to monitor how people manage and respond to their medicines whenever they have contact with them. Every opportunity should be taken to communicate with people about their medicines and support adherence. Constant vigilance is required to pick up any untoward effects of medicines, discuss these with the patient and report to the pharmacist, prescriber or GP.

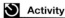 **Activity**

Find out how medication review is undertaken for the people on your mentor's caseload. You will find it helpful to ask your mentor, the GP and the pharmacist about this. With your mentor's guidance, select someone on the caseload who has a complex medication regimen and ask them if you can spend an hour with them discussing why, when and how they take their medication and how it makes them feel. Make a note of this and afterwards search for more information

Continued

and write up your findings. This exercise may help you to complete a practice-based assessment such as a care study or it could be used to evidence learning in your portfolio.

Safe storage of medicines in the community

Medicines can break down and lose their potency prior to the expiry date if they are not stored according to the instructions on the label or in the summary of product characteristics (SPC). Local areas have developed policy and guidelines for the safe and appropriate storage of medicines in the hospital and community. In a hospital setting, the use of locked cupboards, trolleys and fridges to store medicines is well established and part of the ward routine. This is also the case in community settings such as the health centre, care home and community clinic. However, in the home, it can be a very different picture and medicines are often stored in the most inappropriate places.

Case study 4

Safe storage of medicines

Martha King is 86 and lives alone and very independently in a small ground floor flat in the centre of the village. She has little contact with the health service apart from visits to the surgery to see the GP when necessary and to collect her repeat prescription. She takes medicines for hypertension and congestive cardiac failure. She also suffers from joint pain and indigestion and she buys over-the-counter medicines from the pharmacy in the high street to relieve her symptoms. Martha regularly takes six different tablets a day and has difficulty remembering what they are all for and when she should take them. She feels foolish mentioning this to the doctor or pharmacist. She wouldn't like anyone to think she was losing her memory or not able to take her medicines correctly but she does worry that she doesn't always get it right. A while ago, she devised a system to help her remember what to take and she thinks this is working well. This week, the GP has prescribed a course of antibiotics for an ear infection which has been troubling her for some time. This means that Martha is now taking seven different medicines and 21 tablets a day, as shown in Table 12.4. According to the patient information leaflets (PILs), Martha must also remember:

- *not to eat or drink anything containing grapefruit as this is known to increase the effect of Verapamil*
- *to take potassium chloride with fluid during a meal*
- *to take Amoxicillin before meals,*

Martha's system for remembering to take her medicines

Martha keeps all her medicines on the kitchen windowsill. It's always bright in the kitchen in the morning and it's easy for her to read the labels, particularly when it's sunny. She uses three colourful eggs cups and puts into each, the medicines she needs to take at different times of the day. She puts the egg cup containing her morning medicines on the table in the kitchen where she eats her breakfast; the afternoon medicines on the table next to her chair in the lounge where she eats her tea; and keeps the medicines she takes at bedtime next to her bed. Martha spends up to half an hour every morning setting out her tablets. Nevertheless, she thinks it's worthwhile as most days it means she takes all her tablets.

Table 12.4 Martha's medicines

Medicine	Dose	Indication	Total number of tablets
Verapamil	240 mg, 3 times per day	Hypertension	6 × 120 mg tablets
Frusemide	40 mg, once per day	Heart failure	1 × 40 mg tablet
Digoxin	62.5 µg, once per day	Heart failure	1 × 62.5 µg tablet
Potassium chloride (slow K modified release)	600 mg, twice per day	Low blood potassium levels	2 × 600 mg tablets
Amoxicillin	250 mg, 3 times per day	Ear infection	3 × 250 mg capsules
Paracetamol	1 g, twice per day	Arthritic pain	2 × 500 mg tablets
Antacid tablets (calcium carbonate)	1 g, 3 times per day	Indigestion	6 × 500 mg tablets
			21 tablets per day

✎ Activity

1. Martha thinks her system works for her most days but it is far from ideal. Identify the ways in which a system such as this compromises safety.

2. Martha's GP has asked the district nurse to look in on Martha next time she is passing. When he saw her in the surgery this week, he thought she was looking very frail. It's a long time since Martha has had a home visit from a member of the primary healthcare team. What could the district nurse suggest that may help Martha manage her medicines more safely?

The district nurse that visits Martha makes a holistic assessment of her health needs. She is in a very good position to identify the difficulties Martha is having in managing her medicines and they discuss this in detail. The district nurse suggests a home visit by the local pharmacist to review Martha's use of her medicines. She explains that the pharmacist would make an assessment of her current medication and how it is used and may be able to recommend to the GP a reduction in the number of tablets she takes or the number of times a day she needs to take them. Depending on the outcome of the assessment, the pharmacist may offer compliance aids such as a reminder chart or a multi-compartment dosage box prefilled with Martha's medicines at the pharmacy.

All medicines have specific instructions for safe storage according to their properties. However, the following principles apply to all medicines:

- Medicines should be stored in a cool dry place and out of direct sunlight.
  - Avoid windowsills as medicines may be exposed to heat and sunlight
  - Avoid kitchens and bathrooms which may become warm and humid
  - Some medicines require storage in a refrigerator.
- Always keep medicines in their original containers as dispensed from the pharmacy. Do not decant medicines into other containers where they cannot easily be identified, be exposed to air and humidity and be in contact with other medicines. Once removed from child proof containers, they pose a threat to children who may mistake them as sweets.
- All medicines should be kept out of reach and sight of children. Whether children live in the house or not, there is always a risk that children will visit, for example

grandchildren visiting their grandparents' house.

Nurses have a professional responsibility for advising people in the community about the safe storage of medicines as outlined in Standard 6 of the NMC Standards for Medicines Management:

> *Registrants must ensure all medicinal products are stored in accordance with the patient information leaflet, summary of product characteristics document found in dispensed UK-licensed medication, and in accordance with any instruction on the label.*
> NMC (2007: 33)

Safe disposal of medicines in the community

Community nurses must not only adhere to local policy but also legislation relating to the disposal of unwanted medicines. When medicines are no longer required because the prescription has been changed, the medicines reach their expiry date or the patient dies, they should not be destroyed or disposed of in the house. The patient or family should be encouraged to return the unwanted medicines to a pharmacy or the community nurse acting on behalf of the family can do so. In all cases, the medicines are destroyed. Even large amounts of unused and unopened medicines that are still in date cannot be used due to the risk of contamination or degradation due to inappropriate storage. The legislation surrounding controlled drugs allows community nurses according to local policy to destroy and witness the destruction of obsolete, expired or unwanted stocks of controlled drugs.

Summary of learning points from this chapter

This chapter has given a broad overview of medicines management in the community. The principles outlined and the learning activities included are relevant for all nursing students regardless of your field of practice and the community setting in which you are based:

- The importance of medicines management in the community and primary care
- The activities involved in medicines management and the role of patients and practitioners
- The impact of safe and effective medicines management on the quality of care.

References

Barber, N.D., Alldred, D.P., Raynor, D.K., et al., 2009. Care homes' use of medicines study: prevalence, causes and potential harm of medication errors in care homes for older people. Qual. Saf. Health Care 18, 341–346.

Clyne, W., Blenkinsopp, A., Seal, R., 2008. A guide to medications review. NPC, Liverpool.

Department of Health, DH, 2007. Management of medicines – a resource to support implementation of the wider aspects of medicines management for the National Service Frameworks for diabetes renal services and long-term conditions. DH, London.

Department of Health, DH, 2008. Medicines management: everybody's business. DH, London.

Garfield, S., Barber, N., Walley, P., et al., 2009. Quality of medication use in primary care – mapping the problem, working to a solution: a systematic review of the literature. BMC Med. 7, 50.

Howard, R.L., Avery, A.J., Slavenburg, S., et al., 2007. Which drugs cause preventable admissions to hospital? A systematic review. Br. J. Clin. Pharmacol. 63 (2), 136–147.

Latter, S., Blenkinsopp, A., Smith, A., 2011. Evaluation of nurse and pharmacist independent prescribing. Department of Health Policy Research Programme Project 016 0108. DH, London.

National Patient Safety Agency, 2009. Safety in doses: improving the use of medicines in the NHS. NPSA, London.

National Prescribing Centre, 2008. What you need to know about prescribing, the 'drugs bill' and medicines management: a guide for all NHS managers. NPC, Liverpool.

National Prescribing Centre, 2009. Patient group directions: a practical guide and framework of competencies for all professionals using patient group directions. NPC, Liverpool.

NICE, 2009. Medicines adherence – involving patients in decisions about prescribed medicines and supporting adherence. CG76. NICE, London.

Nursing and Midwifery Council, 2007. Standards for medicines management.

NMC, London. Online. Available at: www.nmc-uk.org/Documents/Standards/nmcStandardsForMedicines ManagementBooklet.pdf.

Nursing and Midwifery Council, 2008. The Code: standards of conduct, performance and ethics for nurses and midwives. Online. Available at: http://www.nmc-uk.org/Publications/Standards/The-code/Introduction.

Nursing and Midwifery Council, 2009. Record keeping: guidance for nurses and midwives. NMC, London.

Nursing and Midwifery Council, 2010. Standards for pre-registration nursing education. NMC, London.

Pirmohamed, M., James, S., Meakin, S., et al., 2004. Adverse drug reactions as cause of admission to hospital: prospective analysis of 18,820 patients. Br. Med. J. 329 (7463), 459–460.

Further reading

Barber, P., Robertson, D., 2009. Essentials of pharmacology for nurses. Open University Press, Berkshire.

Blair, K., 2011. Medicines management in children's nursing (transforming nursing practice). Learning Matters, Exeter.

Dougherty, L., Lister, S. (Eds.), 2011. The Royal Marsden Hospital manual of clinical nursing procedures – student edition. eighth ed. Chapter 13 Medicines management. Wiley-Blackwell, Oxford.

McFadden, R., 2009. Introducing pharmacology: for nursing and healthcare. Pearson Education, Harlow.

Mutsatsa, S., 2011. Medicines management in mental health nursing (transforming nursing practice). Learning Matters, Exeter.

Nursing and Midwifery Council, 2006. Standards of proficiency for nurse and midwife prescribers. NMC, London.

Nuttall, D., Rutt-Howard, J., 2011. The textbook of non-medical prescribing. Wiley-Blackwell, Oxford.

Starkings, S., Krause, L., 2010. Passing calculations tests for nursing students (transforming nursing practice). Learning Matters, Exeter.

Tyreman, C., 2011. How to avoid drug errors. Online. Available at: http://www.nursingtimes.net/how-to-avoid-drug-errors/5018923.article (accessed August 2012).

Websites

British National Formulary, http://bnf.org/bnf/index.htm.

The Electronic Medicines Compendium (eMC), www.medicines.org.uk/emc/ contains information about all UK licensed medicines including patient information leaflets (PILs) and summary of product characteristics (SPC).

Medicines and Healthcare Products Regulatory Agency is the government agency which is responsible for ensuring that medicines and medical devices work, and are acceptably safe: www.mhra.gov.uk/home/groups/pl-a/documents/websiteresources/con117389.pdf.

National Institute for Health and Clinical Excellence (NICE), www.nice.org.uk is an independent organisation that provides national guidance on the promotion of good health and the prevention of ill-health.

National Patient Safety Agency (NPSA), www.npsa.nhs.uk/ aims to improve the safety of patient care by informing, supporting and influencing healthcare organisations and individuals working in the health sector.

NHS Choices describes itself as the online 'front door' to the NHS: www.nhs.uk/Pages/HomePage.aspx – the country's biggest health website and gives information to enable people to make choices about their health.

NHS Education for Scotland, Non-medical prescribing website contains resources and information, http://www.nes.scot.nhs.uk/prescribing/index.html.

Oxford University Press Nursing Online Resource Centre gives links to resources that accompany a range of relevant nursing textbooks: http://www.oup.com/uk/orc/nursing/.

Section 4. Consolidating learning

13

Being an effective student: learning in a community setting

CHAPTER AIMS

- To use scenarios to highlight experiences that can challenge nursing students in achieving their learning outcomes during community practice learning

- To invite the student to analyse scenarios, to reflect on similar experiences from practice and consider options and potential actions or outcomes

- To guide the student to use the knowledge and skills from previous chapters and further reading

- To encourage students to discuss challenging situations with their mentor or university tutor

---

Introduction

Most students enjoy a positive and productive learning experience during their community placement. They develop a good rapport with service users and their families, feel part of the multidisciplinary team and benefit from a very wide range of learning opportunities, which enable them

to meet their learning outcomes and personal objectives. There can also be times during practice learning when not everything goes to plan. However, working through a problem or challenge may not only help to resolve difficulties but may also involve very important and positive learning that can be applied to similar situations in the future. Some challenges such as dealing with conflicting opinions or difficult interpersonal relationships are not unique to practice learning in the community but others are. The following scenarios give you an opportunity to think through situations that you may have already experienced or may come across during a community practice learning placement. They may also provide the basis for discussion with your mentor, peers or university tutor.

 Activity

Read through the following four scenarios and try to put yourself in the position of each student. Use the questions to prompt your thinking about:

- how you would feel in a situation like this

Continued

- what it would mean for your learning
- what you could do to resolve or address the issue.

There is no single action or solution and your response will depend on how you view the situation. Some suggestions are provided after each scenario but you may come up with alternatives that are equally relevant. Remember the reflective framework referred to in Chapter 4 will assist you to explore a variety of issues within the scenarios. You may find it helpful to make a note of your thoughts and answers to the questions as you read through the scenarios.

Scenario 1

David: Settling in

I really enjoyed my last placement. I was on a surgical ward in the university hospital with three other students from my year and two third year students who I worked with a lot. The ward was very well organised and the ward routine was like clockwork. My mentor told me exactly what to do and when she wasn't around, there were always other staff to help me. All the students fitted well into the team. I always knew what to do next. As the hospital is next door to the university, it was handy to call in to see my tutor and go to the library. It was easy to meet my learning outcomes and after 6 weeks there, I felt very confident. I was sorry to leave.

I started my community placement this week and I'm not sure if I'm going to enjoy it. I don't know the area, I'm the only student here and my mentor seems to rush around the whole time and not have much time for me. There are so many different people and services and every patient seems to have a completely different

problem. To be honest I don't really know what's going on and what I can learn here.

Discussion points

1. How could David's expectations or pre-conceived ideas about the placement influence his early learning experience in the community?
2. How would you describe his approach to learning in this community placement so far?
3. What could David and his mentor do to enable him to settle in to this new and different learning environment?

Actions for Scenario 1 – David: Settling in

The questions that David could ask himself in relation to maximising his learning opportunities that are listed above could also be asked of him by his mentor. This could be the basis of a discussion with the potential to raise awareness on both parts of what David could do, supported by his mentor to enhance his learning experience and progress towards achieving his learning outcomes.

David had felt very settled in his previous placement in a hospital ward with its controlled environment and set routine. He liked being in close contact with peers and staff members as well as his mentor and being in familiar surroundings in a hospital he knows. He is now in a very different environment, out of his comfort zone and he is feeling daunted and disoriented.

Activity

Look over any notes you have made, think through what you might do in a similar situation and perhaps discuss any potential actions with your mentor or student colleagues before reading the options we have suggested.

Continued

Let's say that David is approaching the first progression point and must meet the NMC requirements to progress to the next part of the programme. There are a number of skills and professional behaviours that he must demonstrate, for example, 'demonstrates safe, basic, person-centred care, under supervision, for people who are unable to meet their own physical and emotional needs' (NMC 2010: 98) and 'acts in a way that values the roles and responsibilities of others in the team and interacts appropriately' (NMC 2010: 101). Learning in practice time is very valuable and it is important that students settle in quickly and use the time available to make sure essential skills are not only mastered but demonstrated to their mentor. What could you learn from this scenario that would help you to meet the NMC requirements and standards of competence for moving through the programme progression points and meeting the criteria for registration?

Discussion point 1

How could David's expectations or pre-conceived ideas about the placement influence his early learning experience in the community?

Nursing in the community is very different from nursing in a hospital setting. If David hadn't expected this, then it is no wonder he feels the way he does. It can take experienced practitioners who move from hospital settings to the community some time to grasp the complexities of nursing in the community and David should not expect to do so in the first few days of his placement. The problem is that feeling insecure and lacking confidence in the value of the placement at the outset can stifle motivation to learn and undermine the whole

experience. Here are some of the things that a student could do beforehand so that they begin their community placement with realistic expectations of the learning environment and the potential for learning and get off to a good start:

- Prepare for the placement, e.g. access information about the placement, make contact with the mentor, talk to students who have been there before, make arrangements to call into the placement, visit the area to see what it's like. More detail about preparing for the placement is given in Chapter 4.
- Develop understanding of the community context, e.g. read over university notes that are relevant to nursing in the community. Chapters 1 and 2 provide an overview of health and social care in the community and the practitioners and agencies that deliver services.
- Appreciate some of the differences between nursing in hospital and community settings. Chapter 3 and Table 3.1 identify and discuss some of the unique characteristics of nursing in the community.
- Think about personal objectives and the types of activities that would assist in meeting the learning outcomes for the placement.

Discussion point 2

How would you describe David's approach to learning in this community placement so far?

David's feelings of insecurity are contributing to an apparently negative approach to learning at this stage in his community placement. He is comparing the beginning of this placement with the end of a previous one where he felt comfortable and confident. Better preparation would have helped him to make a positive start but there are a number of things that he could do now to feel more motivated to learn:

- Accept that early days in a new placement are bound to feel strange and that it is not unusual for students to feel overwhelmed. A positive approach and willingness to get involved and take advantage of the learning opportunities that are available soon enables students to settle into the community environment.
- It is not too late to do the preparatory work and find out about the placement and the community nursing context.
- See the advantages to being the only nursing student, or one of a limited number, in the placement; often one-to-one teaching; undivided attention from specialist staff during observational visits; more choice as there is no competition from other students for learning experiences. Not having peers around to interact with acts as an incentive to get to know the clinical staff, be more involved and feel part of the team.

Discussion point 3

What could David and his mentor do to enable him to settle in to this new and different learning environment?

David is feeling neglected by his mentor, unsure of what he should be doing and what's going on around him. This is in contrast to his previous placement on the surgical ward. Perhaps not enough has been done to recognise David's needs as an individual and maybe he has not made these clear to his mentor. When people have worked in the community for a long time, they can forget what it is like for someone who is unfamiliar with the set up. The important thing at this stage in the placement is for the student and mentor to communicate effectively, understand each other's expectations and agree a plan for student during the placement. Here are some examples of what students and

mentors can do to enable students to settle into the placement effectively:

- Arrange for the student to be introduced to the staff in the placement area preferably on the first day
- Plan a short period of induction or orientation (an example is given in Chapter 3)
- Discuss and agree expectations, e.g. student's role, mentor's role and the role of key staff in the student's learning experience
- Work through the student's personal objectives at a very early stage
- Discuss the student's learning outcomes and the learning opportunities available in the placement that would enable these to be achieved
- Agree a learning contract, including contact times for student/mentor discussion and progress monitoring and feedback.

Moving to any new placement can be difficult at first; not knowing the staff or where to go and what to do. Some students find the community placement challenging, especially if their previous experience has been in a hospital setting. However, community staff will support students to settle in as quickly as possible, particularly when students communicate any concerns or reservations, see the potential for learning and are positive and proactive learners.

Scenario 2

Nikula: Home visiting

My mentor doesn't seem to think I am competent to visit patients on my own and I've been here for 3 weeks now. I've visited quite a few patients on the caseload with different members of the team and I'm familiar with their nursing needs. I spend a lot of time just observing others and going to meet people in different organisations. I was allowed to do a lot on my own in the hospital. I think my skills are being wasted. I could be doing more here.

Discussion points

1. What effect could Nikula's dissatisfaction have on her learning experience?
2. Why has Nikula's mentor ensured there are opportunities for her to spend time in different organisations and observing other practitioners?
3. What could be done to resolve any difference in opinion regarding Nikula's competence and ability to visit patient's independently?

 Activity

Look over any notes you have made, think through what you might do in a similar situation and perhaps discuss any potential actions with your mentor or student colleagues before reading the options we have suggested.

If Nikula was approaching the second NMC progression point (at the end of Year 2), she must demonstrate more independent working, with less direct supervision and make the most of opportunities to extend her knowledge skills and practice (NMC 2010). However, her mentor will only give her the opportunity to do this when she is convinced that Nikula is ready and it is up to Nikula to demonstrate this. What could you learn from this scenario that would help you to meet the NMC requirements and standards of competence for moving through the programme progression points and meeting the criteria for registration?

Actions for Scenario 2 – Nikula: Home visiting

It is not uncommon for students to feel frustrated by not being able to use their skills and knowledge to work independently in the community. Often the student has provided similar clinical care in a hospital setting or already provided care for the patient at home but under supervision of another member of staff. The decision to allow a student to visit patients on their own and provide care when not under supervision is not taken lightly. The mentor uses previous experience, knowledge of the student's capability and competence and professional and clinical judgement to assess each situation. The last thing the mentor wants to do is to put the patient or the nursing student in a difficult or vulnerable position.

Discussion point 1

What effect could Nikula's dissatisfaction have on her learning experience?

Nikula may well be a very competent student. However, she may feel undermined and undervalued, particularly if she does not feel she has had a satisfactory explanation from her mentor as to why she is working under supervision and has not been asked to visit patients on her own. She may feel that some of the learning experiences that have been arranged for her are not as valuable as direct contact with patients. If she fails to take an interest in the broad context of nursing in the community she will miss out on important information to the detriment of patient care. Overall, her feelings of frustration and general approach could have a negative impact on her relationship with her mentor and on her motivation to learn.

Discussion point 2

Why has Nikula's mentor ensured there are opportunities for her to spend time in different organisations and observing other practitioners?

The nursing contribution is just one element of care in the community. Unlike the hospital environment, where service provision is often straightforward and housed under one roof, a wide range of different services and providers in the community work together to ensure that people get the things they need to live as independently and safely as possible. In some areas of practice, e.g. in child protection, health visiting, general practice, social work, education and the police work together as an integrated team. There are also examples where services provided by the voluntary sector for older people add that crucial dimension to the care package that keep them at home and out of long-term care. The better the community nurse's knowledge and understanding of the services that are available in the locality and how to access them, the greater the benefit to people and their carers. Nikula's mentor should be able to assist her in appreciating how insight into the roles and the services provided in the community can be used by nurses in secondary care to enhance admission and discharge planning.

Discussion point 3

What could be done to resolve any difference in opinion regarding Nikula's competence and ability to visit patient's independently?

Communication is the most important aspect of this scenario. Unless Nikula raises her concern, her mentor may be unaware of how she feels. The mentor and student should be able to discuss the issue frankly. This means Nikula understanding the issue from the mentor's perspective in acting in the best interests of people in her care and the student, and the mentor understanding Nikula's frustration.

The mentor should be able to justify her decision based on evidence of Nikula's competence. This will include:

- The record of learning outcomes that the student has already achieved, including those from a previous placement
- Direct observation of the student's practice

- Feedback on the student's performance from other members of staff that have worked with Nikula
- Discussion with Nikula.

In addition, the mentor will be directed by what needs to be achieved in this placement, both identified in the learning outcomes and the student's personal objectives. The mentor and the student should agree any future plans that would help progress the student's practice learning. It would be helpful to document this in the learning contract.

Scenario 3

Mary: Dealing with a difficult situation

Towards the end of my placement, my mentor gave me a small caseload. We had discussed this and both felt that I had developed the competence and confidence required. He had also asked each of the people on the caseload if they were happy for me to visit on my own and gained their consent. The first time I visited Mr Jackson his daughter was there. She was very unhappy, said she didn't know who I was and said she wanted the proper nurse to look after her father. She didn't want to let me in.

Discussion points

1. How would this event make you feel if you were Mary?
2. How would you react and what would you say to Mr Jackson's daughter?
3. What would you do next?

🔌 Activity

Look over any notes you have made, think through what you might do in a similar situation and perhaps discuss any potential actions with your mentor or student colleagues before reading the options we have suggested here.

Continued

There are some useful lessons here for a student at any stage in their programme. However, for entry to the register, NMC expects students to demonstrate that they recognise and act to overcome barriers in developing effective relationships with service users and carers and manage and diffuse challenging situations effectively (NMC 2010).

What could you learn from this scenario that would help you to meet the NMC requirements and standards of competence for moving through the programme progression points and meeting the criteria for registration?

Actions for Scenario 3 – Mary: Dealing with a difficult situation

Visiting people in their own homes is a privilege and usually a pleasure but is not without its challenges. The unpredictable nature of the home visit, which you can read more about in Chapter 3, is one of the reasons why the mentor makes a careful assessment of the student's readiness to visit alone and chooses people on the caseload who the student is competent to care for. Sometimes it is an unexpected deterioration in the patient's condition or even a sudden death that confronts the student visitor and students should discuss with their mentor what they would do in a situation such as this. It is not unusual for carers to feel anxious about their relative and in Scenario 3, Mary is confronted by the patient's daughter. You have been asked to put yourself in Mary's position.

Discussion point 1

How would this event make you feel if you were Mary

You may already be feeling a little uneasy visiting Mr Jackson for the first time on your own. This incident may have left you feeling embarrassed to be confronted at the front door, annoyed by the daughter's interference, when it is her father that you have come to see, insulted by the insinuation that you are not competent to deliver her father's care and concerned for Mr Jackson regarding receiving his care as planned.

First, can you see this incident from Mr Jackson's daughter's perspective? Perhaps Mr Jackson hasn't explained that you are visiting today. She probably knows the community team and is used to them visiting her father. She doesn't know you and potentially you are a stranger in her father's home. She has her father's best interests at heart and maybe doesn't appreciate that you have the knowledge and skills to deliver his care.

Discussion point 2

How would you react and what would you say to Mr Jackson's daughter?

You might not feel very calm but you must be professional and not appear upset or annoyed. Remember that you are there to provide Mr Jackson's care. Ask if you could have the opportunity to introduce yourself; provide identification; explain who you are and that you have visited before with the community team; that Mr Jackson had agreed for you to visit him on your own and that you would be reporting to your mentor when you got back to the health centre.

Discussion point 3

What would you do next?

Mr Jackson's daughter may accept your explanation and be happy for you to care for her father. If you are not given access to the house and Mr Jackson and you are feeling upset by the incident, you should consider contacting your mentor or another member of the community nursing team immediately. It is important to establish that Mr Jackson is safe and receives his care as soon as possible, even if from another member of staff. You will want to discuss the incident with your mentor whatever the outcome, as soon as possible. You might like to use an incident such as this as the basis for a reflective analysis that you could include in your portfolio.

Scenario 4

Kevin: Achieving learning outcomes

I usually get on fine with people and although I'm quite shy it hasn't held me back in any of my previous placements. Apart from my mentor, none of the staff at the health centre talk to me much. In fact I don't think they know my name and refer to me as 'the student', even though I've been here for 4 weeks. I was looking forward to community practice learning. I like working with children and have been thinking about health visiting as a career. It was great when I heard that my mentor was a health visitor. However, I've been very disappointed so far. I haven't spent that much time with my mentor. When I have, I've either sat in the office while she makes phone calls and does paperwork or I've sat in the car while she has made visits that she says wouldn't be appropriate for me to attend. I've done baby clinics and first visits with her but I don't feel I'm getting to see the full picture and the more challenging aspects of the health visitor's role. When there isn't much to do, I get to go home early. I can't see how I can achieve my learning outcomes in the time I have left.

Discussion points

1. How could Kevin's approach be affecting his learning experience and ability to achieve his learning outcomes?
2. How could Kevin maximise his learning opportunities in order to achieve his learning outcomes?
3. What could Kevin and his mentor do at this stage in the placement?

 Activity

Look over any notes you have made, think through what you might do in a similar situation and perhaps discuss any potential actions with your mentor or student colleagues before reading the options we have suggested.

As students progress towards registration, the learning outcomes are increasingly designed to enable you to show that you can make safe and effective use of practice learning. This includes less direct supervision towards the end of the programme (NMC 2010). What could you learn from this scenario that would help you to meet the NMC requirements and standards of competence for moving through the programme progression points and meeting the criteria for registration?

Actions for Scenario 4 – Kevin: Achieving learning outcomes

We discussed in Scenario 1 how important it was for David to get off to a good start, feel part of the team and use time available in the practice placement to best effect. Earlier chapters have emphasised why practice learning in the community is crucial to your development as a nurse of the future, and also the wide range of opportunities for learning that even short placements offer. But in Scenario 4, Kevin does not appear to be making the progress he expected, and is at risk of not achieving his learning outcomes or demonstrating NMC requirements.

Discussion point 1

How could Kevin's approach be affecting his learning experience and ability to achieve his learning outcomes?

A positive, personable and proactive approach is characteristic of an effective learner. Kevin is aware that he is naturally reserved and consequently may have to work a little harder than more confident people at putting himself forward and establishing a rapport with others. If the staff at the health centre do not know his name at this stage of his placement, it suggests that he has not been very forthcoming in making contact, introducing himself, getting to know them and enabling them to get to know him. He is much more likely to have a productive learning experience if people know him and why he is there and he is in a better position to pursue his interests.

Kevin's approach is very passive and non-participative. This can limit his exposure to new situations. Kevin is expecting to learn a lot about health visiting from having direct contact with his mentor. However, so many more agencies are involved in working with children, young people and families. A narrow focus on what he thinks is important may cause him to dismiss or overlook opportunities to learn about much broader and equally important aspects of the role, such as record-keeping, communication and collaboration.

Discussion point 2

How could Kevin maximise his learning opportunities in order to achieve his learning outcomes?

There are number of things that Kevin could do to maximise his learning opportunities but he must take more responsibility for his own learning in order to achieve his

learning outcomes. A student in this situation may find it helpful to ask themselves the following questions:

- Could I have a clearer understanding of how I can achieve the learning outcomes for this placement?
- Am I well enough informed about this aspect of nursing practice? What key background reading could I be doing?
- Am I engaging positively with the people around me or could I be more friendly and approachable?
- Could I be more proactive in seeking out learning opportunities and following up on the things that interest me?
- Do I look enthusiastic and interested?
- Am I relying too much on my mentor for guidance?
- Do I need more support from my mentor or my university tutor?
- Could I be more self-directed and find things to do at the end of the afternoon, rather than going home early?
- Am I open enough to new experiences and see their relevance to my learning outcomes?
- Am I really making the most of my time in this placement?

Viewing every event or interaction as an opportunity to ask questions, offering to assist, requesting follow-up discussion on situations where he has not been included, are all ways that Kevin would significantly increase the potential for learning. He is required to spend a minimum of 40% of his time with his mentor and he should see the remainder not only as a good opportunity to build up a more comprehensive picture of the health visiting role but also to learn about the broader aspects of community nursing practice. There are certainly opportunities for this but they do not only arise from his spending time with this mentor. Students who are motivated, enthusiastic and demonstrate an interest in other people's roles and activities, are generally well accepted and benefit from a wider range of opportunities for learning.

Occasionally, there are situations where patients or families request that students are not present during the visit or at an appointment with the practitioner. There are also occasions where the practitioner feels that the presence of the student could disadvantage the patient or client in some way, e.g. prevent the client from discussing very sensitive issues openly. However, these occasions are rare and even if the student has not been present, in most cases, there is no reason why the student and mentor cannot discuss the issue afterwards and use it as a learning experience. Activities to enhance your practice learning are discussed in Chapter 4.

Discussion point 3

What could Kevin and his mentor do at this stage in the placement?

The midway point in a practice placement is an important time for the mentor and the student to meet to review the student's progress and achievements. Preparation for the meeting is important for both and students should put some thought into how they feel they are doing and any actions that could assist them in demonstrating achievement of the learning outcomes. If a learning contract or plan is in place, then it is useful to review this now also and make any adjustments that would enhance the remainder of the learning experience and enable the learning outcomes to be achieved. If the student or mentor has any concerns they should discuss how these could be resolved, perhaps including the student's university tutor. Often, an action plan can help to clarify what is required and how it can be achieved.

Summary of learning points from this chapter

Situations that students may find challenging in community practice learning often involve communication, conflicting expectations and different approaches to

learning and teaching. These are issues for both the student and the mentor and can usually be resolved by the student and mentor paying attention to the following:

- Effective preparation and orientation to the placement
- Agreeing a learning plan or contract based on shared understanding of expectations
- Frequent reference to the learning outcomes and personal objectives and regular monitoring of progress
- Effective student/mentor relationship and communication
- Being an effective learner/mentor
- Using reflection on and in practice
- NMC Domain 4: Leadership, Management and Team Working.

References

NMC, 2010. Standards for Pre-registration Nursing Education. NMC, London.

Further reading

Arkell, S., Bayliss-Pratt, L., 2007. How nursing students can make the most of placements. Nursing Times 103 (20), 26 Online. Available at: (accessed August 2012)http://www.nursingtimes. net/nursing-practice-clinical-research/how-nursing-students-can-make-the-most-of-placements/199226. article.

Aston, L., Wakefield, J., McGowan, R., 2010. The student nurse guide to decision making in practice. Open University Press, Maidenhead.

Brooks, N., Rojahn, R., 2011. Improving the quality of community placements for nursing students. Nursing Standard 25 (37), 42–47.

Clark, A., Trecarichi, S., Brown, J., 2011. Partnership work in placements. Nursing Times 107 (21), 19–21.

Hart, S. (Ed.), 2010. Nursing study and placement learning skills. Oxford University Press, Oxford.

Holland, K., Roxburgh, M., 2012. Placement learning in surgical nursing: a guide for students in Practice. Bailliere Tindall, Edinburgh.

Levett-Jones, T., Bourgeois, S., 2009. The clinical placement: a nursing survival guide, 2nd ed. Bailliere Tindall, Sydney.

McGarry, J., Clissett, P., Porock, D., et al., 2012. Placement learning in older people nursing: a guide for students in practice. Bailliere Tindall, London.

Sivitar, B., 2008. The student nurse handbook, 2nd ed. Bailliere Tindall, London.

Stacey, G., Felton, A., Bonham, P., 2012. Placement learning in mental health nursing: a guide for students in practice. Bailliere Tindall, London.

Warren, D., 2010. Facilitating pre-registration nurse learning: a mentor approach. British Journal of Nursing 19 (21), 1364–1367.

Websites

Nursing and Midwifery Council, www.nmc-uk. org/.

Nursing Standard, http://nursingstandard. rcnpublishing.co.uk/students.

Royal College of Nursing, http://www.rcn.org. uk/.

14

Developing competence for person-centred nursing in the community

CHAPTER AIMS

- To show how the NMC standards for competence that all nurses are required to achieve for registration underpin safe, effective and person-centred care

- To use a scenario focusing on the care needs and experience of an individual and his family to enable the student to reflect on your learning experience in the community

- To help the student to use your learning experience to best effect in evidencing achievement of your learning outcomes for this placement

Introduction

This final chapter will help you to consolidate your learning from previous chapters and your experience from practice learning in the community. A scenario is used to describe a situation that is not unusual in the community. It illustrates the impact that the needs and experience of one family member can have on the other members of the family.

However, the scenario also illustrates how the four domains of the NMC competency framework underpin nursing practice:

1. Professional Values
2. Communication and Interpersonal Skills
3. Nursing Practice and Decision-making
4. Leadership, Management and Teamwork.

The NMC competencies and essential skills will be evident in the learning outcomes that you have been working towards throughout your placement. Working through the questions associated with each part of the scenario will enable you to relate your responses to these learning outcomes and may be helpful in developing evidence of learning for your portfolio.

Scenario

Margaret and Harry: Part 1 – Introduction to their life and health

Margaret and Harry have been married for 52 years. Harry was the head teacher at the local high school and Margaret was a part-time librarian. They moved to a modern bungalow to be nearer their daughter Alison when her first baby was born 10 years ago. Margaret and Harry had lots of interests: Harry was passionate about his garden and was a member of the local historical society and Margaret ran a book club and was very involved in helping to look after their grandchildren. Margaret and Harry also have two sons who both live in Australia and they have spent extended holidays there.

Five years ago, Harry was diagnosed with Alzheimer's disease. Slowly but surely, their lives have changed as Harry's physical and mental health have deteriorated. It is a while since they have been active in their local community and they have become quite isolated. Harry's short-term memory is now very poor and he is no longer able to go out on his own. He requires supervision most of the time and guidance with most daily activities such as washing, dressing and shaving. Sometimes he becomes extremely frustrated by this and gets angry with Margaret on whom he relies completely.

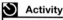 **Activity**

Question 1

- How might Harry be feeling living with dementia?
- What impact do you think caring for Harry would have on Margaret's health and wellbeing?
- If you were visiting Margaret and Harry during your community placement what could you do to understand more about Harry's feelings and Margaret's role?

At the heart of person-centred care is trying to understand the person's perspective and how their condition affects their life and relationships. It may be difficult for Harry to express how he feels at this point in his illness but it may not be difficult to pick up cues. Carers are often very good at this and can interpret behaviour, such as anger and aggression, as fear, frustration and confusion.

Continued

Activity

Access the Alzheimer's Society website, at: http://www.alzheimers.org.uk/ and read about how Alzheimer's can affect the individual and their family.

Discussions throughout the book have made reference to the experiences of carers. Chapter 5 in particular, looks at the impact that caring can have on physical and psychological health.

Let us say that in Margaret and Harry's scenario, Margaret wants to care for her husband; she knows he receives the care he wants and needs, and she wants him to be happy at home. So in this respect, the carer's role brings her pleasure, satisfaction and reassurance. But she is also exhausted, isolated, frustrated and risks developing health problems of her own. In many ways, it is the caring role itself and not what the role involves in terms of the condition or specific needs of the person being cared for that makes the impact. However, caring for someone with dementia has some unique challenges. It is difficult for those on the periphery to fully appreciate the carer's experience. But an empathetic approach of trying to put oneself in the carers' shoes is vitally important in order to offer carers the help and support they need and not what the services they *think* they need.

 Activity

Read the following article to gain some insight into how a nursing student supported a person with dementia and their carer in the community: Roy D, Gillespie M (2011) Who cares for the carers? A student's experience of providing carer support and education. British Journal of Nursing 20 (8):484–488.

If you were visiting Margaret and Harry, the following are some of the ways that could help you understand Margaret's perspective:

- Ask Margaret if you could spend some time with her to ask her about her experience of caring for Harry.
- Ask Margaret if you could spend a day with her to experience 'a day in the life of a carer' (see below).
- It might be difficult for Harry to express his feelings but you could find out more about Alzheimer's disease and other forms of dementia (see Chapter 8 and Further reading at the end of the chapter).
- Learn more about the real life experience of other carers. 'Keeping mum', gives insight into the carer's experience and is an account of Marianne Talbot's own challenges of caring for her mother at home (Talbot 2011).

Professional values underpin this aspect of nursing practice. The NMC generic standard for competence in Domain 1: Professional Values, includes 'safe, compassionate, person-centred, evidence-based care that respects dignity and human rights' (NMC Competencies for entry to the register: NMC 2010: 13).

A day in the life of Margaret and Harry

Margaret describes a typical day in her life which illustrates how caring for Harry affects her health and wellbeing.

> *Harry's sleeping pattern is unpredictable. I seem to just dose nowadays. I'm always listening out for him in case he gets up and gets into difficulty. Last night was a good night and he slept right through. At 6 am I make tea and toast and carry it through to our bedroom. This is the start of our daily routine which I try to stick to as far as possible. Harry finds routine helpful but it doesn't stop him getting confused and upset. Today we had an appointment at the dentist; I explained to Harry that we would drive over for a check-up with Mr Stewart after we had our coffee. I helped Harry to get washed and shaved and I looked out a jacket and shirt and tie for him to wear. Harry became very agitated and angry with me, saying that I was making a fuss. He*

 Activity

Identify the learning outcomes for this placement that are associated with the competencies in NMC Standards Domain 1: Professional Values and the Essential Skills Cluster: Care, Compassion and Communication. Have you made the most of opportunities that nursing in the community provides to develop positive working and therapeutic relationships and nursing practice, which is based on respect for individuals, their values, choices and diversity? What further experience would enable you to evidence learning that relates to your learning outcomes in this area? Discuss with your mentor opportunities to spend a day with a family on the caseload and experience first-hand 'a day in the life of a carer'. This would be an excellent opportunity to develop the skills, knowledge and attitudes required in this domain and evidence your learning in your portfolio.

Access and read the Queen's Nursing Institute publication 'Nursing People at Home', at: http://www.qni.org.uk/docs/RNRS_report_WEB.pdf

The skills that people valued most in the community nurse visiting them at home were competence and confidence and essentially person-centred caring, which involved sensitivity and compassion and demonstrated understanding and support for all members of the family. (QNI 2011)

said that he could go to the dentist as he
was (he was wearing his pyjamas). I
tried to calm him down and talked about
our new grandchild. Alison had baby
Amy last week. He didn't know who I
was talking about and said he doesn't
know an Alison. This made me feel so
upset; such a happy event in our family
and it's passing him by. I returned to the
subject of the dentist and he said I didn't
mention it and why were we going.
This was a difficult start to the day and I
was already feeling tired and stressed.
Eventually Harry was dressed and
we had a coffee in the kitchen. When
I handed him his coat he looked at me
blankly and asked where we were
going. This happens so often but I can't
say I'm used to it.

Harry coped well with the visit to the
dentist. At home over lunch just for a
brief period I saw glimpses of the Harry
I once knew. As things appeared to be
going well I suggested a walk around the
garden which he really enjoys. But he got
tired and became confused. He thought
he was at his parents' home and asked
to go inside to see his mother. When I
tried to explain reality to him he began to
cry. We went back indoors and he fell
asleep. I sat down and fell asleep too
only to waken to hear Harry in the
hallway opening the front door – "thank
you for having me", he was calling, "but
I need to get home". Eventually, he
settled down and after a cup of tea he
fell asleep again. I started to make tea
and Alison came over with the children.
It is good to have some company and to
hear the children's news about school
and their new baby sister. After tea
Harry fell asleep again, but I woke him
up to watch an old film. We have
watched this 20 times or more but he
always enjoys it. At bedtime he asked
what we were going to do today.
I am so tired but this is our daily
routine now.

Scenario

Margaret and Harry: Part 2 – Ongoing health needs and decision-making

Harry had become increasingly confused at
night and on a number of occasions
Margaret had woken up to hear him moving
about downstairs. In the early hours one
morning Margaret heard Harry calling from
the kitchen, sounding distressed. She rushed
downstairs to reach him, slipped in the
hall and fell awkwardly. When she tried to
get up she experienced breathlessness and
chest pain. She managed to phone her
daughter's house and her son-in-law John
immediately came round. He phoned the
emergency services and when they arrived,
they decided to take Margaret to hospital.
Harry was quite safe and John put him
to bed and stayed with him overnight.
Margaret was admitted to hospital and
further investigations confirmed a
diagnosis of angina.

Although Margaret was discharged the next
day, she was advised to rest and it was decided
that Harry would stay with John and Alison for a
few days. This change in circumstances upset
Harry greatly. This resulted in an increase in
emotional outbursts and an increase in
dependency and episodes of incontinence. John
was at home on paternity leave and able to help
supervise Harry and get up with him during the
night. But he was not happy about this. He felt
he should be supporting Alison and spending
time with the new baby and the girls during his
paternity leave and not looking after his father-
in-law. Alison found that she was helping her
father with all his personal care and his complex
medication regime, which she was not familiar
with. Alison tried very hard to maintain the level
of care and support for her father that he seemed
to need. She had had no idea how much her
mother had been doing for him and how
demanding this was. On top of her other
responsibilities, looking after the new baby Amy

and the two girls; she did not know how she would manage when John went back to work if Margaret wasn't fully recovered and able to take care of Harry. John was convinced that the answer was to admit Harry to residential care. Alison did not agree and this was causing friction in their relationship. At this time, Amy was 2 weeks old, and Veronica the health visitor who is well known to the family visits Amy for the first time.

 Activity

Question 2

- What is the purpose of the health visitor's visit at his stage in Amy's development?
- What concerns might the health visitor have?
- What action could the health visitor take regarding Harry's care?

Read the following article to enhance your learning: McAtamney R (2011) Health visitors' perceptions of their role in assessing parent–infant relationships. Community Practitioner 84(8):33–37.

In Chapter 2, there is an overview of the health visitor's role and links to the government programme to promote health in the early years in each UK country.

A home visit and review of all new babies between the ages of 10 and 15 days is an important part of the universal preventative service that health visitors provide.

The home visit gives an opportunity for the following:

- To discuss the baby's feeding and sleeping routine
- For the health visitor to check the baby's weight and length and carry out a general physical assessment
- For the health visitor to assess the mother's general physical and emotional health

- To discuss the general wellbeing of siblings and father
- For the health visitor to provide links with early years services.

In relation to the scenario, we can consider that all assessments of the baby are satisfactory. She is breast-feeding well and sleeping between her feeds. Veronica advises Alison to visit the health centre regularly to routinely monitor Amy's progress.

However, there are a number of issues that could concern Veronica, e.g.:

- *Alison is struggling to give the care and attention that the girls need – they could be feeling left out and may be distressed at seeing their grandad upset and confused.*
- *Alison and John's disagreement about admitting Harry to residential care while Margaret is unwell is causing tension in their relationship and this is upsetting Alison.*
- *She had not been aware until the visit that Alison had been caring for her father. Alison tells her that she is finding this very difficult and that she is exhausted. She does not want to let her mother down as she promised that they would look after Harry until she is able to do so herself. Alison explains that her mother has done everything for Harry since his condition deteriorated last year. Although they have regular contact with the surgery Alison suspects that her mother has not disclosed the full extent of Harry's dependence. In fact Alison hadn't realised it until he came to stay.*

It is not unusual for families to put a brave face on things and give the impression they are managing. They see caring for the family member as their responsibility and feel that asking for help would be admitting failure and an inability to cope. Carers are often concerned and anxious about their relatives being cared for by others, feeling that it will never match their own care. There may also be a fear that an honest expression of feeling exhausted and overwhelmed may result in the services enforcing a decision to admit the family member to institutional care. Of course, this is always a complex and difficult decision to make, and requires the full involvement and support of those concerned.

Veronica's actions regarding Harry's care could include:

- Discussing the situation with John and Alison to explore any short-term actions
- Suggesting that the family discuss the situation with Margaret with a view to referring Harry to the district nurse or community mental health nurse for assessment.

Communication and interpersonal skills are central to this aspect of the scenario, from the health visitor's assessment of the baby and health-promoting behaviour to her ability to listen empathetically and respond sensitively to the family's concerns about Harry. This relates to the competencies required of all nurses in Domain 2: Communication and Interpersonal Skills. (NMC Competencies for entry to the register; NMC 2010: 15).

Scenario

Margaret and Harry: Part 3 – Managing their healthcare and personal needs

The opportunity to talk through the issues and options with Veronica enabled Alison and John to see the situation more clearly and plan what to do. They left things as they were for a further 24 hours to give Margaret time to rest, then Alison talked to her mother. The conversation was difficult to begin with. Margaret realised that Alison and John could only look after Harry for a few days but was adamant that she was now well enough for Harry to come home and for her to look after him herself again. She tried to convince Alison that she could manage without help and that Harry was much happier and more settled if she provided all his care in his own home. Eventually and very reluctantly, she agreed to talk to their GP about Harry's medication and whether this could be

---

 Activity

Identify the learning outcomes for your community placement that are associated with the competencies in the NMC Standards: Domain: Communication and Interpersonal Skills and the Essential Skills Cluster: Care, compassion and communication (NMC 2010). How confident do you feel, depending on the stage of your education programme, in responding effectively in situations where people are anxious or distressed? Observe other members of the primary care team in these situations and use learning from this experience, your knowledge of communication theory and reflection on previous experience from practice, to develop your own skills further. Take opportunities to be involved and if you are at the end of your programme, manage situations where the interaction is distressing. This will require support from your mentor and other members of the team.

Read the following article, which discusses situations which students find challenging in practice and the supportive interventions that can be used by mentors to support them: Cooke M (1996) Nursing students' perceptions of difficult or challenging clinical situations. Journal of Advanced Nursing 24 (6):1281–1287.

simplified and improved. Alison felt that at least this was a start. She told Margaret that she would contact the practice to make an appointment. Harry was to return home the following day.

Alison contacted the surgery immediately and spoke to Harry's GP, Dr Sinclair. She ended up disclosing the full story as she thought Dr Sinclair was not aware of the extent of Harry's dependence on Margaret for day-to-day care. Dr Sinclair was very concerned about Margaret's ability to manage and particularly in the light of her recent diagnosis. He said he would request that the district nurse visited the next day.

Initially, Margaret was not at all happy that the GP had referred them to the district nursing service and told Alison that it was not necessary and that she would talk to Dr Sinclair herself. But Alison managed to help her see it from the perspective of her own health and the risk of being unable to look after Harry if she took on too much now. Alison thought she detected relief in her mother's expression once the decision was made to see the district nurse. The next morning, John brought Harry home and the district nurse telephoned to make an appointment to visit in the afternoon.

When the district nurse visited, she made a full assessment of Harry's health needs, from a family-centred perspective and discussed with Margaret and Alison the possible options and interventions which could assist Harry and support the family at this time.

The purpose of the district nurse's assessment would be to identify Harry's health and care needs and working with him, probably through Margaret's knowledge of his personal preferences, finding out what he wants and needs and what would make most difference to his health and wellbeing. This type of approach focuses on the outcomes that the person wants to achieve rather than what the service dictates or the practitioner thinks would be best. Inextricably linked with Harry's needs are Margaret's and the district nurse would be assessing these also.

Options for Harry's care in the future based on the district nurse's assessment could include:

- Appointment with the GP to review Harry's medications (see Chapter 12, Medicines management)
- Develop an Anticipatory Care Plan (see Kennedy et al 2011)
- Referral to an occupational therapist to assess the home for aids and home adaptations to make life easier and safer for Harry and Margaret. This could include assistive technology such as bed and chair occupancy sensors to alert Margaret if Harry has got up during the night
- Referral to the community mental health nurse or specialist dementia service for assessment and support

 Activity

Question 3

■ What would the district nurse's assessment aim to do?

■ What options for Harry's future care could be discussed?

Read the following articles to inform your answers:

1. Hope T (2009) Ethical dilemmas in the care of people with dementia. British Journal of Community Nursing 14(12):548–550
2. Roy D, Gillespie M (2011) Who cares for the carers? A student's experience of providing carer support and education. British Journal of Nursing 20(8):484–488
3. Access the signs and symptoms section of the Alzheimer's Society website, at: http://www.alzheimers.org.uk/site/scripts/documents.php?categoryID=200341.

- Referral to the local authority for assessment for day care or carer assistance with washing and dressing
- Short-term respite care
- Contact with local voluntary groups for people with dementia and their carers.

(Refer to Chapter 2 for information about services and the roles of community practitioners that could support Margaret and Harry.)

The nurse's competence in NMC Standards: Domain 3: Nursing Practice and Decision Making (NMC 2010) is essential in this part of the scenario. The NMC states that, *'all nurses must assess and meet the full range of essential physical and mental health needs of people of all ages who come into their care'* and *'must make person-centred evidence based decisions in partnership with others involved in the care process to ensure high quality care'* (NMC 2010: 17).

Scenario

Margaret and Harry: Part 4 – Conclusion: outcome of shared decision-making

Margaret had not realised how isolated they had both become and how much more could be done to improve not only Harry's wellbeing but also her own. She recognised that her devotion to Harry was blurring her ability to see what was best for him. A long chat and ongoing support from the community mental health nurse and information from national dementia organisations helped her to understand what she could do to help Harry.

Margaret and Harry's life is now quite different. Harry attends a day centre, two mornings a week, where he enjoys singing, reminiscing and reciting the poetry he used to teach many years ago. He can meet with the

---

Activity

Review your learning outcomes and identify those which are associated with NMC Standards: Domain 3: Nursing Practice and Decision Making and Domain 4: Leadership, Management and Team Working plus the Essential Skills Cluster: Organisational aspects of care (NMC 2010).

Reflect on your learning in this area to date and in the light of the issues that have been raised in the scenario, could your skills be developed further? For example, would you be able to explain to Margaret and Harry what a local authority assessment for day care or home care assistance would entail? How could you arrange to find out more about this? To what extent have you been involved in anticipatory care planning? What are the opportunities for gaining more experience in this important area of practice in the community? How could you evidence this learning in your portfolio?

Read the following articles to inform your answers:

1. Kennedy C, Harbison J, Mahoney C et al (2011) Investigating the contribution of community nurses to anticipatory care: a qualitative exploratory study. Journal of Advanced Nursing 67(7):1558–1567
2. Staff nurse Claire O'Brien values her student portfolio and urges other student nurses to do the same. The short article is available at: http://nursingstandard. rcnpublishing.co.uk/students/study-skills/techniques-and-advice/student-nurses-should-keep-a-record-of-achievement

community mental health nurse there and although Margaret drops him off, he is driven home by the local voluntary action drivers. This gives Margaret two free mornings, one of which she spends at Alison's house and looks after Amy so that Alison can have some free time. The other morning Margaret is now able to attend a book club which meets in members' houses. This gets her out of the house, socialising with others and taking an interest in reading again. Harry's medication has been reviewed by his GP, the number of tablets has been reduced and the regime has been simplified to twice daily. Minor adaptations to the home have improved his mobility. Margaret is now better informed about the sorts of activities that Harry finds helpful and stimulating and is better able to cope when he is anxious or upset. Her worst fears for Harry's care when she is no longer able to look after him have been alleviated by having an anticipatory care plan in place. This has been agreed by the family and sets out Harry's care trajectory including supported care at home for as long as possible.

Despite the family's initial concerns about residential care, it was suggested that a week of respite care twice a year would be enjoyable for Harry and a break for Margaret, allowing her to have a short holiday. Harry has already spent a week in the local private care home which has worked out very well and appears to suit Harry. He has enjoyed the company of the other residents, the activities and the attention from the carers.

Alison and John have settled into life with the new baby and the children have adapted well to having a new sister. Alison has been able to get involved with a mother and toddler group and regularly takes Amy to the baby clinic. She continues to assist her mother with Harry's care when required but this is infrequent now that Margaret is not trying to cope without other help.

This case study touches on the complexity of caring in the community for clients and their families who have significant emotional and physical needs. A single event, Margaret's fall, led to a series of events

which not only highlighted but also resolved difficulties and challenges that the family had not faced up to before. The case study helped to demonstrate how the competences that are required for entry to the register underpin the nurse's role. All registered nurses continue to develop all of the knowledge, skills and attitudes that the NMC requires at the point of registration but community nurses, perhaps more than most constantly adapt and develop them to fit a wide variety of situations and settings. Increasingly, newly registered nurses are being appointed straight into community posts and are supported within community nursing teams to continue to develop their competences for safe, effective and person-centred care in the community.

◆ Activity

Read the following article, which discusses how students valued their final placement in a community setting to build confidence, develop professionalism in relationships and learn to manage care prior to registration: Anderson EE, Kiger A (2008) 'I felt like a real nurse' – Student nurses out on their own. Nurse Education Today 28(4):443–449.

Summary of learning points from this chapter

This chapter aimed to prompt thinking and reflection on your community learning experience to date in relation to achieving your learning outcomes. We used a scenario to help you to apply learning from your community placement and from previous chapters of the book in an exercise to assess a family's situation and propose some potential actions or solutions. We then added some fairly direct questions for you to ask yourself about your learning in practice, *'have I got the most from my community placement? Is there a learning experience that I missed? Is there something that I would like to pursue in more depth?'*

Conclusion

Our intention, throughout the book, has been to help you get the most from your community placement by explaining the context and describing what to expect from the rich variety of learning opportunities available in this setting. Most importantly, we have aimed to develop your skills and confidence as an independent and proactive learner, not only as a nursing student in a community practice context but also as a nursing student in any practice or other learning environment. These are the skills that will support your continuing professional development in the future as a registered nurse and promote effective life-long learning throughout your career.

References

Anderson, E.E., Kiger, A., 2008. 'I felt like a real nurse' – Student nurses out on their own. Nurse Educ. Today 28 (4), 443–449.

Cooke, M., 1996. Nursing students' perceptions of difficult or challenging clinical situations. J. Adv. Nurs. 24 (6), 1281–1287.

Hope, T., 2009. Ethical dilemmas in the care of people with dementia. Br. J. Community Nursing 14 (12), 548–550.

Kennedy, C., Harbison, J., Mahoney, C., et al., 2011. Investigating the contribution of community nurses to anticipatory care: a qualitative

exploratory study. Journal of Advanced Nursing 67 (7), 1558–1567.

McAtamney, R., 2011. Health visitors' perceptions of their role in assessing parent–infant relationships. Community Practice 84 (8), 33–37.

NMC, 2010. Standards for pre-registration nursing education. NMC, London.

Roy, D., Gillespie, M., 2011. Who cares for the carers? A student's experience of providing carer support and education. British Journal of Nursing 20 (8), 484–488.

Talbot, M., 2011. Keeping mum: caring for someone with dementia. Hay House, London.

Further reading

Baker, J.D., 2012. The nurse explains: dementia. Alzheimer's disease and vascular dementia, 4th ed. John Baker, London.

Department of Health, 2009. Healthy Child Programme: pregnancy and the first five years of life. DH, London.

Evans, D., Coutsaftiki, D., Patricia Fathers, C., 2011. Health promotion and public health for nursing students. Learning Matters, Exeter.

Hart, S. (Ed.), 2010. Nursing study and placement learning skills. Oxford University Press, Oxford.

Hindle, A., Coates, A., 2011. Nursing care of older people. Oxford University Press, Oxford.

Holland, K., Hogg, C., 2010. Cultural awareness in nursing and health care: an introductory text, 2nd ed. Hodder Arnold, London.

Lindon, J., 2010. Understanding child development: linking theory and practice, 2nd ed. Hodder Education, London.

Naidoo, J., Wills, J., 2010. Developing practice for public health and health promotion (public health and health promotion practice), third revised ed. Bailliere Tindall, Edinburgh.

NMC, 2009. Guidance for the care of older people. NMC, London.

QNI, 2011. Nursing people at home; the issues, the stories, the actions. QNI, London.

Reed, A., 2011. Nursing in partnership with patients and carers. Learning Matters, Exeter.

Royal College of Nursing, 2012. The RCN's UK position on health visiting in the early years. RCN, London.

Websites

Age UK is a voluntary organisation, which has brought Age Concern and Help the Aged into one. It works to improve later life for everyone by providing life-enhancing services and support: www.ageuk.org.uk.

Alzheimer's Society is the leading support and research charity for people with dementia, their families and carers: www.alzheimers.org.uk.

Alzheimer Scotland, www.alzscot.org/.

Carers UK, www.carersuk.org/.

DIPEx charity. Healthtalk online is the website of the DIPEx charity. It shares people's experiences of over 60 health-related conditions and illnesses: http://www.healthtalkonline.org/.

Mumsnet is an independently funded website, which is run by parents for parents and enables knowledge, advice and support to be shared: www.mumsnet.com.

Queen's Nursing Institute publication 'Nursing People at Home', http://www.qni.org.uk/docs/RNRS_report_WEB.pdf.

The Good Practice Guide for carers and young carers. http://www.scotland.gov.uk/Publications/2010/07/23153853/0.

The Scottish Government Modernising Nursing in the Community Website, http://www.mnic.nes.scot.nhs.uk/.

The Social Care Institute for Excellence (SCIE) is a charity set up by the Department of Health. It disseminates evidence and good practice in social care and produces resources and tools to support practitioners and service users: www.scie.org.uk/Index.aspx.

Subject Index

Subject Index